An
American
Physical
Therapy
Association
Monograph

Balance

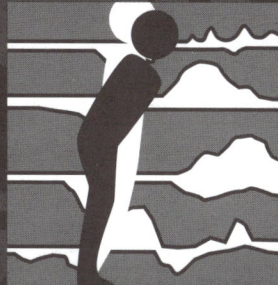
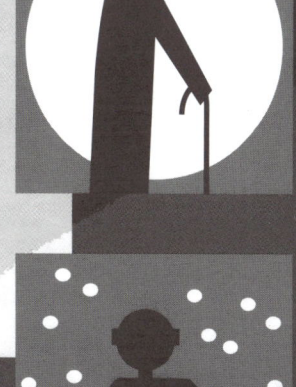

This monograph is a compilation of articles originally published in the January, April, May, June, August, and September 1997 issues of *Physical Therapy* and June 1997 issue of *PT—Magazine of Physical Therapy*.

ISBN 1-887759-17-4

©1997 by the American Physical Therapy Association. All rights reserved.

For more information about this and other APTA publications, contact the American Physical Therapy Association, 1111 North Fairfax Street, Alexandria, VA 22314-1488.
[Order No. P-146]

Table of Contents

3	Preface
5	Professional Issues
7	Balance Strategies: 2000 and Beyond
21	Physical Therapy Special Series on Balance
23	Editor's Note/Jules M Rothstein
24	Guest Contributors and Reviewers
26	Introduction/Richard P Di Fabio
28	Aging and the Mechanisms Underlying Head and Postural Control During Voluntary Motion/Richard P Di Fabio, Alongkot Emasithi
46	Light Touch Contact as a Balance Aid/John J Jeka
58	The Role of Limb Movements in Maintaining Upright Stance: The "Change-in-Support" Strategy/Brian E Maki, William E McIlroy
78	Locomotion in Patients With Spinal Cord Injuries/Volker Dietz, Markus Wirz, Lars Jensen
87	Postural Perturbations: New Insights for Treatment of Balance Disorders/Fay B Horak, Sharon M Henry, Anne Shumway-Cook
104	Case Report: Rehabilitation of Balance in Two Patients With Cerebellar Dysfunction/Kathleen M Gill-Body, Rita A Popat, Stephen W Parker, David E Krebs
123	Update: Balance Retraining After Stroke Using Force Platform Biofeedback/Deborah S Nichols
129	Advances in the Treatment of Vestibular Disorders/Susan J Herdman
146	The Role of Vision and Spatial Orientation in the Maintenance of Posture/Michael G Wade, Graeme Jones
156	Evaluation of Postural Stability in Children: Current Theories and Assessment Tools/Sarah L Westcott, Linda Pax Lowes, Pamela K Richardson
173	Balance Control During Walking in the Older Adult: Research and Its Implications/Marjorie H Woollacott, Pei-Fang Tang
189	Additional Physical Therapy Articles
191	The Effect of Multidimensional Exercises on Balance, Mobility, and Fall Risk in Community-Dwelling Older Adults/Anne Shumway-Cook, William Gruber, Margaret Baldwin, Shiquan Liao
203	The Effect of Tai Chi Quan and Computerized Balance Training on Postural Stability in Older Subjects/Steven L Wolf, Huiman X Barnhart, Gary L Ellison, Carol E Coogler, Atlanta FICSIT Group
214	Invited Commentary/Fay B Horak
215	Author Response
217	Predicting the Probability for Falls in Community-Dwelling Older Adults/Anne Shumway-Cook, Margaret Baldwin, Nayah L Polissar, William Gruber
225	Case Report: The Individualized Treatment of a Patient With Benign Paroxysmal Positional Vertigo/Cheryl D Ford-Smith
233	Evaluation of Health-Related Quality of Life in Individuals With Vestibular Disease Using Disease-Specific and General Outcome Measures/Lori J Enloe, Richard K Shields
247	Use of the "Fast Evaluation of Mobility, Balance, and Fear" in Elderly Community Dwellers: Validity and Reliability/Richard P Di Fabio, Rebecca Seay

Preface

In the Editor's Note that prefaces *Physical Therapy*'s Special Series on Balance, Jules Rothstein asks, "Are the balance strategies that we have all come to understand 'real'?" In this monograph, which includes peer-reviewed articles published in *Physical Therapy* and interviews published in *PT—Magazine of Physical Therapy*, physical therapists and researchers from other disciplines explore new concepts and models, provide rationale for developing and testing new approaches, and raise important questions about the clinical meaningfulness of balance strategies.

Professional Issues

COVER STORY
by Jan P Reynolds

Balance Strategies: 2000
AND BEYOND

"Are the balance strategies that we have all come to understand 'real'?" The answer to that question, posed by *Physical Therapy* Editor Jules Rothstein in the Journal's special series on balance (May and June issues), will have important implications not just for physical therapy but for health care worldwide in the 21st century. More people are living longer with a variety of conditions—from stroke to Parkinson's disease to brain tumors—that are associated with balance problems. And more people simply are living longer, developing balance problems that occur as a result of the aging process. From the Far East to Scandinavia, there is one overarching concern: Falls among the elderly. As health care systems everywhere increasingly demand optimal patient outcomes with fewer visits, the management of patients with balance problems will hinge on knowing which strategies are "real" and which are not—and whether, as Rothstein says, "fascination with clinical devices [is] taking precedence over common sense."

One Area That Has Evidence

Few areas of physical therapy practice have received as much attention in the peer-reviewed literature as balance. Why? "One reason is that multiple disciplines have been involved in studying balance for a long time," says Rothstein. "There are known relationships between pathologies and symptoms. In fact, there is an entire treatment approach based on applying mechanical forces to the defective labyrinthine system. The conditions are well defined, and we have distinct classifications of patients."

> "Are the balance strategies that we have all come to understand 'real'?"

Find out where the current research in balance may lead clinical practice—and where current clinical practice may lead research.

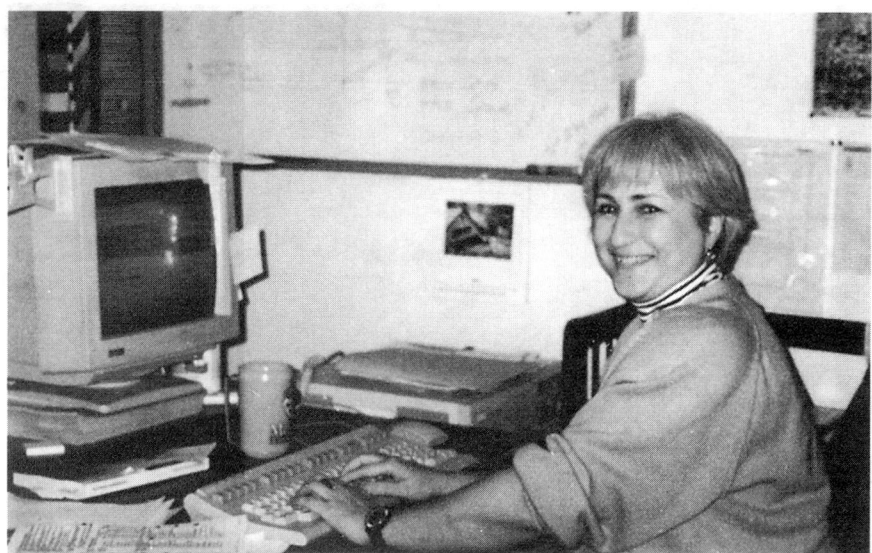

Today, Katherine Berg, PhD, is studying a population of community-dwelling seniors, comparing outcomes obtained using measures such as the Berg Balance Scale to outcomes obtained using the SF-36.

Lewis Nashner, ScD, the biomedical engineer credited with pioneering research in postural control mechanisms and etiological and clinical measures of balance performance, has watched the profession make tremendous in-roads during the past decade. He had his first collaboration with physical therapists in the late 1970s.

"I had come from the aeronautical world to teach neurophysiology at the University of Oregon. Anne Shumway-Cook [cover] visited our laboratory. She needed a sponsor for her doctoral thesis work on human motor control, an area in which very little research had been done. Together, we obtained one of the first research grants awarded by the Foundation for Physical Therapy. Other researchers, such as Marjorie Woollacott and physical therapist Fay Horak, also came on the scene."

Have most of the questions that drove balance research in the 1970s and 1980s been answered? "In research, questions are never fully answered, which is both good and bad!" says Nashner. "Our understanding of vestibular disorders certainly has grown. Back in the '70s, if surgery or drugs didn't work, there was nothing more to do for these patients. The medical community is known for being conservative, and that conservatism has impeded reimbursement, but today most clinicians in the United States and Canada accept the concept of vestibular rehabilitation. My own area of research interest has turned to applying basic science to improve clinical care," adds Nashner, who today is President of NeuroCom® International, a producer of balance systems based in Clackamas, Oregon. "We still don't know enough about the capacity of aging people and people with specific conditions to learn balance and motor control skills." Although the United States and Canada continue to lead the way in balance research, Nashner is impressed with the studies now being conducted in countries such as Australia, Great Britain, and Sweden.

"Even though the economics of medicine differ dramatically from country to country, the questions and concerns are much the same: What treatments are most cost effective? What programs will best help maintain function in an aging population?"

The Research Explosion

From university-based balance research laboratories to centers on aging to the multiple sites involved in the National Institute on Aging's FICSIT (Frailty and Injuries: Cooperative Studies on Intervention Techniques) Project, physical therapists have helped develop an understanding of what Pam Duncan, PhD, PT, described as "a complex motor control task, requiring integration of sensory information, neural processing, and biomechanical factors."[1] What's changed since the landmark Balance Forum held at APTA's Annual Conference in Nashville, Tennessee, 8 years ago this month?

"The forum provided a great deal of emerging information about the physiological and biomechanical factors that contribute to balance," says Duncan, editor of *Balance: Proceedings of the APTA Forum*,[1] and currently Director of Research, Center on Aging, University of Kansas Medical Center. "The focus was on basic science. Since then, there has been an explosion of major epidemiological studies on falls in the elderly, of studies on intervention programs, and of research into the factors that contribute to instability. We understand so much more about the aging process. We have a wealth of information on epidemiology and clinical intervention—now we just have to *apply* it."

The explosion in research also has resulted in an explosion in standardized measures, notes Duncan, adding, "There is no longer any reason for a therapist to grade balance as 'good,' 'fair,' or 'poor.'" Clinical assessment instruments, often described as "low tech," include the Tinetti performance-oriented assessment of mobility,[2] the "Get Up and Go" Test,[3] the Berg Balance Scale,[4] the Duke Mobility Scale,[5] and the Functional Reach Test.[6] There also has been a steady development of "high-tech" tools, such as the BalanceMaster® and Smart Balance-Master® (NeuroCom®) and the Balance System™ (Chattanooga Group).

High Tech vs Low Tech

Debate on the value of high tech versus low tech, especially in an era of managed care and cost containment, is ongoing. For Emory University's Steven Wolf, PhD, PT, FAPTA, the bottom line is that "there still are no data to suggest that the use of high-tech equipment is justified or prudent." Wolf, who coauthored "The Effect of Tai Chi Quan and Computerized Balance Training on Postural Stability in Older Subjects" with Barnhart, Ellison, Coogler, and the Atlanta FICSIT Group (*Physical Therapy*, April 1997), believes that "the use of sophisticated equipment to evaluate balance may be a primarily academic phenomenon. In daily practice, clinicians use clinical measures and common sense when dealing with balance disorders. The use of balance machines would be an extravagance."

What about outside the United States and Canada? Susan Herdman, PhD, PT, a balance researcher based at the University of Miami School of Medicine in Coral Gables, Fla, reports that overseas physical therapists are not as reliant on high-tech tools, possibly because those tools "have not been as available outside Canada and the United States—although that's changing." Funding for such equipment is limited, both in terms of practice and research, says Wolf. "In many countries, there is only one research lab for the whole of physical therapy, and most of the physical therapist educators haven't been exposed to balance systems. How can they prepare future therapists to use them? The required levels of sophistication and resources don't exist—and, in fact, may not be necessary."

Today, most clinicians across the globe recognize the armamentarium of low-tech balance assessment tools. That hasn't always been the case, says physical therapist Katherine Berg, PhD. "It's a big step toward consistency in the way we conduct research and manage patients. People are still developing and using their own tools in isolation, however, which continues to make it difficult to collect the standardized data that could help us determine what treatments work best with what types of patients."

Berg may be best known for the balance scale developed as part of her master's thesis.[4] A 1994 survey[7] found that instrument to be "the most commonly used 'outcome measure' of any kind, with the exception of manual muscle testing," says Berg, who has been surprised by the extent of the scale's use. Thorbahn and Newton[8] recently discussed the use and limitations of the scale in predicting falls in elderly persons. Now Assistant Professor (Research) in the Department of Community Health and Center for Gerontology and Health Care Research at Brown University in Providence, Rhode Island, Berg currently is involved in a study of community-dwelling seniors, comparing outcomes obtained using measures such as the

FICSIT: What Have We Learned About Balance?

The National Institute on Aging's FICSIT Project (Frailty and Injuries: Cooperative Studies on Intervention Techniques) was "the first attempt of its type," says Robert Whipple, MA, PT, Project Administrator, FICSIT–Farmington. Whipple is Director of the Balance and Gait Enhancement Laboratory, University of Connecticut Health Center, Farmington, Conn.

"A key intent of the NIA was to assemble a diversity of approaches toward fall prevention," explains Whipple. "The participants' identity wasn't known until the awarding of the grants, and the creation of a common database compatible with the goals of each site could not proceed until the players met together. Coming to closure on common outcome measures of motor function was particularly thorny, given the wide variety of site-specific objectives, interventions, subject populations, and instrumentation. Of necessity, a 'lowest common denominator' of measures was chosen, such as gait velocity, hand-grip strength, sit-to-stand time, and timed narrow-based stances."

Sites ranging from San Antonio to Seattle to Atlanta looked at semifrail community dwellers, nursing home residents, and healthy community dwellers. Interventions varied, says Whipple, "from Mary Tinetti's [New Haven] targeted risk factor approach (eg, medication use, transfer deficits, environmental hazards, weakness, imbalance) to Maria Fiatarone's [Boston] use of high-intensity resistance exercise to Steven Wolf's [Atlanta] and Leslie Wolfson's [Farmington] use of tai chi and high-tech balance strategies."

Whipple believes that some of the most clinically meaningful results of FICSIT will come from the studies involving tai chi. The Atlanta group found that tai chi reduced fall risk and slowed preferred walking speed. "A tantalizing question," says Whipple, "is whether people fell less because they slowed down or because their balance improved. My money's on the latter. Walking slowly may actually be a specialized balance skill,[1] and work in progress from the Pepper Foundation in Tallahassee [personal communication, F Sullivan-Fahs] suggests that tai chi may help improve both single-leg stance and isokinetic strength.... It's conceivable that tai chi systematically incorporates many different balance skills, but it's unlikely that it's a panacea for poor balance. The Farmington results[2] suggest that low-intensity follow-up tai chi training was able to preserve previously attained strength—but only certain aspects of balance." Whipple, who spoke on FICSIT at the Hong Kong Hospital Authority conference held in March, notes with irony that the physical therapists he met in Hong Kong "feel such an urgency to accept high-tech medical models that they're at risk of minimizing the value of a potent balance-enhancing approach—tai chi—that is a part of their own cultural heritage."

Whipple emphasizes that many different areas of balance deserve physical therapists' attention. "For example, Kaye's group found that in optimally healthy oldest-old subjects, aged 85 to 100 years, single-leg stance time and visual tracking were dramatically reduced,[3] although almost no decay was seen in tolerance for an unstable surface[4].... The relationships between all of the different balance deficits and falling are unknown. FICSIT was an important start, but so far all we know from a meta-analytic study[5] of the common database is that time to first fall was significantly reduced through either tai chi training or a multiple-risk abatement strategy. Much work clearly remains to be done."

References
1 Leiper CI, Craik RI. Relationships between physical activity and temporal-distance characteristics of walking in elderly women. *Phys Ther.* 1991;71:791-803.
2 Wolfson L, Whipple R, Derby T, et al. Balance and strength training in older adults: intervention gains and tai chi maintenance. *J Am Geriatr Soc.* 1996;498-506.
3 Kaye JA, Oken BS, Howieson DB, et al. Neurologic evaluation of the optimally healthy oldest old. *Arch Neurol.* 1994;51:1205-1211.
4 Panzer V, Kaye J, Edner A, Holme L. Standing postural control in the elderly and very elderly. In: Woollacott M, Horak F, eds. *Posture and Gait, Volume II.* Eugene, Ore: University of Oregon; 1992:220-223.
5 Province MA, Hadley EC, Hornbrook MC. The effects of exercise on falls in elderly patients: a preplanned meta-analysis of the FICSIT study. *JAMA.* 1995;273:1341-1347.

Berg Balance Scale with outcomes obtained using the SF-36.[9]

"Not Fall Prevention, *Disability* Prevention"

In March, Berg was an invited speaker at the Hong Kong Hospital Authority's international balance conference, which included a workshop attended by physical therapists and a multidisciplinary symposium of physicians, physical therapists, occupational therapists, and nurses.

"In Hong Kong as elsewhere, the health care community is very concerned with reducing the number of falls," says Berg. "I spoke on the need for a *framework* for fall prevention. That is, clinicians and researchers both should think about balance in the context of ability; opportunity, such as environment; and judgment, in terms of safety. The goal really isn't fall prevention. The goal is disability prevention."

A number of fall prevention clinics exist in Hong Kong hospitals, with a few using balance systems, says Berg. "People in the Far East are asking the same kinds of questions we're asking in North America," she says. "When is the use of high-tech equipment necessary or best practice? Many clinicians assume that equipment by its very nature will be more reliable. But the results of some studies, such as one by Liston and Brouwer,[10] question that assumption. Equipment has limitations. For the patient who is lower functioning and can't perform tests with eyes closed, for instance, clinical measures may be more useful than the high-tech tools, whereas for healthier populations, the high-tech tools may be more useful. This is just one more area that needs research."

Lewis Nashner agrees that high tech "isn't for every patient. It's not for patients with relatively straightforward problems that are likely to resolve on their own or with generic treatment programs. Technology is most appropriate in chronic, multifactorial cases requiring treatments customized to the specific needs of the individual patient." Nashner believes that high tech has the potential to "contribute quantitative measures that will supplement clinical measures of balance performance and quality-of-life measures. It also could help PTs maintain a high quality of care even in a time when they aren't allowed to spend as much time with patients as they once did. Just as more patients will be doing 'self-therapy' with home equipment, more PTs will be using machines in evaluation."

Jon F Peters, PhD, Director of International Marketing and Sales at NeuroCom, says that several balance systems have been installed in Australia, Japan, Korea, and Hong Kong. "NeuroCom went overseas in 1988 with the EquiTest™, the diagnostic system that is the predecessor to Balance-Master. We didn't expand into physical therapy and rehabilitation in those markets until a few years later." In the Far East, he says, a number of researchers have been schooled in the United States and so "are generally sophisticated when it comes to the use of high tech. But when it comes to *purchasing* high tech from the United States, they are more reluctant. They want to know whether major North American universities are currently using a particular piece of equipment. If it isn't being used here, they suspect—perhaps with some justification—that a company is trying to exploit them. There also are concerns that the existing databases created with balance systems are based on predominantly US populations." Nonetheless, the international market is still growing, says Peters. Systems produced by a number of companies are being installed throughout Europe, the Middle East, and Mexico, in addition to the Pacific Rim.

Vestibular Rehabilitation vs Balance Training

When it comes to balance disorders, countries may differ not just in the use of high tech but in the type of diagnosis. Susan Herdman offers one example from the vestibular arena.

"Therapists in the United States identify some patients as having benign paroxysmal positional vertigo, a condition that therapists in Europe would diagnose as cervical vertigo," she says. "That diagnosis is rarely used here. I believe that US therapists have some patients with dizziness—not necessarily vertigo—that is being produced as a result of neck disorders, not as a result of vestibular problems." Joint receptors in the upper cervical region may project to the vestibular nuclei, Herdman suggests. "That might be one mechanism; altered somatosensory cues could be another," she adds.

Differences in scope of practice from country to country affect the therapist's role in treating balance problems. Some of those differences relate to whether a patient's problem has its source in the vestibular system. "I've observed that most physical therapists in most countries treat balance problems related to conditions such as hemiplegia," says Jon Peters. "In many countries, however, the treatment of vestibular disorders is still not well accepted. In some nations, health care providers simply do not have the funding to treat these complicated disorders. In the United States, a patient with vestibular problems might be referred to a physical therapist by a physician, who would leave treatment up to the therapist; in Germany, for instance, the therapist typically might never even see this type of patient."

Ming-Hsia Hu, PhD, PT, Associate Professor in the School of Physical Therapy at National Taiwan University, concurs, explaining that physical therapists in Taiwan traditionally have not treated patients with vestibular disorders. "The National Health Insurance Plan has a reimbursement 'price list' for physical therapy services, and balance training is on that list. But treatment of vestibular disorders is a different story. Physical therapists in Taiwan are just beginning to be educated in this area."

Last year, Hu led six physical therapy staff members, in cooperation with an otorhinolaryngologist, in an investigation of treatment for dizziness in older adults. "We showed positive outcomes associated with physical therapy, and since then we have been receiving referrals from otorhinolaryngologists—via physiatrists, as is the requirement in Taiwan."

Hu has become a resource not just for physical therapists, but for members of other disciplines in Taiwan. "Several OTs are completing balance control research projects," she says, "and engineering researchers in at least two different research labs are designing local versions of balance training and evaluation tools. They all are seeking out the expertise of physical therapists."

A therapist licensed to practice both in Taiwan and the United States, Hu first became interested in balance "when my grandmother fell in front of me so quickly that I could not catch her. I also found myself falling in situations when my classmates did not. I wanted to understand how balance mechanisms worked. My master's degree, which I received at the University of North Carolina at Chapel Hill, involved analysis of hemiplegic gait. When my advisor, Carol Giuliani, and I hypothesized that balance, not gait per se, was the problem for the subjects in the study—I was hooked!"

Hu and eight other members of the Taiwan Physical Therapy Association have formed a geriatrics special interest group, which recently submitted two grant proposals to investigate the potential benefits of home health physical therapy. (There currently is no reimbursement for home health physical therapy in Taiwan.) Several members of the special interest group are conducting research on fall prevention programs.

"My own 3-year study is on the effects of a systems approach to balance training—an approach based on the concept that movement emerges from an interaction between the individual, the task, and the environment—to reduce frequency of falls and improve balance among elderly people in Taipei. The study is being supported by the National Health Research Institute of the Ministry of Health." Hu has recruited 160 subjects so far, assigning them to five exercise classes. The first class recently returned for a 6-month follow-up.

In her research, Hu primarily uses the Smart BalanceMaster® and a portable system, the Balance Performance Monitor® (SMS Health Care), which, she says, "is easy to use. I found it cited in some studies. It's being used here as a training tool in the clinic, whereas the BalanceMaster® is used primarily for evaluation. Many researchers in Taiwan use multiple evaluation tools, as Woollacott and I recently

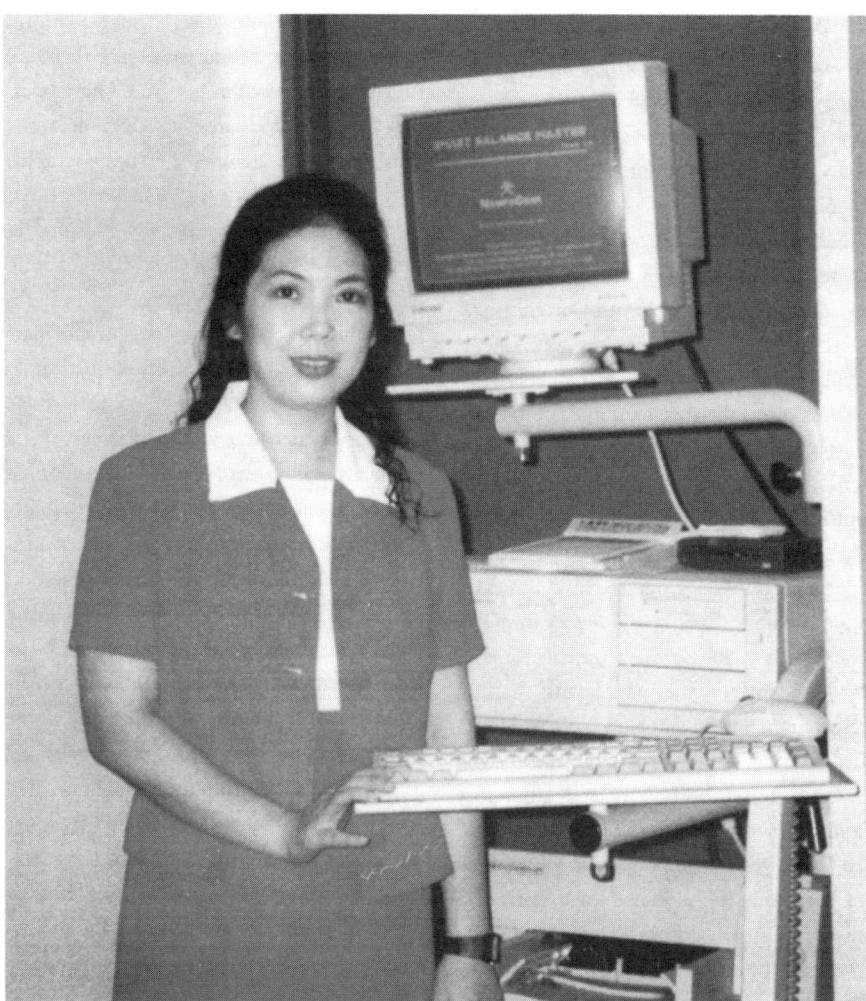

"I am convinced that once physicians realize what physical therapists can do for patients with vestibular disorders, they will refer these patients to us," says Ming-Hsia Hu, PhD, PT of Taipei, Taiwan.

discussed in *Reviews in Clinical Gerontology*.[11] They use both high-tech balance testing and clinical measures such as the Tinetti test and the Berg scale. In most clinics, however, evaluation still is done primarily through visual observation, with therapists grading balance as 'good,' 'fair,' or 'poor' and quantifying duration in terms of how long the patient can maintain balance under different situations, such as standing on one leg on foam with eyes closed or doing the tandem walk. Occasionally, videotape systems are used in the clinic as well."

Taiwan, notes Hu, is about one third the size of the state of Oregon, with about 21 million people. "How many high-tech systems does my country really need? At Chung-Chung University in southern Taiwan, there are three gait labs within 3 minutes' walking distance, and each is equipped with three-dimensional motion analysis systems and forceplates. But what about the hundreds of clinicians who need to begin collecting evaluation data? They need simple, durable, relatively inexpensive systems." To help develop what she calls 'moderate tech,' Hu is working with Taiwan's National Engineering Research Institute.

"Physical therapists in the smaller cities and smaller hospitals just aren't as familiar with computers as most therapists, and most people, in the United States are," Hu says. "In Lo-Dong, a medium-sized city in northeastern Taiwan, one of the two hospitals owns a $30,000 balance system—but no one knows how to use it! It just sits there. Such a waste. This is one example of why I advocate moderate tech. Equipment has to be *very* easy to use."

"What Are We Really Testing?"

In Sweden and other Nordic countries, balance problems are "attracting more and more attention," says Charlotte Håger-Ross, PhD, Department of Rehabilitation Medicine at University of Umea in Umea, Sweden. "My own research focuses on sensorimotor control of the upper extremity, specifically reactive control of grasp stability, which I believe involves components similar to those of balance control when patients are subjected to unpredictable disturbances. The nature of the task, the use of sensory input, and the regulation of motor output all play a factor in balance." Håger-Ross is organizing a Nordic postgraduate course for physical therapists this summer on contemporary research and theory in motor control, to include a focus on balance control. "Many of the participants have a research interest in falls among the elderly.... In Sweden, therapists are conducting research using both advanced laboratory equipment and more clinically related tests."

Three years ago, physical therapist Helga Hirschfeld, PhD, joined forces with Elisabeth Olsson, PhD, head of the Department of Physical Therapy at the Karolinska Institute in Stockholm, to establish the Motor Control and Physical Therapy Research Laboratory. "It's the first of its kind in a physical therapy setting in Europe," says Hirschfeld, who began her career as a specialist in neurologic rehabilitation working primarily with children. "I am the director of the laboratory, supervising five doctoral students and eight projects that are looking at integration of posture, including anticipatory and compensatory postural adjustments, and voluntary movement during everyday motor tasks in adults and children with and without disabilities. Our patient groups come from neurologic and orthopedic clinics." Hirschfeld is focusing on the neurobiomechanical mechanisms related to the initiation of the task, such as weight transfer and center-of-pressure and center-of-mass coordination. Her research team is presenting several papers at the International Society for Posture and Gait symposium in Paris, France, this month.

"In Sweden, we don't have the debate on high tech versus low tech. Karolinska Hospital has a movable balance platform that was constructed at the Royal Technical University; it's used in research. Our laboratory has six forceplates, a four-camera system, and a 16-channel electromyographic testing system, and the Ear-Nose-Throat Department at the University Hospital in Linkoping uses the EquiTest™ for treating patients with vestibular disorders. But high-tech equipment is not available to most therapists. In clinical practice, evaluation is performed using a variety of low-tech tests.

"For us, debate centers on what clinical balance tests are *really* testing. In one project, we are investigating whether instability during one-legged standing in children with what we call 'developmental coordination disorders' is related to impaired postural control. As discussed at the Society for Neuroscience meeting last November in Washington, DC, many clinical tests score one-legged standing for 'static balance.' That is, in a task-oriented approach, PTs have the child practice one-legged standing in different situations, such as during stair climbing or kicking, with a focus on increasing the amount of time that the child is able to stand on one leg without large body movements—'static balance.' We propose that the apparent instability reflected by those large movements may actually be an appropriate postural response strategy for maintaining equilibrium and compensating for inadequately programmed movement of the lifting leg. If this is true, PTs should focus on the programming of weight transfer and leg lift—that is, on feedforward control—in clinical practice."

At Umea University's Department of Geriatric Medicine, physical therapist researchers Lillemor Lundin-Olsson, Lars Nyberg, and Jane Jensen want to develop instruments—ultimately, a fall risk index to include such items as "stops walking when talking"—that will be applicable in the clinic. Their focus: fall risk factors in patients with stroke who are receiving "in-hospital rehabilitation" and in elderly people in sheltered living programs.

"We hope to start a project on prevention of falls," reports Lundin-Olsson. "We also plan a study on balance and divided attention, for which we'll use both low-tech tools and tools in a virtual reality lab." Many therapists in Sweden, says Lundin-Olsson, use tests such as "one-legged standing or 'homemade' tests. As a lecturer, I teach about tests such as the Functional Reach Test; however, these tests don't seem to be meeting the needs of our established therapists. Something must be lacking. Our profession needs to study, in a structured way, what therapists are really seeing.... The Swedish version of the Berg scale has been received with great interest, although the scale does have a ceiling effect. We would like to see the observation of safe and unsafe performance added to the timed "up and go" test: A short time does not necessarily indicate a safe performance!"

Lundin-Olsson and her colleagues are most encouraged—and challenged—by Mary Tinetti's work on fall prevention. "We need to find good fall prevention models for different target groups. We also need to know more about how patients experience balance—and how that influences treatment results."

A Global Consensus on Balance Strategies?

"In Sweden," says Lundin-Olsson, "we have a tradition of assessment and treatment of body awareness, and that applies to balance control. In fact, a body awareness scale was developed by Roxendahl.[12] Our hope is that physical therapists all over the world will come to view balance assessment and treatment in the context of the interactions among body, mind, tasks, and environment. Sooner or later, a consensus among PT researchers will be sorted out."

A burning issue in balance—and in all other areas of practice—is the need for computerized databases, says Katherine Berg. "We need to be able to compare rehabilitation databases on balance, gait, and mobility to find out whether measures overlap or can be 'crosswalked.' Does a score of 46 on the Berg balance test correspond to a score of 18 on the Tinetti test, for instance? Once we know that kind of information, we can compare apples with apples. Then, we can take a look at balance worldwide. For instance: Each country has a different health care system. Let's use that to find out what works and what doesn't! In Australia, patients with stroke receive 8 weeks of inpatient rehabilitation, no questions asked. In other countries, they may receive much less. If data show that similar patients in other countries who receive less inpatient rehabilitation achieve the same outcomes as do patients in Australia, think of how that could revolutionize patient management!"

Steven Wolf believes that "there now are 'global research concepts' in the balance arena" that ultimately will result in better information for clinicians. As Chair of the Abstracts Committee of the 1995 Congress of the World Confederation for Physical Therapy, Wolf reviewed abstracts from several countries and found a universal growing awareness of the impact that physical therapists have on the behavioral components of balance. But there still is a critical gap, says Fay Horak, PhD, PT, "between how posture control scientists around the world understand neural control of balance and motor learning and how clinicans around the world view balance and how to train or rehabilitate it. In my experience, scientists view balance as an emergent property of a complex, multicomponent, sensorimotor system, whereas clinicians often think of it as a single set of automatic reactions. The implications for how to assess and treat balance disorders based on these different assumptions about neural control of balance are immense."

Pam Duncan, who recently attended a World Health Organization conference in Florence, Italy, finds that "therapists worldwide are extremely knowledgeable about current balance research, though they may not be quite as aggressive in their treatment approaches as we are here in the States.... I always like to say that impaired balance is a necessary but not sufficient reason to fall. Whether a patient falls is very complicated and has to do with the type of medication the patient is taking, the cognitive skills, the task, the environment, and the willingness to take a risk. Balance, that is, postural control, is only one component that can contribute to falls, as is vestibular disorders. In fact, I believe the number of patients with primary vestibular disorders is actually quite small." Clinicians everywhere, says Duncan, need to understand the conceptual model of balance; evaluate the factors contributing to instability, including sensory function, motor function, and reaction time; select from a battery of standardized tests; and intervene, taking into account such factors as medication and environment and referring to other health professionals as necessary for vestibular problems.

Duncan points out that "not a single FICSIT trial was completed in less than 10 weeks. The implications are that some patients require very intensive programs—and that we have to convince insurers that those programs will decrease disability. We have to articulate research findings in a way that makes sense to managed care."

Although Duncan is optimistic about the future of balance rehabilitation, she reinforces that there is a great deal of work to be done. "We have the international community of basic science researchers who focus on postural control, we have the geriatricians, we have the physical therapists, and we have the vestibular researchers. Each group is making tremendous progress on its own. The next step is to integrate their work."

Changing the Way PTs Treat

Richard Di Fabio, PhD, PT, editor of *Physical Therapy*'s special series on balance, agrees with Duncan and Berg that "we have numerous tools that enable us to detect balance dysfunction. Many of them involve low technology that is suitable for use in many clinical settings. The biggest problem we face today comes *after* the evaluation. What do we do to improve equilibrium, postural stability, or gait?" Di Fabio believes that the Journal series will provide the catalyst and the foundation for changing the way therapists view and treat balance dysfunction.

"Even though there are many different ways to study postural control, the articles in the series have some common themes that give us a glimpse into the future," explains Di Fabio. "You cannot escape the conclusion, for instance, that sensory input and expectation have a profound influence on balance. The response to a test in a lab, however, might be different from the response to a balance challenge in the real world. This makes total sense—in fact, it seems blatantly obvious. The surprise is that so many of our treatment methods are based on the results of tightly controlled lab experiments that prohibit natural motion! Today, lab experiments are being developed with less restriction of natural movements. Research on balance is moving toward a more holistic approach to the patient, and the Journal series begins to address that transition." PT

Jan P Reynolds is Contributing Editor to PT and Managing Editor of the Journal.

References

1. *Balance: Proceedings of the APTA Forum, Nashville, Tenn, June 13-15, 1989.* Alexandria, Va: American Physical Therapy Association; 1990.
2. Tinetti ME. Performance-oriented assessment of mobility problems in elderly patients. *J Am Geriatr Soc.* 1986;34:119-126.
3. Mathias S, Nayak ULS, Issacs B. Balance in elderly patients: the "Get-up and Go" test. *Arch Phys Med Rehabil.* 1986;67:387-389.
4. Berg K, Wood-Dauphinee S, Williams JT, Gayton D. Measuring balance in the elderly: preliminary development of an instrument. *Physiotherapy Canada.* 1989;41:304-311.
5. Hogue CC, Studenski S, Duncan PW. Assessing mobility: the first step in preventing falls. Funk SG, Tornquist E, Champagne MT, et al. *Key Aspects of Recovery: Improving Nutrition, Rest, and Mobility.* New York, NY: Springer Publishing Co; 1990.
6. Duncan P, Weiner DK, Chandler J, Studenski S. Functional reach: a new clinical measure of balance. *J Gerontol.* 1990;45:M192-197.
7. Cole B, Finch E, Gowland C, Mayo N. *Physical Rehabilitation Outcome Measures.* Toronto, Ontario, Canada: Canadian Physiotherapy Association and Canada Health and Welfare Department; 1994.
8. Bogle Thorbahn LD, Newton RA. Use of the Berg balance test to predict falls in elderly persons. *Phys Ther.* 1996;76:576-585.
9. Ware JE, Sherbourne CD. The MOS 36-item short-form health survey (SF-36), 1: conceptual framework and item selection. *Med Care.* 1992;30:473-483.
10. Liston RA, Brouwer BJ. Reliability and validity of measures obtained from stroke patients using the BalanceMaster. *Arch Phys Med Rehabil.* 1996;77:425-430.
11. Hu MH, Woollacott MH. Balance evaluation, training, and rehabilitation of frail fallers. *Reviews in Clinical Gerontology.* 1996;6:85-99.
12. Roxendahl G. *Body Awareness Therapy and the Body Awareness Scale. Treatment and Evaluation in Psychiatric Physiotherapy.* Gothenburg, Sweden: University of Göteborg; 1985.

"The response to a test in a lab...might be different from the response to a balance challenge in the real world," says Richard Di Fabio. "The surprise is that so many of our treatment methods are based on the results of tightly controlled lab experiments that prohibit natural motion!" One of the most exciting aspects of *Physical Therapy*'s special series, says Di Fabio, was "conveying the bigger picture through a blend of work by clinicians and researchers from across the globe." For highlights and author insights, turn the page.

E-mail From: JOURNAL AUTHORS

To: PT Readers
From: Journal Authors
Subject: "New Perspectives on Balance"

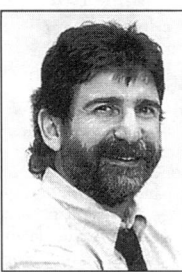

Richard P Di Fabio, PhD, PT (University of Minnesota, Minneapolis), and **Alongkot Emasithi, PT**

Aging and the Mechanisms Underlying Head and Postural Control During Voluntary Motion

Head control is essential for regulating the quality of sensory input for balance! In situations in which there is a decrease in sensory input, precise adjustments of head position might make the difference between standing and falling. Just imagine trying to walk in a dark room with a "floppy" head. The head serves as the "reference" for upright posture. Our article helps clarify the mechanisms that influence head stability.... As people grow older, the way in which they stabilize the head during activity seems to change. This topic will be studied more in the future to determine whether head control strategies are related to falling in older persons.

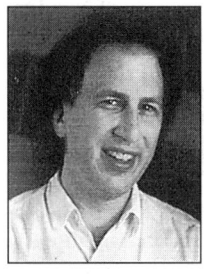

John J Jeka, PhD (University of Maryland at College Park)

Light Touch Contact as a Balance Aid

Have you ever noticed how your patients use light touch contact for balance? Countless clinicians have approached me after I've given presentations at conferences, saying, "Patients are always touching their spouses' sleeves." And PTs have told me that when they instruct their patients not to use a cane anymore because they're strong enough to do without it, those patients often insist that they do need it. That may be because the subtle touch contact with a cane gives people the orientation they need.... As a therapist, you may view canes and other aids solely as biomechanical supports, but now we have evidence to suggest that the use of a cane gives patients important sensory information. [See page 36 for more on the collaboration between Jeka and physical therapist Lisa DePasquale.]

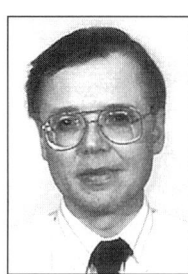

Brian E Maki, PhD, PEng, and **William E McIlroy** (Sunnybrook Health Science Center and University of Toronto)

The Role of Limb Movements in Maintaining Upright Stance: The Change-in-Support Strategy

Physical therapists help me see research's clinical relevance—or lack thereof. This feedback is particularly important in guiding us to examine motor control issues that have practical importance, to increase the chances that our results may actually end up helping people maintain a more mobile and independent lifestyle.... Over the last 25 years or so, unfortunately, the focus of much of the balance research has been limited to a rather narrow subset of postural behavior: the ability to maintain upright stance without moving the feet or arms. Although some of the postural reflexes and reactions that enable us to accomplish this task are undoubtedly important in providing an early defense against loss of balance, there are other postural behaviors that are of equal, if not greater, functional importance in our daily lives. In particular, the ability to maintain balance by using rapid stepping or grasping reactions appears to be used in preference to other types of reactions, such as the "hip strategy." The hip strategy may allow us to balance when standing on the edge of a cliff, for instance, but if we have the option, our natural reaction to unexpected loss of balance is to take a step or grasp onto something. It therefore seems unlikely that training of the hip strategy will provide much functional benefit. We hope that clinicians will begin to focus more on the ability to control rapid compensatory limb movements.

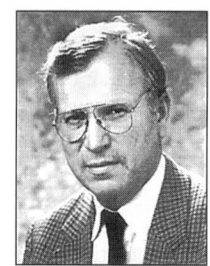

Volker Dietz, MD, and **Markus Wirz, PT,** and Lars Jensen, DM (University Hospital Balgrist, Zurich, Switzerland)

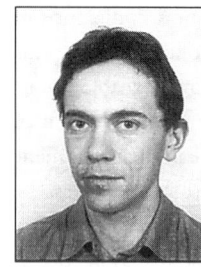

Locomotion in Patients With Spinal Cord Injuries

There are three points we'd like you to think about as you treat patients: 1) you can assess effects of physical therapy through biomechanical and electrophysiological recordings; 2) you should always consider functional movements such as locomotion for therapy, not just reflexes and muscle tone in a passive state; 3) some of the neuromuscular changes due to spinal or brain motor lesions, such as increased muscle tone, can be advantageous to the patient if they provide body support during stepping movements. These changes could be incorporated into physical therapy; however, research is needed to determine effectiveness. In the future, partial regeneration of the lesioned spinal cord tract fibers, combined with locomotor training, may improve functional mobility, even for patients with almost complete paraplegia!

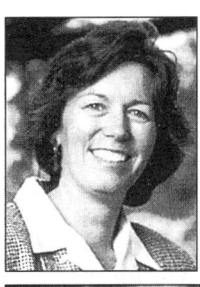
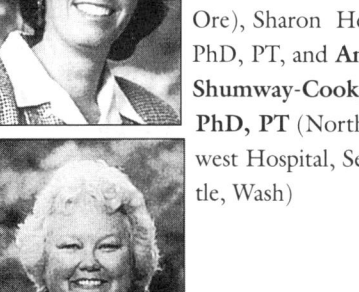

Fay B Horak, PhD, PT (RS Dow Neurological Sciences Institute, Portland, Ore), Sharon Henry, PhD, PT, and **Anne Shumway-Cook, PhD, PT** (Northwest Hospital, Seattle, Wash)

Postural Perturbations: New Insights for Treatment of Balance Disorders

Research in postural perturbation has taught us that balance is a motor skill that can improve with practice.... When Anne Shumway-Cook and I first began studying balance disorders in the laboratory, we were flabbergasted to find out that most of our clinical assumptions about balance disorders did not hold up to clinical testing. For instance, patients with complete absence of vestibular function had normal postural responses! Patients with spasticity in ankle extensors showed later and smaller—rather than earlier and larger—postural responses to ankle stretch! Furthermore, patients with Parkinson's disease did not have late postural responses, as clinicians often assumed, and, although levadopa certainly improved patients' ability to move, it did not improve their responses to postural perturbations. Experimental testing of our clinical assumptions about postural control has forced us to reconsider how the brain controls movement and has inspired new approaches to the rehabilitation of balance and motor disorders.

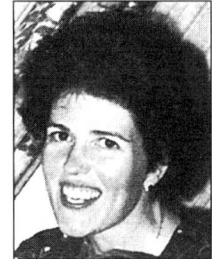

Kathleen M Gill-Body, PT, NCS (MGH Institute of Health Professions and Massachusetts General Hospital, Boston), Rita A Popat, PT, NCS, Stephen W Parker, MD, and David E Krebs, PhD, PT

Case Report: Rehabilitation of Balance in Two Patients With Cerebellar Dysfunction

Patients often say things that make me stop and think. One patient with a balance disorder, who had been in a wheelchair for many months and walked with a cane at the end of rehab, said, "Thanks for giving me back my own set of wheels".... Patients with cerebellar dysfunction can be quite challenging to treat because of the myriad of symptoms, the scarcity of research to support a definitive treatment approach, and the unclear relationship between their specific impairments and their functional limitations. And, as we all know, in today's health care environment we have marked limitations on the number of physical therapy visits that a patient is allowed to receive, which makes it compulsory to have a clear, hypothesis-driven approach to patient management. In our case report, we laid out our hypotheses and closely followed two patients to monitor their responses to treatment. Although not every PT can evaluate each patient before and after treatment to the extent that we did, we encourage you to step back occasionally to examine your own assumptions. Based on the data in this case report and on other pilot data, we plan to do a randomized controlled trial—the next step in the process!

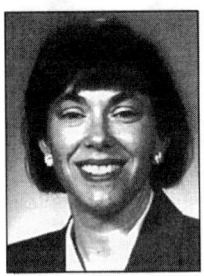

Deborah S Nichols, PhD, PT (The Ohio State University, Columbus)

Update: Balance Retraining After Stroke Using Force Platform Biofeedback

In researching balance retraining for the Update—which is a kind of "mini literature review"—I encountered very negative views about the use of force platform biofeedback, views that are held by many clinicians and researchers despite the fact that many studies have documented significant improvements in function associated with this type of training. I hope my article will give you a better expectation of what benefits may be possible from force platform biofeedback and how to best design a treatment protocol to achieve those benefits. I also emphasize the limitations of this type of treatment, so that you can be more realistic about what outcomes to expect. In my own work, I will continue to look at biofeedback as a treatment protocol for the relearning of postural control and the relative contributions of this type of treatment to functional outcomes, such as activities of daily living, ambulation, and standing reach, in patients with neurological injury. Many of the limitations described in my article may reflect the type of equipment that is available and the training protocols used—not the treatment itself.

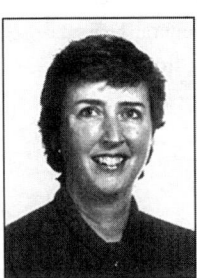

Susan J Herdman, PhD, PT (University of Miami School of Medicine, Coral Gables, Fla)

Advances in the Treatment of Vestibular Disorders

In this article, I outlined the advances in use of vestibular exercises during the past 5 years based on the direct outcome of controlled studies on the use of exercises. During the next 5 years, we can expect that there will be a better understanding of the stimulus to induce otolith—utricle and saccule—adaptation. From that, clinical tests will be developed for assessing otolith function, and exercises will be developed specifically for improving otolith-related deficits, including exercises that incorporate virtual reality systems. In the next 5 years, I plan to use a computerized system that my colleagues and I have developed to measure dynamic visual acuity to distinguish healthy vestibular function from unilateral and bilateral vestibular loss. I'll be using the test to determine whether vestibular rehab techniques improve visual acuity during head movements and decrease the patient's oscillopsia [perception of visual blurring]—with the ultimate goal of determining underlying mechanisms and who is likely or not likely to recover. I hypothesize that oscillopsia can change cadence and gait pattern as well as result in increased fear of falling. Also, like all PTs, I've become increasingly aware of the need to measure functional outcomes. Some of the measures we use, such as static balance, don't translate into what happens when the patient walks. I encourage you to take a look at the work that Sue Whitney, PhD, PT, has done on validity and reliability of balance tools when used with patients who have vestibular disorders.

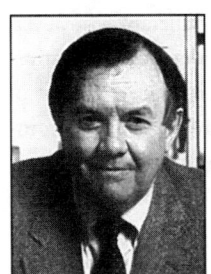

Michael G Wade, PhD, and Graeme Jones (University of Minnesota, Minneapolis)

The Role of Vision and Spatial Orientation in the Maintenance of Posture

Several of my past and present graduate students in kinesiology began as physical therapy clinicians. They've brought a rich clinical background to our program. But I've noticed that they have a very traditional medical background in areas such as locomotion and gait. There's been an interesting marriage in our program between those students with a strong research background and those students who are very well prepared clinically. I believe that PTs have been taught a few "golden rules" that need to be questioned when it comes to theories of coordination and control, information processing, and dynamical systems. Only recently have PTs begun to address these areas in clinical practice; Crutchfield and Barnes were among the first. I'd like to see a closer academic tie between kinesiology and physical therapy, and this special series supports the development of that tie.

Sarah L Westcott, PhD, PT (Allegheny University of the Health Sciences, Philadelphia, Pa), **Linda Pax Lowes, PhD, PT, PCS**, and **Pamela K Richardson, PhD, OT**

Evaluation of Postural Stability in Children: Current Theories and Assessment Tools

Balance is a complex issue that can be evaluated in many ways, which is why it's important to know the reason why you're doing an assessment. You need to be aware not only of the available assessments but of the reliability and validity of those assessments. The evaluation of balance can be simplified by thinking of it as being produced through the cooperation of many systems.... Evaluation of balance in children is difficult due to problems with controlling both the environment and the children themselves. Much variability exists in children's responses, which makes it difficult to find consistent test results over time. Because of this, many of the existing tools related to measurement of balance in children have only marginally acceptable psychometrics. A focus of future studies should be to define the pertinent variables associated with balance that are most stable over time. And with the shift to a greater focus on functional changes with treatment, we need to develop assessments of "functional balance."

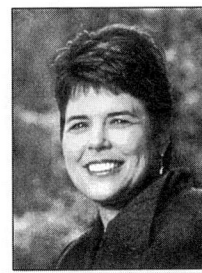

Marjorie H Woollacott, PhD, and Pei-Fang Tang, PhD, PT (University of Oregon, Eugene)

Balance Control During Walking in the Older Adult: Research and Its Implications

What's surprised me lately is that balance control during perturbed gait is very different from that during normal gait. The locus of balance control in normal gait is at the hip and is aimed at the control of the stability of the head-arms-trunk segment. However, in perturbed gait, such as a slip, the locus of control is in the leg and thigh, with hip and trunk muscles contributing very little to balance in the early phase of recovery. If the leg and thigh muscles are too weak to control balance by themselves, the hip and trunk muscles are recruited. Clinicians should be aware of this relationship.... On the surface, balance control seems like such a simple task, doesn't it? But without it, a person can't perform other tasks with agility, coordination, and grace. To assess balance control, we need to use the framework of both proactive and reactive balance control mechanisms in assessment and treatment. If we know that attention is a critical issue and that attention to a secondary task may cause a deterioration in balance control, we can add secondary tasks to locomotor assessments and treatments in the clinic. In our laboratory, Pei-Fang Tang is developing an instrument for assessing the various sensory contributions to functional mobility, and Anne Shumway-Cook is currently working with us to design assessment and treatment approaches that incorporate attentional demands. Anne suggests that clinicians ask the person to talk, to carry or manipulate an object, or to turn the head from side to side while simultaneously walking. If the patient slows down, deviates from his or her normal path, or stops when performing the secondary task, that's valuable information.... I encourage clinicians to work with researchers to write grants for the development of more assessment instruments. The time has never been more right.

Multisensory Integration:
What Could It Mean for Designing Physical Therapy Treatment Programs of the Future?

"It was an accident!" says Richard Di Fabio, Journal Special Series Editor. "I found John Jeka when I was reviewing one of his papers for *Perception and Psychophysics*. I thought, 'Here's a scientist in a very different field who might have something important to tell physical therapists.'" Jeka, an Associate Professor in the Department of Kinesiology at the University of Maryland at College Park, recently received funding from the National Institute on Aging to pursue how touch is integrated with other senses to give humans their overall sense of orientation in space.

When people lose their vestibular system, explains Jeka, "they rely on vision and the somatosensory system of the feet. But they have tremendous difficulty moving from a solid surface to a wet, spongy surface such as grass. It can even make them nauseous. Why? What's different about that somatosensory system? It could be that individuals with an impaired vestibular system have a limited ability to adapt to a wide range of disruptions. But we don't really know what that means, because we don't understand the properties of *healthy* adaptation.... When people with bilateral vestibular loss assume a heel-to-toe stance, they fall over immediately. We've found that with light touch, such as with a cane, their postural stability can be normal, as though they had an intact system." In addition to static balance testing, Jeka is using sensory immersion in his research.

Working with Jeka as part of her master's thesis is physical therapist LCDR Lisa DePasquale, PT, ECS. "I started out taking classes on motor control parttime. Then I took some of John's classes on postural control, and I got hooked." Jeka had previously worked with Jim Lackner, PhD, at Brandeis University's Ashton Graybiel Spatial Orientation Laboratory, which conducted research (funded by the National Aeronautics and Space Administration) on movement control and sensory influences during weightlessness. Jeka also worked with David Krebs, PhD, PT, researching vestibular disorders using the postural paradigm.

"John approaches his research from a basic and applied science perspective," says DePasquale. "I was excited when he suggested using the touch paradigm in an applied science approach using a patient model to investigate how patients with bilateral vestibular loss recover their postural control."

Patients in this project range in age from 35 to 72 years and have been diagnosed with vestibular loss associated with conditions such as peripheral lesions or systemic infections that required heavy-duty antibiotics resulting in ototoxicity. "These individuals need a wide base of support, and they

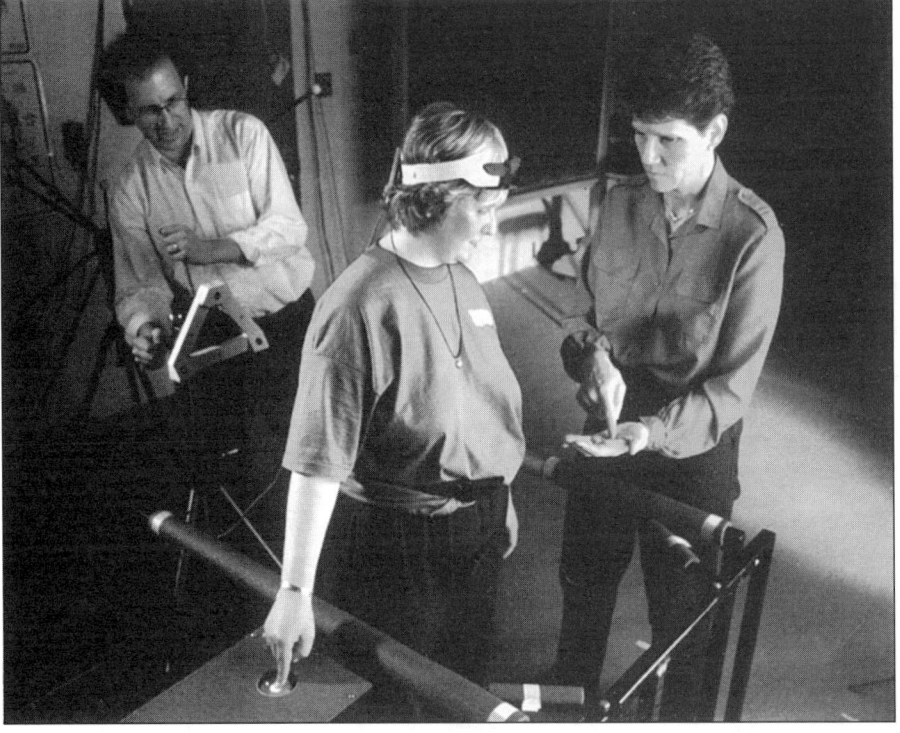

For Lisa DePasquale, an electrophysiologic certified specialist, the vestibular system is a brand new horizon. "The impact of a total systems approach is fascinating. So many components are involved.... The people in my research peer group at University of Maryland have always done didactic research involving healthy subjects. When I said, 'Let's do something that could have a direct impact on the kinds of patients that physical therapists see every day,' they got really excited." In this photo: DePasquale instructs Bonnie Jo Chittum, who has bilateral vestibulopathy, in how to use the touch bar, while John Jeka, PhD, adjusts the head-tracking device that will monitor head movement during static balance testing.

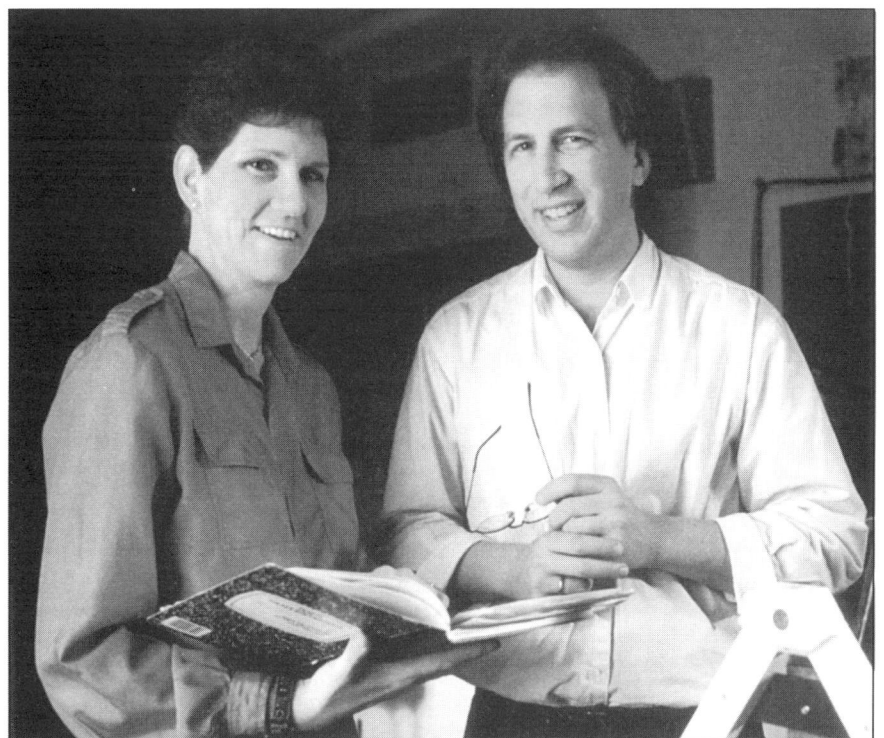

"The information we gather should help clinicians structure individualized treatment programs," says John Jeka, who will be presenting preliminary data this summer in Paris at the International Society for Posture and Gait symposium. Working with physical therapist Lisa DePasquale has helped Jeka "bridge the gap between basic science and clinical intervention."

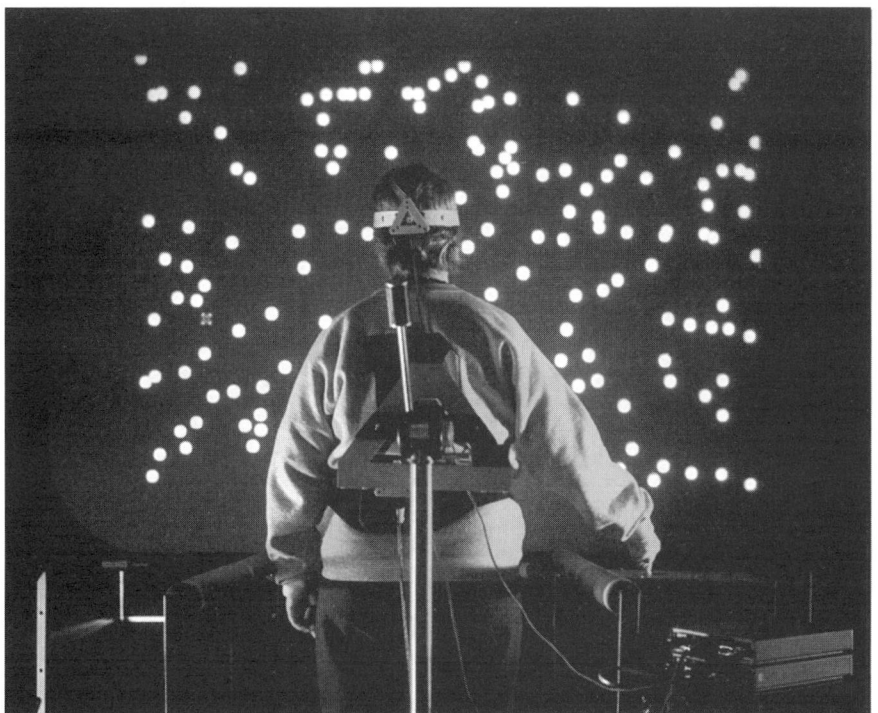

"It took John Jeka and his student team 2 years to get this project up and running," says DePasquale. "They had to refine the computer program so that the perturbations would be added in the correct sequence." Subjects stand in a random-dot visual field created on a back-projected screen and touch a bar that moves. "We think it gets at multisensory integration below the cortical level.... It's a kind of virtual reality," says Jeka, who originally considered using virtual reality helmets but decided against them in part because "the helmet prevents the wearer from seeing the real environment, which can be frightening to people if they lose their balance. The helmets also have relatively small visual displays that wouldn't allow complete sensory immersion." Jeka considered using a moving room that is hung from the ceiling (moving rooms have been used in postural control research) but found that it was too difficult to keep the room stable. "We're looking at vision and touch simultaneously in the context of standing posture to understand how the senses are integrated," says Jeka. "In some situations, a particular sense may dominate; in others, the senses may cooperate."

have a great deal of apprehension about walking on grass or sidewalks. Many subjects have said, 'I have difficulty walking—but I'm willing to help out with your study.'"

One of DePasquale's roles is to "keep the focus on the patient model. I give the research team a clinical perspective. I'm a clinician at heart, and I know that this study could have important implications for the way physical therapists design treatment programs. Even a patient with an ankle sprain, for instance, could benefit from a therapist's understanding of postural control—understanding not only what's happening at the level of the joint in terms of swelling and hypomobility, but taking a dynamical systems perspective." There is another benefit to being involved in this project, adds DePasquale. "It's teaching me a way of thinking. Putting data through power analysis prepares you for clean, organized decision making in the clinic."

Physical Therapy Special Series on Balance

Editor's Note

Illuminating Balance

Few areas of physical therapy practice have drawn as much attention in recent years as the treatment of persons with balance disorders.

In a world that demands evidence-based practice, this is an area in which evidence does exist—and an area in which there is cutting-edge application of theories and concepts. It also is an area in which dogma seems to be growing and fascination with clinical devices may be taking precedence over common sense. Balance needs illumination, and, in that spirit, the Journal is delighted to present this special series.

Assembled under the leadership of Special Series Editor Richard Di Fabio, PhD, PT, the series contains a wide-ranging selection of articles. The content illustrates an ongoing difficulty for those who treat patients. At what point do concepts that we use in practice take on lives of their own and become immune to challenge? Are the balance strategies that we have all come to understand "real"? Are they ubiquitous? Do we need to expand our horizons to think of balance in new ways? This series offers differing views. The contrasts are testimony to the vibrancy of this area of practice and to the robustness of the research.

This special series sets a new precedent: We have included an Update and a Case Report related to the central theme. The series not only provides vital information at all levels—from basic sciences to applied clinical sciences—it also demonstrates the ongoing effort of this Journal to publish articles that are relevant for all readers. Whether you are a clinician who only rarely treats patients with balance problems, a clinician specializing in balance disorders, or a researcher in the field, this series has material you can use *now*.

As Editor, I am grateful to Dr Di Fabio; to Alan Jette, PhD, PT, former Deputy Editor of the Journal, who assisted in the effort; to the reviewers; and to the authors, many of whom are publishing specifically for physical therapists for the first time.

Jules M Rothstein, PhD, PT, FAPTA
Editor

Special Series Contributors

The following individuals contributed articles to the balance special series.

Richard P Di Fabio, PhD, PT
Professor and Director
Doctoral Graduate Studies
Program in Physical Therapy
Dept of Physical Medicine
 and Rehabilitation
University of Minnesota
Minneapolis, Minn

Volker Dietz, MD
Professor, Doctor, and Chair/Head
 of Paraplegiology
Swiss Paraplegic Centre
University Hospital Balgrist
Zurich, Switzerland

Alongkot Emasithi, PT
University of Minnesota
Minneapolis, Minn

Kathleen M Gill-Body, PT, NCS
Assistant Professor
Graduate Programs in Physical Therapy
MGH Institute of Health Professions
Boston, Mass

Neurologic Clinical Specialist
Physical Therapy Services
Massachusetts General Hospital
Boston, Mass

Sharon M Henry, PhD, PT
Research Associate
RS Dow Neurological Sciences Institute
Portland, Ore

Susan J Herdman, PhD, PT
Associate Professor
Div of Physical Therapy
Dept of Orthopaedics and Rehabilitation
University of Miami School of Medicine
Coral Gables, Fla

Fay B Horak, PhD, PT
Senior Scientist and Professor
RS Dow Neurological Sciences Institute
Portland, Ore

John J Jeka, PhD
Assistant Professor
Dept of Kinesiology
College of Health and Human Performance
University of Maryland at College Park
College Park, Md

Lars Jensen, DM
Bioengineer
Swiss Paraplegic Centre
University Hospital Balgrist
Zurich, Switzerland

Graeme Jones
School of Kinesiology and Leisure Studies
College of Education and
 Human Development
University of Minnesota
Minneapolis, Minn

David E Krebs, PhD, PT
Associate Professor
MGH Institute of Health Professions
Boston, Mass

Director
Biomotion Laboratory
Massachusetts General Hospital
Boston, Mass

Instructor
Harvard Medical School
Boston, Mass

Lecturer
Massachusetts Institute of Technology
Cambridge, Mass

Linda Pax Lowes, PhD, PT, PCS
Assistant Professor
Texas Woman's University
Houston, Tex

Brian E Maki, PhD, PEng
Senior Scientist
Sunnybrook Health Science Centre
Toronto, Ontario, Canada

Associate Professor
University of Toronto
Toronto, Ontario, Canada

William E McIlroy, PhD
Senior Scientist
Sunnybrook Health Science Centre
Toronto, Ontario, Canada

Associate Professor
University of Toronto
Toronto, Ontario, Canada

Deborah S Nichols, PhD, PT
Director & Associate Professor
Physical Therapy Div
School of Allied Medical Professions
The Ohio State University
Columbus, Ohio

Stephen W Parker, MD
Chief of Otoneurology
Massachusetts General Hospital
Boston, Mass

Assistant Professor of Neurology
Harvard Medical School
Boston, Mass

(continued on next page)

Rita A Popat, PT, NCS
University of Massachusetts
Amherst, Mass

Pamela K Richardson, PhD, OT
California Children's Services
Santa Barbara, Calif

Anne Shumway-Cook, PhD, PT
Research Coordinator
Dept of Physical Therapy
Northwest Hospital
Seattle, Wash

Pei-Fang Tang, PhD, PT
Adjunct Assistant Professor
Dept of Exercise and Movement Science
and Institute of Neuroscience
University of Oregon
Eugene, Ore

Michael G Wade, PhD
Professor and Director
School of Kinesiology and Leisure Studies
College of Education and
Human Development
University of Minnesota
Minneapolis, Minn

Sarah L Westcott, PhD, PT
Assistant Professor
Allegheny University of the Health Sciences
Philadelphia, Pa

Markus Wirz, PT
Swiss Paraplegic Centre
University Hospital Balgrist
Zurich, Switzerland

Marjorie H Woollacott, PhD
Professor
Dept of Exercise and Movement Science
and Institute of Neuroscience
University of Oregon
Eugene, Ore

Special Series Reviewers

The following individuals were reviewers for the articles appearing in the balance special series.

Dennis Brunt, EdD, PT
University of Florida
Gainesville, Fla

Rebecca L Craik, PhD, PT, FAPTA
Beaver College
Glenside, Pa

Volker Dietz, MD
University Hospital Balgrist
Zurich, Switzerland

Kathleen M Gill-Body, PT, NCS
MGH Institute of Health Professions
Boston, Mass

Susan R Harris, PhD, PT, FAPTA
University of British Columbia
Vancouver, British Columbia, Canada

Fay B Horak, PhD, PT
RS Dow Neurological Sciences Institute
Portland, Ore

Gregory M Karst, PhD, PT
University of Nebraska
Omaha, Neb

Marie Koch, PT
Quinnipiac College
Hamden, Conn

David E Krebs, PhD, PT
MGH Institute of Health Professions
Boston, Mass

Carl G Kukulka, PhD, PT
University of Florida
Gainesville, Fla

Irene R McEwen, PhD, PT, PCS
University of Oklahoma
Oklahoma City, Okla

Michael J Mueller, PhD, PT
Washington University
St Louis, Mo

Roberta A Newton, PhD, PT
Temple University
Philadelphia, Pa

Deborah S Nichols, PhD, PT
The Ohio State University
Columbus, Ohio

Carol A Oatis, PhD, PT
Beaver College
Glenside, Pa

Mark W Rogers, PhD, PT
Northwestern University
Chicago, Ill

Richard K Shields, PT
The University of Iowa
Iowa City, Iowa

Stephanie A Studenski, PT
Kansas University Medical Center
Kansas City, Kan

Introduction to Special Series

New Perspectives on Balance

Is there any activity that does not require the control of posture? The corrections of posture that are characteristic of a healthy nervous system provide stability and allow us to initiate motion and to move without falling—all with no conscious awareness. Disorders of postural control alter the efficiency and effectiveness of our actions, so it is easy to understand why the improvement of balance is a primary goal for many people receiving rehabilitation.

This special series is devoted to the exploration of new concepts in the control of postural stability and balance, such as the use of touch receptors in the fingertips and hand to provide spatial orientation for balance, the management of altered reflex activity in a way that enhances mobility, and a scientific rationale for selecting the most effective exercises to treat disorders of the vestibular system. Assessment of balance deficits is addressed across the life span, from pediatric to geriatric populations.

Our authors describe theories that address sensory influences on balance, the role of reflexes in postural control, and some of the relationships between perception and action that influence spatial orientation and equilibrium. The discussion of clinical implications throughout this series suggests new treatments that could be developed, tested, and applied in practice. There also is some new evidence to support old theories: Certain procedures described long ago, such as the Alexander technique, may deserve another look. Models of motor control have been introduced in this special series as a way to study integrated behaviors in natural environments. These models depart from more traditional approaches that were designed to study the isolated influences of sensory stimulation on postural reflexes.

The divergent perspectives and methodologies used to study postural control have produced some divergent findings. Investigations that use perturbations of balance to study postural control, for example, have provided a way to understand how the central nervous system manages multiple sensory inputs and prior experience to stabilize the body. This methodology forms an essential component of the research that has popularized the "ankle," "hip," and "stepping" strategies outlined in many clinical assessments of balance—strategies that represent different ways to regain balance following disturbances of equilibrium.

[Di Fabio RP. Introduction: new perspectives on balance. *Phys Ther.* 1997;77:456–457.]

Richard P Di Fabio

Questions are raised in this special series about the neural organization of balance strategies and about the usefulness of evaluating the responses to these strategies. Are some strategies clinically meaningful, or simply an artifact of the constraints of laboratory experiments? Alternative models that test subjects performing natural movements with few constraints have produced results that challenge our current views about balance strategies. This work provides the backdrop for a debate concerning the way we assess balance strategies in the clinic.

Perhaps the most important contribution of this special series is the rationale that the authors provide to develop and test new approaches for the rehabilitation of postural control. Age, the type of and amount of practice, the nature of the task (eg, self-initiated motion versus a reaction to an external disturbance of balance), and the availability of sensory inputs can alter how a person maintains equilibrium, but what are the best ways to address these factors when planning a treatment program to improve postural stability? Specific examples of the methods now being used to treat balance dysfunction in persons with stroke or cerebellar disease are provided in the Case Report and Update.

This collection of articles represents a new beginning. As the work of these authors is applied to the clinical environment, our views about the control of posture will be modified and refined. Another renaissance of balance research is on the horizon, and I am convinced that the next generation of "new perspectives" on balance will originate with this special series.

RP Di Fabio, PhD, PT, is Professor and Director of Doctoral Graduate Studies, Program in Physical Therapy, Department of Physical Medicine and Rehabilitation, University of Minnesota, UMHC, Box 388, 420 Delaware St SE, Minneapolis, MN 55455 (USA) (difab001@maroon.tc.umn.edu).

Aging and the Mechanisms Underlying Head and Postural Control During Voluntary Motion

The quality of sensory information that is necessary for balance and postural stability will depend to a great extent on head stability as the body moves. How older persons coordinate head and body motion for balance during volitional activities is not known. The purposes of this article are to present a basis for understanding the influence of aging on head control during voluntary motion and to discuss some data that demonstrate how elderly people might control head movement to improve gaze and the quality of vestibular inputs. A "top-down" or "head-first" control scheme is proposed as the mechanism that elderly people without disabilities use to maintain head position during self-initiated motion. This type of control ensures that the angular position of the head in space remains relatively constant—through the use of a head-stabilization-in-space (HSS) strategy—regardless of the magnitude or direction of displacements in the body's center of force. The HSS strategy is thought to reduce potential ambiguities in the interpretation of sensory inputs for balance and is derived primarily from a geocentric (orientation to the vertical) frame of reference. Egocentric (orientation of the head with respect to the body) or exocentric (orientation to objects in the environment) frames of reference, however, refine the control of head stabilization. Preliminary research suggests that elderly people use the HSS strategy to control head pitch during difficult balance tasks. These findings, if supported by more definitive studies, may be useful in the treatment of patients with balance disorders. The treatment of patients with balance dysfunction is discussed within the conceptual framework of a "head-first" organization scheme. [Di Fabio RP, Emasithi A. Aging and the mechanisms underlying head and postural control during voluntary motion. *Phys Ther.* 1997;77:458–475.]

Key Words: *Balance, Head control, Posture, Sensory integration.*

Richard P Di Fabio

Alongkot Emasithi

The quality of sensory information that is necessary for balance and postural stability depends to a great extent on head stabilization as the body moves. Some investigators have proposed that a "top-down" or "head-first" control scheme is used to ensure that the head remains stable, with respect to the direction of looking, during body movement.[1-4] Head stability allows gaze (the direction of looking) to be properly oriented.[1-4] This orientation is supposedly accomplished by modifying head position in anticipation of displacements in the body's center of force (COF)* so that the angular orientation of the head in space remains relatively constant. Anticipatory control of the angular displacement of the head is referred to as a head-stabilization-in-space (HSS) strategy (Fig. 1).[6] This strategy differs from a response that fixes the head to the trunk, because the HSS allows adjustments of head position that are independent of trunk motion (Fig. 1).[6,7]

Stabilizing the head in advance of body motion is thought to improve the interpretation of vestibular inputs for balance,[6,8] particularly when visual and somatosensory inputs are distorted or incongruent.[6] Sensory inputs that yield conflicting perceptions of motion are considered to be incongruent. For example, visual cues are incongruent with vestibular inputs when vision conveys the sense of motion in the environment but vestibular information indicates that the body is stationary with respect to gravity. Asymptomatic elderly persons have demonstrated the ability to use multiple sensory inputs for balance as long as two of three primary modalities—visual, vestibular, or somatosensory inputs—are available.[9,10] Changes in the sensorimotor system with aging have been well documented,[11-13] but these changes have not been studied with respect to head stabilization in older persons. Age-related changes

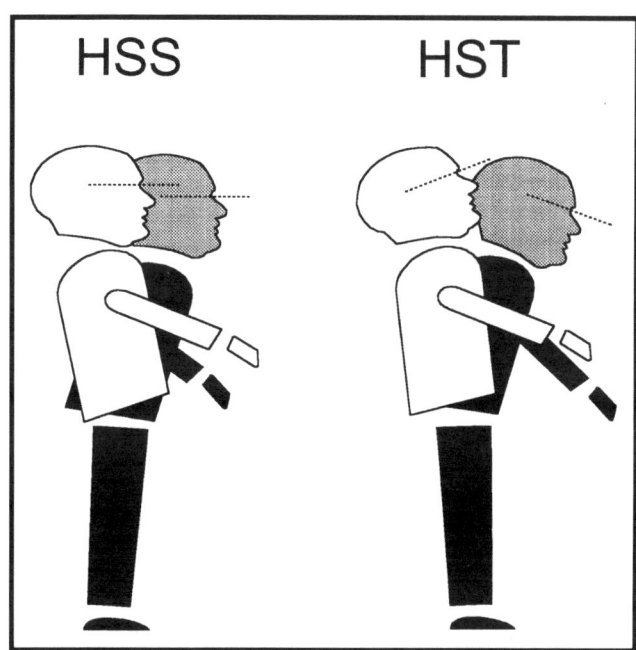

Figure 1.
Illustration of head-stabilization-in-space (HSS) and head-stabilization-on-trunk (HST) strategies for controlling head motion. Head pitch orientation (depicted by the horizontal dotted line through the orbit) is maintained during HSS. In contrast, during HST, head position cannot be regulated independently from the trunk.

---

* *Center of force* is the location of the vertical ground reaction force vector measured by a force platform and is equal and opposite to a weighted average of all of the downward forces acting on the force plate.[5]

RP Di Fabio is Professor and Director of Doctoral Graduate Studies, Program in Physical Therapy, Department of Physical Medicine and Rehabilitation, University of Minnesota, UMHC Box 388, 420 Delaware St SE, Minneapolis, MN 55455 (USA) (difab001@maroon.tc.umn.edu). Address all correspondence to Dr Di Fabio.

A Emasithi, PT, is a doctoral student in the Department of Physical Medicine and Rehabilitation and the Department of Kinesiology, University of Minnesota.

in the vestibular ocular reflex[14] (VOR), for example, could distort visual input during activities of daily living such as walking. A deficient VOR impairs the ability to fix eye position while the head is moving.[15] One way to partially compensate for a deficient VOR is to stabilize the head in a way that nullifies the effect of body motion. The HSS, therefore, would provide one compensatory strategy that elderly persons might use to improve gaze.

Whether the HSS strategy is used by elderly people to stabilize gaze during movement or whether the natural changes in sensory processing with age alter the head stabilization strategy is not known. Hirasaki et al[16] studied the influence of various locomotor activities on compensatory head pitch motions (counteracting vertical translations of the body during gait) in subjects over 60 years of age, but the influence of sensory inputs on head control was not addressed in the experimental design. Although some authors have addressed the control of head stabilization during support-surface perturbations[8,17–20]; during voluntary motions such as walking, hopping, or running[1,2,6,21–23]; and during rotations of the entire body,[24,25] the populations studied were primarily younger than 60 years of age. Balance in elderly persons has been assessed using altered sensory environments,[9,26–29] platform perturbations,[26,27] and voluntary motion to test the limits of stability,[30,31] but there have not been systematic investigations addressing the integration of sensory inputs for head control in aging populations.

The purpose of this article is to present a theoretical basis for understanding the influence of aging on head control during voluntary motion. In addition, a discussion of some preliminary research findings that demonstrate how elderly individuals might utilize a head control strategy to improve gaze and the quality of vestibular inputs for balance will be provided. The discussion of theory is organized into four content areas: (1) frames of reference for balance and head control, (2) sensory influences on each frame of reference, (3) development of head control strategies, and (4) presentation of a conceptual model of head control mechanisms. A presentation of the results of some preliminary studies that demonstrate head stabilization strategies in older persons follows the discussion of theory.

Theoretical Mechanisms Underlying Head Control During Voluntary Motion

Frames of Reference for Balance and Head Control

A frame of reference for balance is a standard against which a change in posture is measured.[32,33] There are three frames of reference that are relevant to the discussion of head and postural control.[32–34] An *egocentric* reference frame provides spatial coordinates for limb and body-segment positions (eg, head position relative to the trunk), whereas an *exocentric* reference gives information about body position with respect to the environment (eg, visual localization of an object that is extrinsic to the subject). A *geocentric* reference system maintains posture with respect to gravity (vertical orientation). Berthoz[32] and Paillard[33] suggested that the relative importance of each frame of reference was organized in a hierarchy, with the egocentric and exocentric frames of reference derived from a geocentric reference system.

Frames of reference for head and postural control, in theory, have several common characteristics.[32,33] Each frame of reference is produced by the transformation of sensory input to spatial perception. In addition, each reference system contributes to the development of an overall body schema or template for balance, and the frames of reference enable the prediction of displacements of the COF.

Transformation of sensory input. Information from visual, vestibular, and proprioceptive systems are transformed in each frame of reference to contribute to aspects of postural control that are not sensor-specific. For example, there is no single dedicated sensor in the nervous system that measures the "margin of postural stability" during stance.[35] This variable can only be derived from an interpretative process within the central nervous system (CNS) that utilizes sensory inputs to estimate the configuration of the support surface, the magnitude and sequence of postural muscle activity, and the location of the center of gravity.[35] The "sense" of the limit of postural stability, therefore, is a perception based on one or more frames of reference for balance.

Contribute to a body schema. Head and Holmes defined *body schema* as "a combined standard against which all subsequent changes of posture are measured."[36] They emphasized that the body schema is a template for postural control that influences spatial orientation of the body "before a change of posture enters consciousness." From a theoretical perspective, the body schema can be viewed as the collective influence of the egocentric, exocentric, and geocentric frames of reference for balance.

Enable the prediction of movement. A primary goal of postural regulation is to stabilize the head with respect to the vertical.[32,33] To provide effective control of head position during movement, the geocentric frame of reference enables anticipation or prediction of COF displacements that are induced by voluntary motion.[32,34] The geocentric frame of reference is thought to use somatosensory, proprioceptive, and vestibular inputs for "feed-forward" control of head stabilization. In the context of a "top-down" or "head-first" control model,[4,6] feed-forward means that corrections of head position occur in advance of a voluntary change in body position. A feed-forward mechanism is a preprogrammed (predetermined) response that appears to be formed through experience with self-initiated goal-directed activity.[34] Sensory input in a feed-forward mode is used primarily for "knowledge of response" to make appropriate adjustments in subsequent anticipatory postural actions.[37] This interative process is thought to develop various frames of reference that make up the template (body schema) to control head and trunk orientation for balance.[35,37,38]

Sensory Influence on the Frames of Reference for Balance and Head Control

The literature reviewed in this section highlights three issues. First, a geocentric frame of reference is essential for generating anticipatory control of head position during voluntary motion. Distortions or absence of sensory input results in an improvement of feed-forward stabilization of the head as long as the geocentric reference is intact.[6] Second, the frames of reference for balance are not based on the input from a single sensory modality. Each frame of reference is derived from multiple sensory inputs.[33,35,39–43] Third, there are interactions among the frames of reference that contribute to the internal representation of a body schema and the overall perception of head, trunk, and limb orientation.[32,33,35,44] The contribution of various sensory modalities to each frame of reference for head stability and postural control will be reviewed.

Vestibular influence on the geocentric frame of reference.

The labyrinth provides two types of information about head kinematics: (1) orientation of static head posture with respect to gravity and (2) detection of head acceleration.[45–53] The vestibular inputs that sense static head posture provide the backdrop for anticipatory or "feed-forward" control of head position[4,6] by continuously monitoring the orientation of the head.[45,46] The otolith organs provide an invariant reference for head position with respect to earth-vertical.[47] An example of this static gravitational reference can be illustrated by the ocular counter-rolling reflex. When the head is tilted to the side, the eyes counter-rotate to nullify the effects of head motion[51,53] and maintain vertical orientation of the visual scene (Fig. 2). Vestibular input, therefore, is used for repositioning of the eyes based on changes in head orientation (a more detailed review of visual-vestibular interactions is beyond the scope of this article, but the reader should refer to the article by Herdman in this special series and to a review by Cohen and Henn[54]).

Vestibular inputs also influence trunk and limb stability when head position changes. The functional linkage

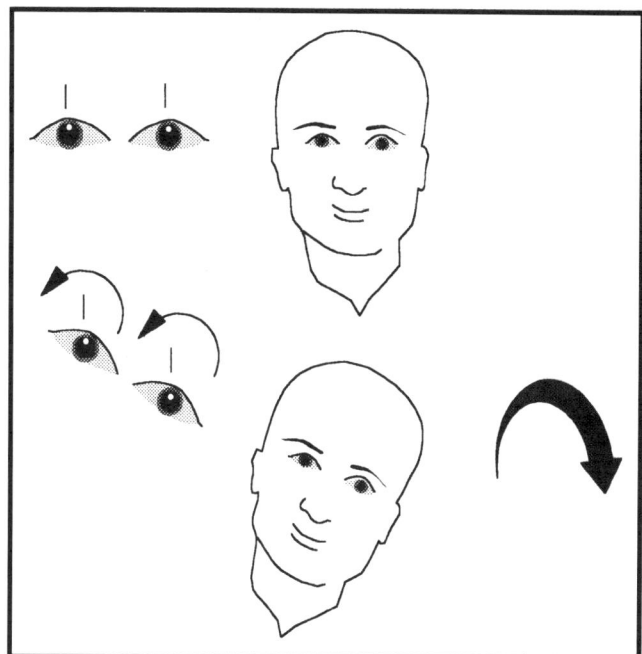

Figure 2.
Ocular counter-roll reflex. (Top) Head and eye position in the baseline condition. (Bottom) Tilt of the head results in stimulation of the otolith receptors. The eyes counter-rotate to nullify the effects of head tilt and stabilize the visual scene.

between head orientation and lower-extremity muscle activity was demonstrated by Zangemeister et al.[55] They used a backward head tilt to enhance the influence of the otolith end organs during gait for five subjects without impairments (mean age=27 years). Zangemeister et al[55] found that tibialis anterior muscle discharge markedly increased during the entire walking cycle and also showed a phasic burst of activity at mid-stance. This pattern of tibialis anterior muscle activity was thought to represent a feed-forward postural adjustment mediated by the otolith organs in anticipation of the COF displacements (beyond the base of support) that normally occur during gait.

When vestibular input is absent, there is a loss of postural stabilization that normally occurs prior to self-initiated voluntary motion. The loss of anticipatory postural control following vestibular dysfunction is manifest by the loss of feed-forward control of the head.[56–61] Deficits in the anticipatory control of head position occur in persons without vestibular dysfunction who are exposed to microgravity and in patients with bilateral vestibular dysfunction. Astronauts returning to Earth from orbit in space experience difficulty coordinating head and trunk motion during gait, and as a result they experience temporary postural instability.[22] Reschke et al[22] have suggested that the absence of gravity results in recalibration of the otolith gravity receptors so that the ambiguities between the sense of linear motion during gait and the sense of gravity contribute to a loss of feed-forward head control. Bronstein[56] studied six patients with vestibular loss (32–73 years of age) and six subjects without vestibular impairment (18–62 years of age) who were seated in a chair and rotated in random directions while the subjects attempted to fixate on a visual target. The subjects without vestibular impairment were able to anticipate changes in the direction of chair rotation and corrected head position in advance of the changes in trunk (chair) position. In contrast, subjects with bilateral vestibular deficits did not show this feed-forward adjustment in head position.[56] Other researchers have shown that subjects with bilateral vestibular deficits have larger head displacement amplitudes, angular velocities, or gaze velocities (motion of the eyes with respect to the head) in the dark during hopping or running[57–59] and walking in place[60,61] compared with subjects without vestibular impairment.

Somatosensory influence on geocentric frame of reference. Because bilateral vestibular dysfunction results in a loss of anticipatory head control, it is reasonable to conclude that vestibular inputs that monitor the resting position of the head appear to be necessary to establish feed-forward control of head position. Vestibular inputs, however, may not be sufficient to completely form or elaborate the geocentric reference because other sensory inputs are known to lead to modification of head position with respect to the vertical. Somatosensory (cutaneous, joint, and pressure receptors) as well as muscle proprioception from spindle afferents, for example, can shape the geocentric reference for balance and head stabilization.[3,35,39–41,62]

Evidence that somatosensory inputs to the CNS influence the geocentric frame of reference for head stability was provided in separate investigations by Pozzo et al,[3] Young and Standish,[39] and Jeka and colleagues.[40,41] Pozzo et al[3] observed that during a self-initiated jumping motion, there was an unbroken trajectory of head rotation in the sagittal plane in spite of the impact of foot-floor contact. They suggested that physical contact between the foot and the floor provided the capacity to predict a perturbation of gaze and provide anticipatory neck muscle contraction to correct impending head displacement.[3] Light touch from the fingertip may also provide somatosensory input to the CNS that contributes to head stabilization.[39–41] Young and Standish[39] showed that visually induced postural sway was attenuated in seven of nine subjects without vestibular impairment when light tactile pressure (insufficient to stabilize posture) was applied to the shoulder. Jeka et al[41] found that sighted individuals with eyes closed had a decrease in head and COF displacement when only light fingertip contact (<2.0 N) was placed on a cane during tandem stance. Postural sway in subjects with congenital blindness also improved with touch cues gained by fingertip contact, but head stability did not improve.[41] These results suggested that persons with congenital blindness were unable to integrate somatosensory information to control head displacement.[41] As noted, considerable sensory processing must occur to transform tactile information to orientation information. Head stability, therefore, appears to depend on a geocentric frame of reference that integrates vestibular inputs with somatosensory inputs from both upper- and lower-extremity load-bearing surfaces to stabilize the head with respect to the vertical.

Mittelstaedt[63] has argued that the geocentric reference is strongly influenced by somatic gravity receptors originating from the viscera within the trunk. There is preliminary evidence suggesting that somatic gravity receptors exist in monkeys[64] and in humans,[65] but further study is needed to reproduce these findings and to determine the influence of these receptors on the control of head stabilization.

Influence of vision on the geocentric frame of reference. Visual input (retinal information) does not appear to be needed for head stabilization.[1,3,4,6] The alteration of visual inputs by darkness or stroboscopic illumination actually improved head stabilization in space during hopping and running,[1,3] locomotion,[6] and stance within a tilting visual enclosure.[43] Collectively, these results suggest that in the absence of normal visual input, a feed-forward mode of head stabilization may control head position in a precise way so that the remaining sensory inputs (ie, vestibular and somatosensory) can provide optimal orientation information.

Influence of gaze and muscle proprioception on egocentric and exocentric frames of reference. Gaze is the intended direction of looking and occurs as a result of eye muscle activation. Factors that determine gaze are the position of the eyes in the head and the position of the head in three-dimensional space. Gaze contributes to both the exocentric and egocentric frames of reference. The "egocentric" component of gaze exists because the muscles that control eye movements provide proprioceptive feedback that is used to control the spatial orientation of the head and trunk.[66,67] Gaze is also "exocentric," because there is evidence that spindle afferent information from muscles surrounding the eye help localize visual targets in the environment.[68] The influence that gaze has on the egocentric and exocentric frames of reference for balance, therefore, is thought to be related to proprioception provided by the ocular muscles (the term "proprioception," as used here, refers specifically to muscle spindle afferent information).

Alteration of the egocentric and exocentric frames of reference can be studied by applying vibration to a muscle or tendon.[44,62,66–71] Vibration alters the perception of limb localization[44,66,67,69,70] (distorting the egocentric frame of reference) as well as the localization of objects viewed in the environment (distorting the exocentric frame of reference).[68,71] A classic example of altering the egocentric frame of reference was provided by Goodwin et al,[69] who showed that vibration of the Achilles tendon in restrained standing subjects can create the illusion of forward body sway. If subjects are not restrained, stimulation of the Achilles tendon results in a corrective body sway backward, because the CNS acts to correct the perceived body tilt.[66,67,70] Several investigators[66,67,70] have reported that vibration of the extraocular inferior rectus muscles or the sternocleidomastoid muscles of freely standing subjects with eyes closed induces the same corrective postural response that is observed with soleus muscle vibration. A proprioceptive linkage between the head, trunk, and lower extremities that controls head and body orientation was proposed to explain the analogous postural effects of muscle vibration at these different sites.[66] For each vibrated muscle, corrective body sway was presumed to be related to a perceived change in the egocentric frame of reference.[66,67,70]

Alterations in the exocentric frame of reference have been studied with subjects in a sitting position or by restraining standing subjects from swaying during muscle vibration. In these conditions, subjects not only experience an illusion of sway, as described earlier, but also a perception that fixed visual targets are moving.[66,68] Distortion of the exocentric frame of reference was demonstrated by Roll et al.[68] They studied 10 subjects without vestibular impairment during a task involving pointing toward a fixed visual target.[68] The subjects were seated in the dark and were instructed to point toward the lighted target once the light was extinguished. Low-amplitude vibration of the eye or neck muscles changed the direction of pointing to correspond to the direction of head motion that would have stretched the vibrated muscle (ie, pointing drifted upward during vibration of sternocleidomastoid muscles or the extraocular inferior rectus muscles). Similar findings with other neck muscles were reported by Biguer et al.[71] Roll et al[68] and Biguer et al[71] presumed, therefore, that spindle afferent input to the CNS from the vibrated muscle altered the localization of visual targets because of a change in the exocentric frame of reference.

In summary, feed-forward control of head position occurs against the backdrop of a constant geocentric reference. Vestibular information signaling static head tilt with respect to gravity is necessary to enable anticipatory stabilization of the head, but somatosensory and proprioceptive inputs are also needed to refine the head stabilization response and the geocentric reference for balance. Minimizing head motion when sensory information is absent or distorted is desirable, because head stabilization can reduce the ambiguity of sensory inputs for balance. This "protective mechanism" might account for the improvement in head stabilization during the distortion or absence of visual input. Proprioceptive inputs from ocular and postural muscles appear to have an influence on geocentric, egocentric, and exocentric frames of reference for balance. There appears to be a "functional synergy" between eye, limb, and trunk muscles that influences the control of head and trunk orientation.

Development of Anticipatory Head Control Strategies

Hayes and Riach[37] proposed that sensory inputs serve three purposes in a feed-forward control system for balance: (1) identification of the initial stance conditions (ie, position, orientation, and motion of the body), (2) provision of immediate information about the feed-forward response once it has been initiated (ie, knowledge of response if balance was maintained), and (3) provision of feedback that is used over the long term to improve the effectiveness of subsequent feed-forward responses. The visual and vestibular end organs are located in the head. The quality and "usability" of these sensory inputs for identifying initial conditions depends, therefore, to a great extent on the strategy used to control head position prior to voluntary motion.

Assaiante and Amblard[6] reported that children 3 to 6 years of age used an HSS strategy while walking on flat ground (Fig. 1). This strategy involves the correction of head position in advance of the rhythmic body oscillations produced during gait. When an equilibrium task became more difficult for these children (ie, walking on a narrow beam), there was an increase in head-trunk stiffness that resembled a head-stabilization-on-trunk (HST) strategy (Fig. 1). The HST strategy reduces the need for anticipatory correction of head position because the head and trunk tend to move as a single unit. Adults, by comparison, showed a preference for the HSS strategy, particularly during difficult equilibrium tasks.[6]

The inability of children under 6 years of age to adopt the HSS strategy during difficult equilibrium tasks suggests that the neural signals that specify head position with respect to the base of support are not fully integrated by the CNS at this age. There is evidence showing that infants just beginning to walk independently attempt to use sensory feedback to develop head-trunk control.[72] Ledebt et al[72] reported a marked improvement in head-trunk control during the first 10 to 15 weeks after the onset of independent walking. The delay between the initiation of walking and the improvement in head-trunk coordination was attributed to the devel-

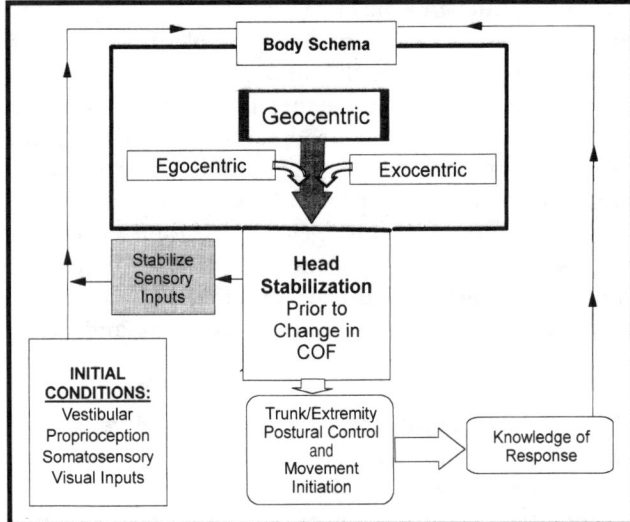

Figure 3.
Proposed conceptual model of head control during voluntary motion. COF=center of force.

opment of neural processing to integrate sensory inputs for equilibrium during ambulation.[72] Feed-forward postural adjustments may develop in parallel with the maturation of sensory feedback processes.[37] Whether the degradation of sensory processing attributed to aging, in turn, degrades the mechanisms that produce anticipatory head stabilization during voluntary motion is not known.

Conceptual Model of Head Control During Voluntary Motion

Head stabilization as the body moves is partly an expression of righting reflexes, the passive elastic and viscous properties of muscle and connective tissue surrounding head and neck body segments, and "higher-order" sensory mechanisms.[73] The body schema and frames of reference for head stability are higher-order sensory mechanisms that must play a dominant role in the control of head position during voluntary motion, because the ability to anticipate the location of the center of gravity and correct head position in advance of a change in body posture requires the integration of multiple sensory inputs. Head control, therefore, cannot be viewed simply as a vestibular reflex or a passive tissue response.

The higher-order mechanisms that link sensory inputs to the control of head stabilization have not been delineated. Schor et al[74] speculated that feedback provided by muscle proprioceptors and somatosensory information contributes to the voluntary and reflex responses that underlie head control. Light-touch cues, for example, could increase the efficiency of head stabilization through the cervicocollic reflex, because this reflex relies on peripheral somatosensory inputs to monitor the position of the head with respect to the body.[74] In parallel with this reflex "loop," a neuronal network facilitating the interaction between ankle somatosensory inputs with information from proprioceptors along the vertical axis of the body—including information from neck, trunk, and eye muscles—could also influence head displacement prior to the initiation of voluntary motion.[66,67,75–77]

We are proposing a preliminary conceptual model that uses a template for head stabilization based on the body schema (Fig. 3). The body schema for head and trunk orientation is influenced by vestibular and other sensory inputs. The amplitude and direction of anticipatory stabilization of the head will depend on the initial conditions established by sensory input to the body schema. Angular orientation of the head in space in this model is corrected at a subconscious level after a change in one or more frames of reference, but in advance of the conscious initiation of voluntary motion. Head stabilization in turn reinforces the body schema in a feedback loop by minimizing an immediate change in eye position (stabilizing retinal input), the position of the vestibular end organs, and the position of the neck (stabilizing neck somatosensory and proprioception inputs). Head control, in this model, is influenced by sensory inputs through the frames of reference for balance, rather than directly by individual sensory modalities. Once the head is stabilized, trunk and extremity postural control follows. This action creates sensory feedback and "knowledge of response" that can be used to modify the body schema for subsequent action.

The geocentric frame of reference in this model is at the top of a hierarchy with respect to the other frames of reference.[32,33] The geocentric frame of reference is necessary, but not sufficient for feed-forward control of the head. Other frames of reference (ie, egocentric or exocentric) are needed to fully form the response for anticipatory head stabilization. The invariant gravitational reference provided by the geocentric system provides a protective mechanism that ensures angular stability of the head during difficult balance tasks.[6] Task difficulty is determined by mechanical factors (eg, stance on a narrow surface,[6,19] stance on a compliant support surface,[9] single-leg stance[29]) or by the availability or quality of sensory information (ie, balance while walking in the dark or with stroboscopic illumination).[6] The HSS strategy (Fig. 1) is a feed-forward control strategy that, theoretically, will be useful during difficult balance tasks because the precise control of angular head displacement optimizes the quality of available sensory inputs that will contribute to proper orientation of the body (Fig. 3).

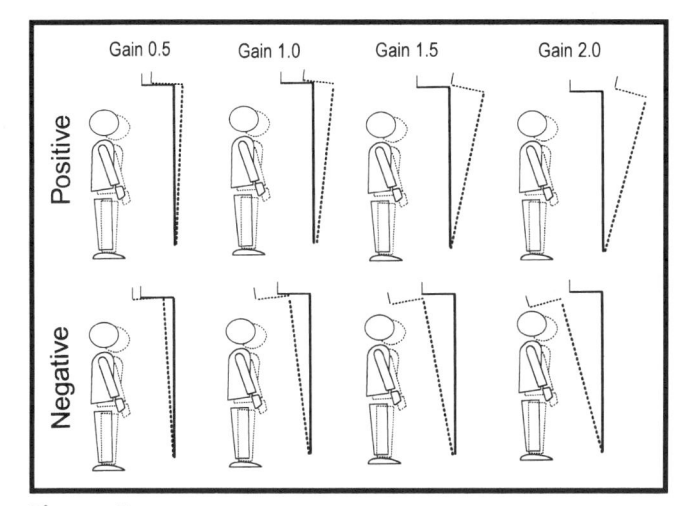

Figure 4.
Effect of gain magnitude and polarity on sway-driven displacement of the visual surround. The subject is swaying forward an identical amount in each frame. Positive sway gains tilt the surround in the same direction as displacement of the center of force (COF) in the sagittal plane. Negative sway gains tilt the surround in the opposite direction of COF displacement.

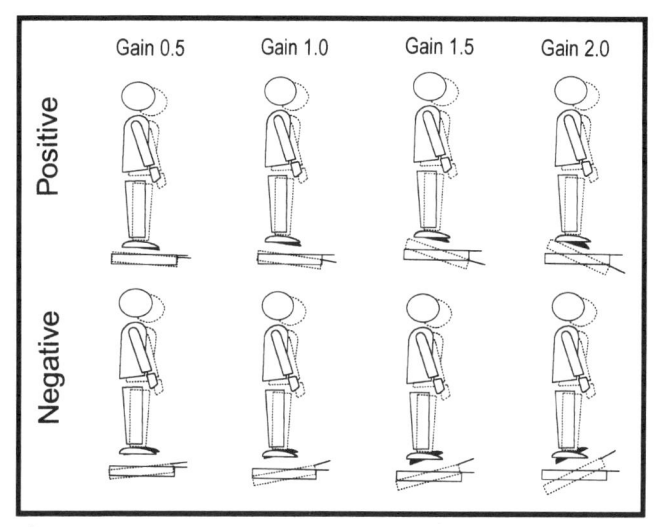

Figure 5.
The effect of gain magnitude and polarity on sway-driven displacement of the stance platform. The subject is swaying forward an identical amount in each frame. Positive sway gains tilt the platform in the same direction as displacement of the center of force (COF) in the sagittal plane. Negative sway gains tilt the platform in the opposite direction of COF displacement.

Demonstration of Head Stabilization Strategies in Older Persons

Experimental Paradigm and Research Questions

We have completed several experiments[43,78,79] that begin to examine the ability of elderly people to produce head stabilization strategies that might protect gaze and stabilize sensory inputs for balance. The experimental paradigm that we utilized involved balance tasks that have different levels of difficulty (Figs. 4 and 5). Subjects stood on a movable force platform and faced a visual enclosure (described in more detail later). The level of difficulty was controlled by changing the coupling—referred to as the "gain"—between body sway and simultaneous tilt of the platform or visual surround. For example, any displacement of the COF at a gain of +2.0 will create a tilt of the visual surround (away from the subject) or a tilt of the platform (toes down) that will be four times larger than a tilt at a gain of +0.5 (Figs. 4 and 5). Changing the polarity of the gain to negative reverses the direction of the surround or platform motion (ie, as the COF moves forward, the surround is tilted toward the subject or the platform is rotated toes up). Balance in the negative gain conditions was more challenging than balance in the positive gain conditions, because the environment in a negative gain condition moved completely opposite the direction of body sway. Greater frequency or amplitude of corrective balance responses in the negative gain conditions compared with the positive gain conditions (described in the "Findings" section) confirmed the relative difficulty of the negative gain conditions. It was possible, therefore, to evaluate head stabilization using a spectrum of task difficulty by altering the stability of the support surface (platform tilt) or by distorting visual input (surround tilt).

We studied two research questions: (1) Do elderly people use the HSS strategy to control head position during more difficult balance tasks? and (2) Do the head stabilization strategies used by elderly people differ, descriptively, from those strategies implemented by younger persons? With regard to the first research question, many elderly people without vestibular symptoms (ie, those without a history of falling, frequent dizziness, or vertigo) have difficulty interpreting sensory inputs that provide conflicting information about spatial orientation.[9,10,26] For this reason, it seemed reasonable to propose that older persons would need to enhance their ability to use sensory inputs that contribute to each frame of reference for balance, particularly in conditions with sensory incongruence. We hypothesized that elderly persons would rely on the HSS strategy to optimize the quality of sensory input for balance.

In formulating the second research question, we considered previous findings that postural stability decreases with age.[80-82] To compensate for age-related deterioration in postural stability, elderly individuals without vestibular symptoms may develop greater control of head position compared with younger individuals. This strategy would allow elderly to efficiently use sensory inputs that contribute to each frame of reference discussed earlier. We hypothesized, therefore, that elderly persons without vestibular symptoms would have greater head stabilization compared with younger persons.

Table 1.
Pretest/Posttest and Block Randomization of Tester-Selected Gain Across Sensory Conditions

	Sensory Condition[a]	Gain	No. of Trials
Pretest	EO-FPS	0	3
	EC-FPS	0	3
Gain-block randomization			
A	SM, EO-PM, EC-PM	+0.5	3
		−0.5	3
B	SM, EO-PM, EC-PM	+1.0	3
		−1.0	3
C	SM, EO-PM, EC-PM	+1.5	3
		−1.5	3
D	SM, EO-PM, EC-PM	+2.0	3
		−2.0	3
Posttest	EO-FPS	0	3
	EC-FPS	0	3

[a] Eyes open (EO-FPS) and eyes closed (EC-FPS) with a fixed platform and visual surround; gain blocks A–D systematically randomized and presented during sensory conditions with surround motion (SM), platform motion with eyes open (EO-PM) and eyes closed (EC-PM).

The methods used to study these research questions are outlined in the Appendix, and the experimental conditions are summarized in Table 1.

Outcome Measures

Head stability was analyzed by comparing the peak-to-peak head motion with the peak-to-peak displacement of the COF in the sagittal plane for each trial. The ratio of head motion to COF displacement was referred to as the *head mobility score* (HMS). An HMS was calculated for sagittal translation of the head (head-x HMS) and for rotation of the head in the sagittal plane (pitch HMS).

The HMS provided an index for detecting relative changes in head-body coupling. Larger HMS values indicated that the head was moving greater distances with respect to the COF, as compared with a lower HMS. The relative extent of head stabilization in space between experimental conditions, therefore, could be compared using the HMS ratios. A pitch HMS of 0.5, for example, means that the peak-to-peak pitch rotation of the head per unit of COF displacement was half as much as a pitch HMS of 1.0. The head is relatively more stable in space with respect to body motion, therefore, with a lower HMS.

Data analysis. Each subject served as his or her own control. Baseline values for head-x and pitch HMS were evaluated using paired t tests for each age group (pretest versus posttest). For the experimental conditions, trials with positive gains were paired with the corresponding trial utilizing a negative gain of the same absolute value. Paired t tests were done for each dependent variable (head-x and pitch HMS) in each sensory condition (surround motion [SM], eyes open–platform motion [EO-PM], and eyes closed–platform motion [EC-PM]). The experimentwise error rate was adjusted using a Bonferroni correction for multiple comparisons ($P<.025$).

Findings

Baseline measurements. Baseline HMS measurements in stance on a fixed platform and fixed visual surround with eyes open (EO-FPS) and eyes closed (EC-FPS) did not differ from pretest to posttest measurement for elderly subjects or for younger subjects (Fig. 6). The increase in peak-to-peak COF displacement at the posttest measurement compared with the pretest measurement (Fig. 6) was offset by a parallel increase in head

Table 2.
Head-x and Pitch Head Mobility Scores for Each Age Group and Gain Polarity During Visual Surround Motion (SM) and With Eyes Open (EO-PM) and Eyes Closed (EC-PM) During Stance on a Movable Platform

		Under 50 Years of Age				Over 65 Years of Age			
		Positive Gain		Negative Gain		Positive Gain		Negative Gain	
Condition	Motion	X̄	SD	X̄	SD	X̄	SD	X̄	SD
SM	Head-x	1.54	0.42	1.37[a]	0.33	1.51	0.28	1.31[a]	0.29
	Pitch	1.80	0.96	1.44[a]	0.85	1.41	0.63	1.14[b]	0.53
EO-PM	Head-x	1.05	0.31	1.10	0.37	1.27	0.39	1.07[b]	0.25
	Pitch	0.99	0.58	1.48[c]	0.79	1.40	1.29	0.85[b]	0.27
EC-PM	Head-x	1.27	0.29	1.24	0.19	1.40	0.30	1.21[a]	0.23
	Pitch	0.64	0.56	0.91[c]	0.54	0.67	0.35	0.76	0.29
No. of trials		60		60		24		24	

[a] Significantly lower compared with positive gain; $P<.025$.
[b] Trend for lower head mobility score compared with positive gain; $.025<P\leq.07$.
[c] Significantly greater compared with positive gain; $P<.025$.

displacement. The net result was that the head-x and pitch HMS ratios remained relatively constant from pretest to posttest measurement.

Head stabilization response to sway-driven tilt of visual surround. There were decreases in head-x and pitch HMS (Tab. 2 and Fig. 7) for younger subjects in the negative, more challenging gain conditions compared with the positive gain conditions. Elderly subjects also showed a decrease in head-x HMS (Tab. 2), and there was a nonsignificant finding that pitch HMS decreased in negative gain compared with positive gain conditions ($t=-1.92$, $df=23$, $P=.067$; Tab. 2 and Fig. 8), although the probability value for the decrease in pitch HMS was close to being significant.

Head stabilization response to sway-driven tilt of the platform: eyes open. In young subjects, there was no change in the head-x HMS for positive versus negative gain during EO-PM (Tab. 2). The pitch HMS for young subjects, however, increased during negative gains compared with positive gains (Tab. 2 and Fig. 9). In contrast, elderly subjects showed a reduction in the head-x HMS and a nonsignificant reduction of the pitch HMS (Tab. 2 and Fig. 9) in negative gains compared with positive gains ($t=-2.31$, $df=23$, $P=.03$), although the probability value for the reduction of pitch HMS was close to being significant. The frequency and amplitude of corrective adjustments in the COF were greater for the negative gain conditions (see "Elderly Subjects," Fig. 9) compared with the positive gain conditions. Head pitch remained stable in spite of the COF fluctuations.

Head stabilization response to sway-driven tilt of the platform: eyes closed. Young subjects showed no change in head-x HMS, whereas elderly subjects had a decrease in this variable (Tab. 2 and Fig. 10). There were small increases in the pitch HMS for younger subjects in negative versus positive gains, but there was no change in the pitch HMS for elderly subjects (Tab. 2). The frequency of corrective adjustments in the COF for the negative gain conditions (for both young and elderly subjects; Fig. 10) was greater compared with the frequency for the positive gain conditions. Head pitch remained stable for all subjects in spite of these frequent COF adjustments.

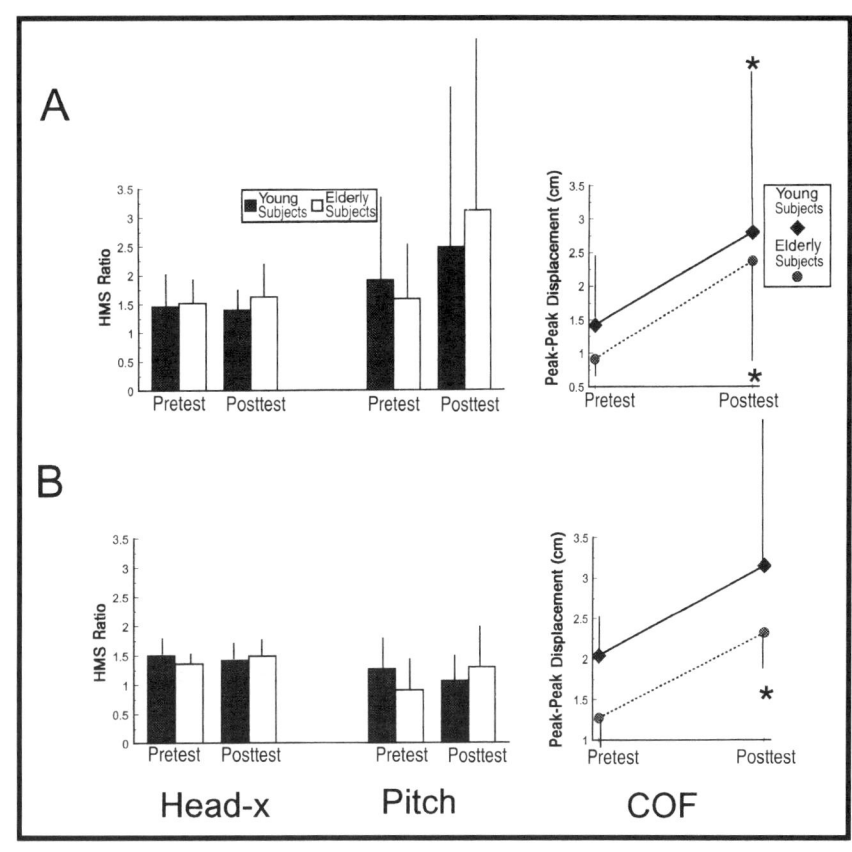

Figure 6.
Pretest and posttest measures of baseline conditions during stance on a fixed platform within a fixed visual surround: (A) eyes open and (B) eyes closed. Head-x and pitch head mobility scores (HMS) remain relatively constant (no statistically significant difference) from pretest to posttest measurement. Statistically significant increases in the magnitude of the center of force (COF) during the posttest measurement compared with the pretest measurement are indicated by the asterisk (*).

Discussion

There are no specific sensors in the body that signal the sequence of limb motion, the position of the center of gravity, or the dimensions of a support surface.[35,62] The control or spatial perception of these variables requires a body schema—an internal representation of the head and body orientation—that serves as a template for balance and equilibrium. The body schema can be viewed as the collective expression of egocentric, exocentric, and geocentric frames of reference (Fig. 3). Anticipatory head stabilization that accompanies voluntary motion occurs because these frames of reference for balance enable the prediction or anticipation of a change in the position of the COF. Stabilization of the head in a feed-forward manner, in turn, optimizes the quality of sensory inputs that are used for equilibrium.[3,4,6,22]

Minimizing head motion during more difficult balance tasks is desirable because head stabilization can reduce the ambiguity of sensory inputs that contribute to the body schema. In our preliminary studies, we demon-

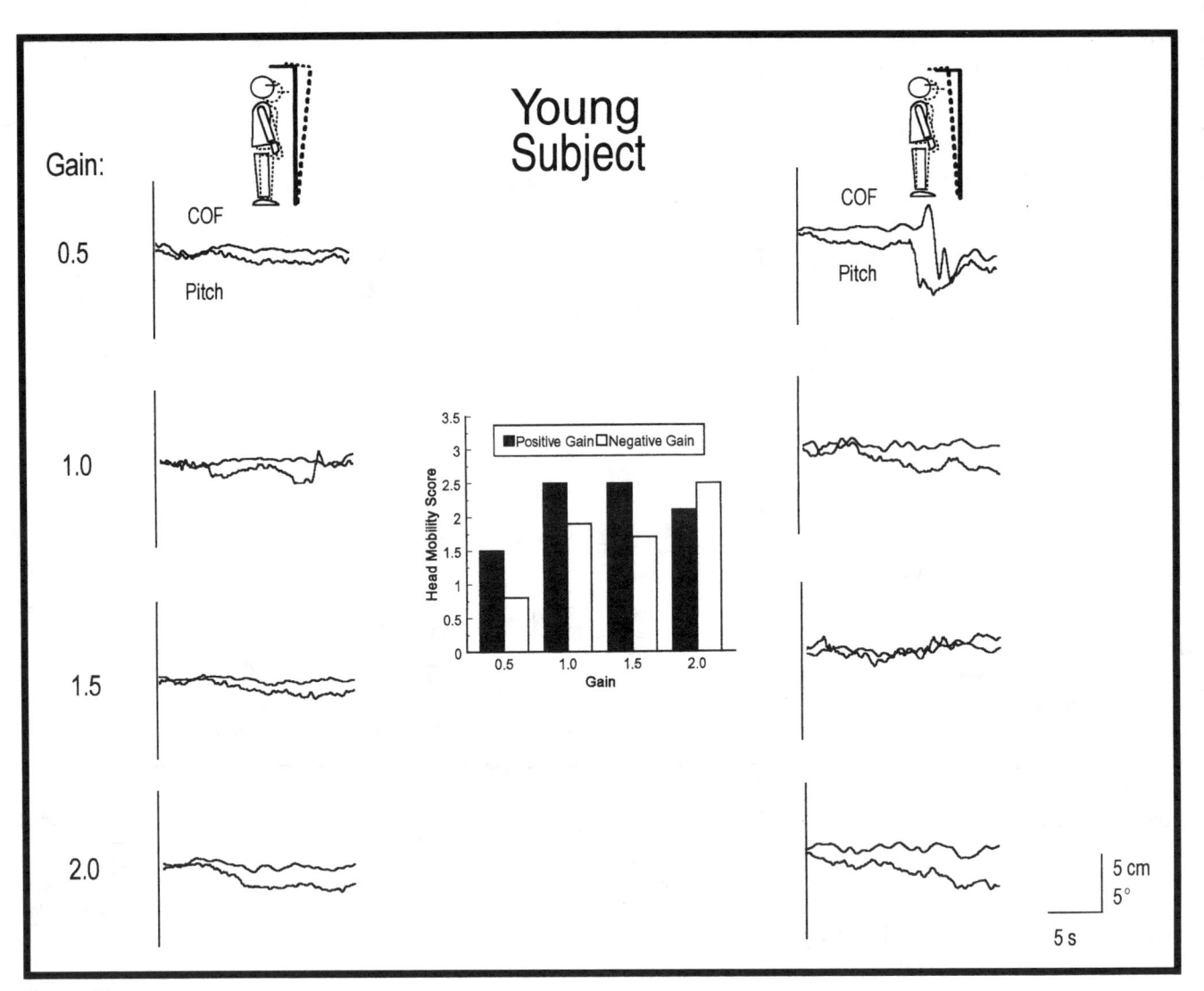

Figure 7.
Head pitch and center-of-force (COF) tracings for one young (32-year-old) subject during stance coupled with sway-driven tilt of the visual surround. Each data frame represents the first trial at the gain shown. Positive gains are in the left column, and negative gains are in the right column. The bar graph in the middle of the figure depicts the head mobility scores for each trial in the figure.

strated that elderly subjects without vestibular symptoms restrained head motion to a greater extent in conditions where mechanical compliance of the force platform or distortion of visual inputs was most disruptive to equilibrium (eg, in the negative gain conditions; Figs. 8–10). The HSS strategy in older persons was apparent from the tight control of head pitch when the balance tasks were most challenging. This finding means that older persons could use a HSS strategy to control head position during active balance tasks as an effective way to stabilize the head in a feed-forward manner during a wide range of COF displacements (Figs. 8–10). Confirmation of these preliminary results awaits further testing, but the observations in this study appear to demonstrate the theory that elderly persons might use an HSS strategy to stabilize the head.

Age-related differences in processing proprioceptive inputs have been reported by Quoniam et al,[70] who showed that vibration-induced postural sway was slower and had less amplitude for 26 elderly subjects (60–83 years of age) than for 9 younger subjects (20–44 years of age). This finding implies that elderly persons underestimate the dysequilibrium that is signaled by the proprioceptive systems. The reduction of corrective sway amplitude and velocity for the elder subjects might also suggest that elderly persons process incongruent sensory inputs less efficiently than do younger persons, and therefore have a greater need to constrain body tilt during balance activities. The results from our preliminary study support this idea. Specifically, during conditions that distorted proprioceptive inputs from the lower extremities (EO-PM and EC-PM), elderly subjects showed either an attenuation of the pitch HMS (EO-PM) or no change in the pitch HMS from positive to negative gain conditions. The mean pitch HMS for the elderly subjects never increased during the transition from positive to negative gains (Tab. 2). In contrast, younger

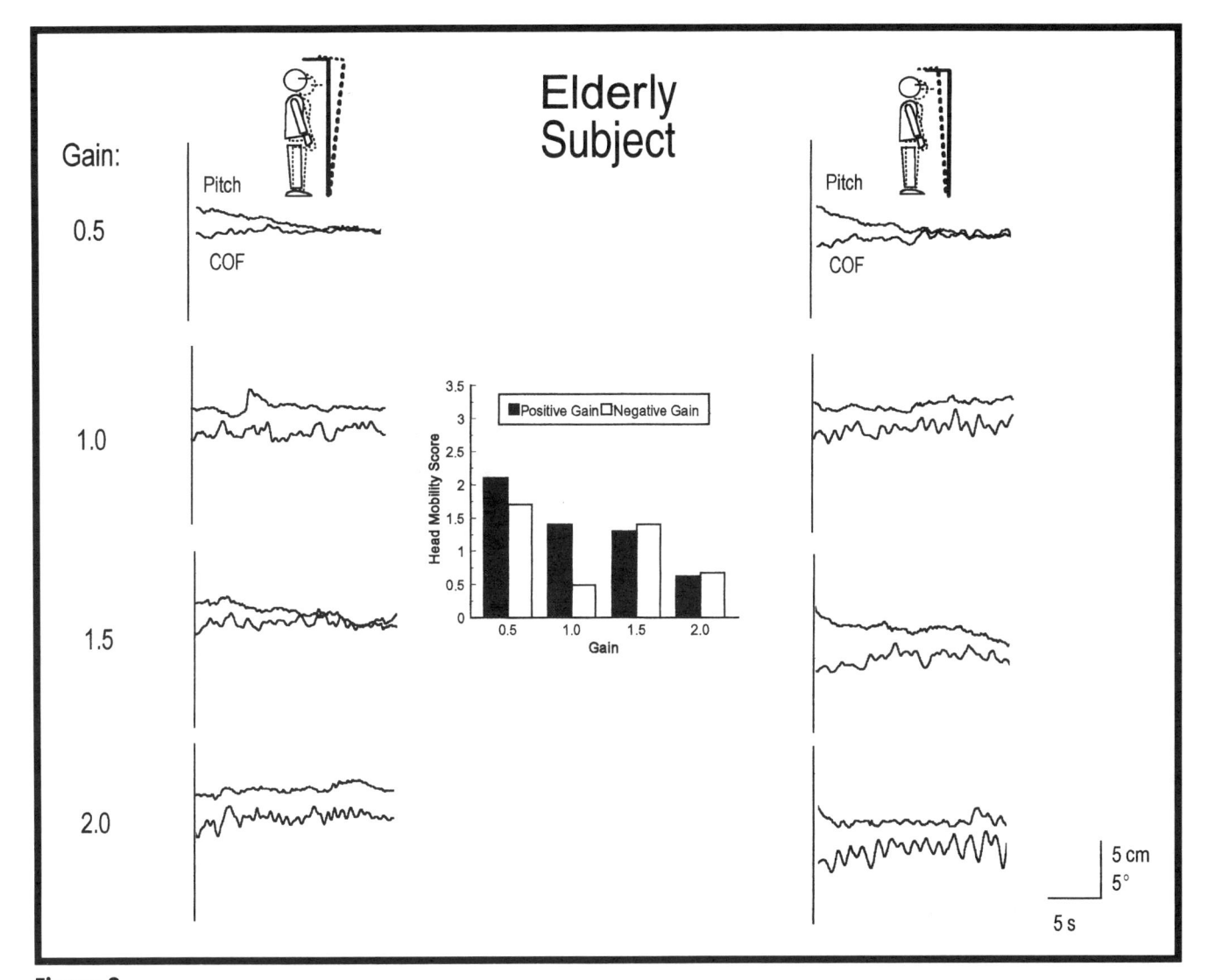

Figure 8.
Head pitch and center-of-force (COF) tracings for one elderly (72-year-old) subject during stance coupled with sway-driven tilt of the visual surround for positive and negative gains. Each data frame represents the first trial at the gain shown. Positive gains are in the left column, and negative gains are in the right column. The bar graph in the middle of the figure depicts the head mobility scores for each trial in the figure.

subjects increased the pitch HMS, and this increase occurred most markedly in EO-PM (Tab. 2 and Fig 9). The implication of the preliminary findings is that elderly persons without vestibular symptoms may actually constrain head motion to a greater extent than younger persons in an attempt to optimize the quality of visual and vestibular inputs for balance. Additional research is necessary to further evaluate this theory.

The adjustments in head position prior to initiation of voluntary movement are not likely to influence body stabilization because of the relatively low mass of the head.[7] By contrast, anticipatory postural adjustments in the *limbs* (ie, activation of the thigh muscles to stabilize the knee prior to rapid ankle plantar flexion while standing) appear to stabilize the body in preparation for movement initiation.[83–90] A complete discussion of anticipatory postural adjustments in the limbs is beyond the scope of this article. Feed-forward control of head position and limb position are important for successful balance behavior, but for different reasons. Head stabilization may optimize the quality of sensory inputs used by the CNS to activate postural muscles for balance (Fig. 3), whereas the preparatory muscle activation in the limbs ensures postural stability during task initiation.[7,83–90] The "functional synergies" between eye, limb, and trunk muscles that were described earlier may provide a fundamental mechanism that could enhance the coordination of head stabilization with the preparatory limb stabilization that occurs prior to initiation of voluntary movement.

The postural control mechanisms underlying self-initiated voluntary motion[1,3,6] may be different from those controlling balance during a reaction to external perturbation.[8,17–20] Shupert et al,[19] for example, found

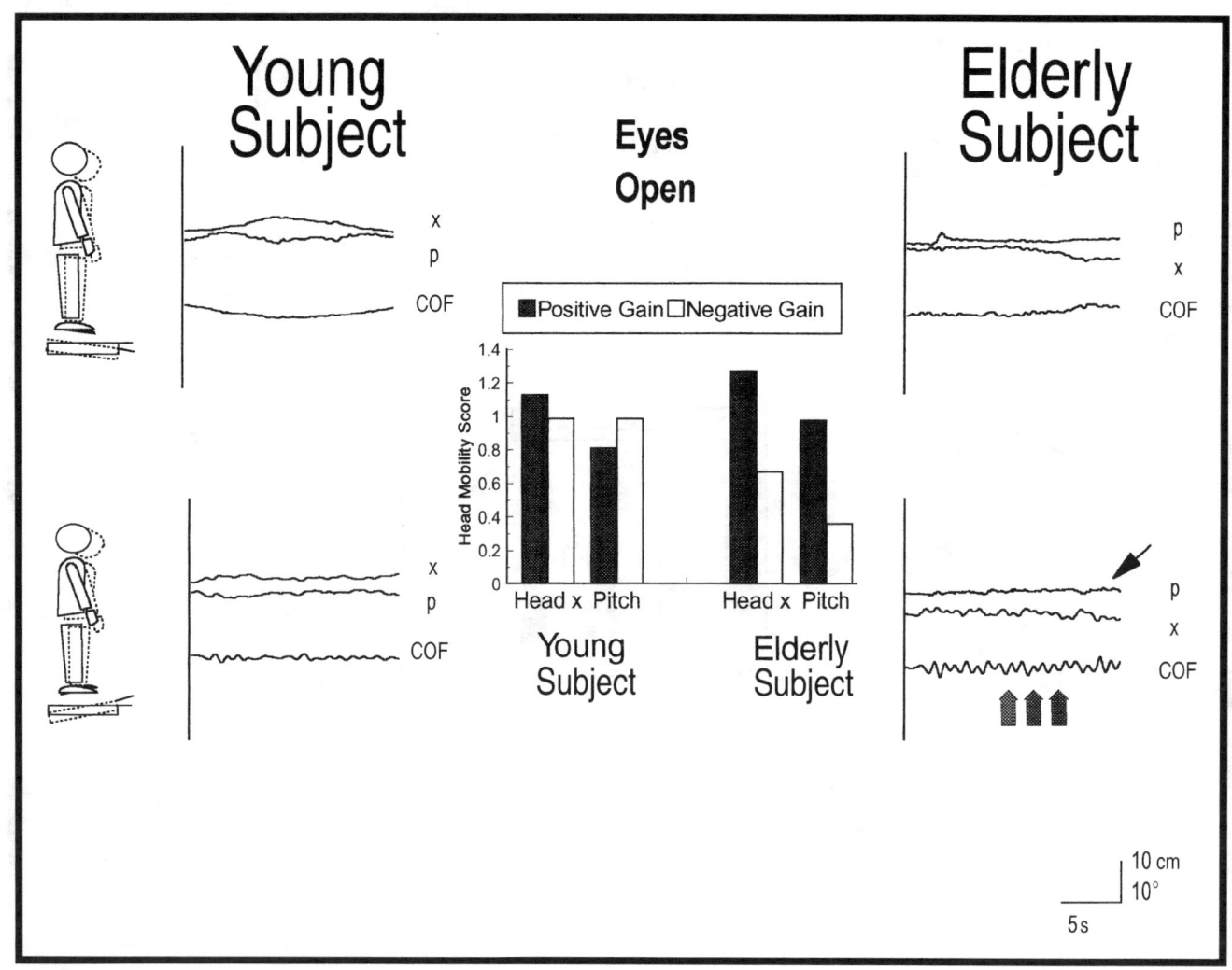

Figure 9.
Eyes open–sway induced platform motion: Head-x (x), pitch (p), and center-of-force (COF) tracings for one young (32-year-old) subject and one elderly (72-year-old) subject during stance coupled with sway-driven tilt of the platform (top row is positive gain of 1; bottom row is negative gain of 1). The bar graph in the center of the figure depicts the head mobility scores for each trial illustrated. Note the precise control of pitch (single arrow) in the elderly subject even when the COF is frequently adjusting in the negative gain condition to maintain stance (recordings highlighted by triple arrows).

that head motion did not appear to be coordinated with ankle or hip motion when subjects reacted to perturbations of stance on a flat surface or a transverse beam. These authors suggested that changes in the neck angle were passively propagated up the body following lower-extremity reaction to support surface displacement (ie, primarily viscoelastic rather than active control of head position). This reactive response to perturbation was different from the anticipatory head stabilization that has been reported for self-initiated voluntary motion.[1,3,6] More work is needed to clarify how aging influences the mechanisms controlling head stability during "reactive" postural adjustments compared with goal-directed voluntary movements.

Clinical Implications
Balance during voluntary motion requires that patients gain precise control of head motion. In persons with neurologic dysfunction, it is possible that disruption of sensory integration may alter anticipatory head stabilization and lead to balance dysfunction during self-initiated motion. Many types of treatment have been advocated for patients with deficits in the ability to integrate sensory information for balance.[29,91] These treatments often involve practicing standing while the therapist alters the availability or congruence of sensory inputs. Patients who rely on "support surface" cues for orientation, for example, are asked to practice balance and walking on compliant surfaces such as foam or moving surfaces. The goal is to train patients to become proficient with balance in progressively more difficult conditions by altering or distorting available sensory information (a more detailed review of the treatment procedures is provided by Shumway-Cook and McCollum[91]). These procedures, however, do not specifically

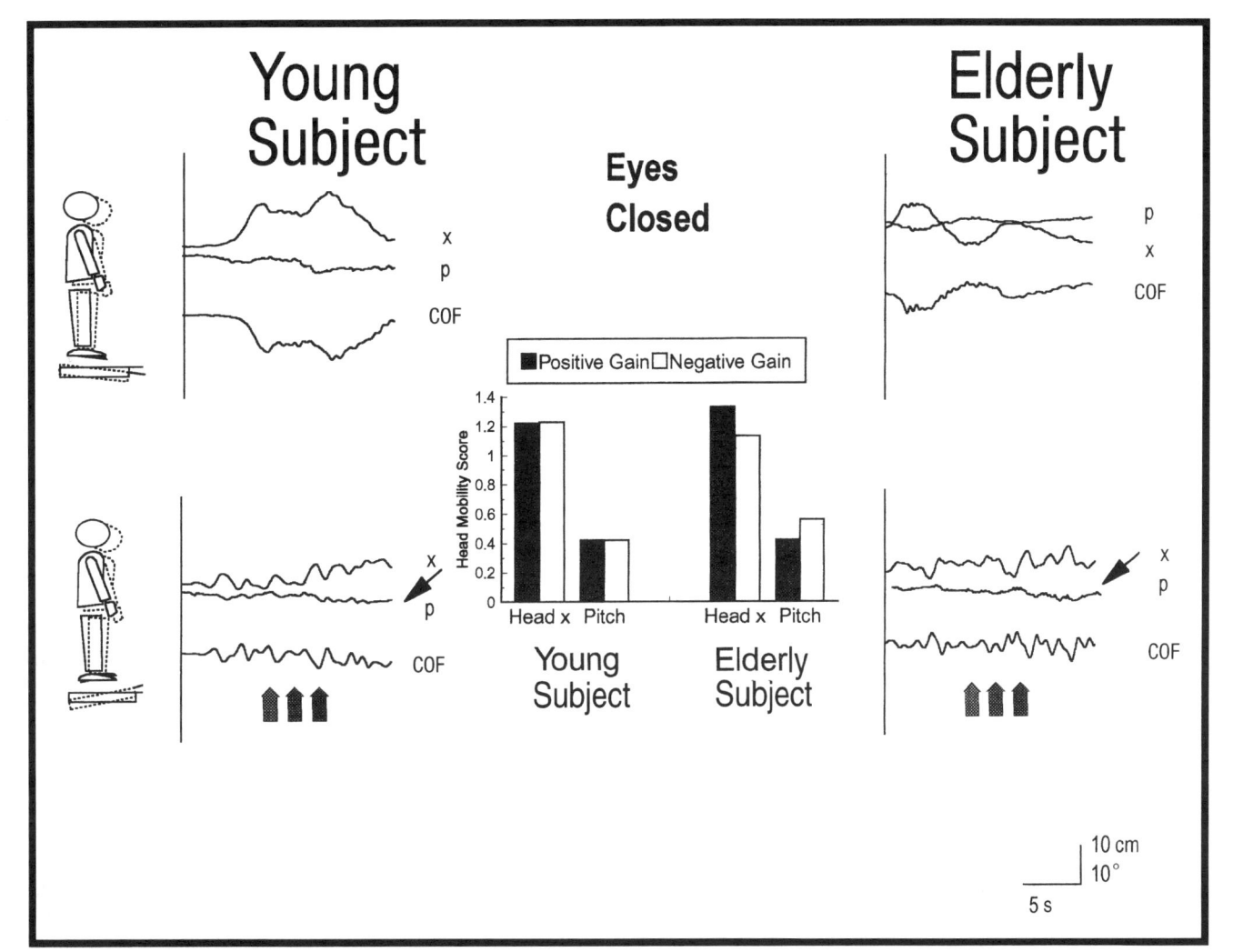

Figure 10.
Eyes closed–sway induced platform motion: Head-x (x), pitch (p), and center-of-force (COF) tracings for one young (32-year-old) subject and one elderly (72-year-old) subject during stance coupled with sway-driven tilt of the platform (top row is positive gain of 1; bottom row is negative gain of 1). The bar graph in the center of the figure depicts the head mobility scores for each trial illustrated. Note the precise control of pitch (single arrow) especially in the negative gain condition (both young and elder subjects) compared with frequent corrections in the COF needed to maintain stance (recordings highlighted by triple arrows).

address the control of head motion as a distinct feature in the treatment protocol.

Some interventions have been described that focus on the control of the head as a means of facilitating overall postural control.[92] The "Alexander Technique," for example, involves positioning the head prior to voluntary motion as a way of integrating the flow of head and body action (reviewed by Jones[92]). Jones[92] found that the coordination of head-body motion observed during activities such as walking, stair climbing, or raising from a chair was altered when the position of the head was modified prior to the beginning of the task. He suggested that changes in head posture would facilitate more efficient movement patterns.[92] There has been little recent attention to this procedure in the literature, but some of the concepts advanced by Alexander (eg, that head control will influence overall postural stability) are supported by the "top-down" or "head-first" scheme of postural organization described in our review.

Although balance is often disrupted following a lesion of the CNS, loss of head control has not been specifically addressed in many patient populations that require physical therapy. It is known that certain CNS deficits alter anticipatory postural adjustment. For example, when subjects with stroke perform a rapid voluntary sway, the number of response defaults (the number of times that postural muscles are not recruited) is greater than for subjects who are not disabled.[93] When a postural response is initiated, "anticipatory" activation of the paretic limb occurs closer in time to the intended movement. Patients with hemiplegia appear to be unable to fully integrate anticipatory, feed-forward components of balance to execute a voluntary motion.[94] Furthermore, prior knowledge of the task constraints—

usually in a nonchoice reaction-time paradigm—does not improve the onset or timing of feed-forward postural adjustments[84,93,95] or change the sequence of postural muscle activation following stroke.[96] Therapy aimed at head control during voluntary motion may improve anticipatory postural responses in the lower limbs of patients after strokes, but this idea warrants further study.

Conclusions

Voluntary, self-initiated movement involves feed-forward, anticipatory control of head position. The mechanism of head stabilization seems to rely primarily on a geocentric frame of reference, but can be refined by egocentric or exocentric frames of reference. Increasing the difficulty of balance tasks might increase the dominance of an HSS strategy in older persons. The HSS strategy will theoretically optimize the use of sensory inputs for balance. There is some support for addressing head stabilization within the context of a "top-down" or "head-first" control scheme, and alternative treatments for balance dysfunction might be developed using this theoretical framework. The development of treatment strategies that address head control during voluntary motion seems to be justified from the theoretical constructs and preliminary findings reported here. The implementation of new treatments based on the "head-first" model will require additional study.

Acknowledgments

We sincerely appreciate the help of Jennifer Suarez and Danielle R Di Fabio for their assistance with manuscript preparation.

References

1 Pozzo T, Berthoz A, Lefort L. Head stabilization during various locomotor tasks in humans, I: normal subjects. *Exp Brain Res.* 1990;82:97–106.

2 Bloomberg JJ, Reschke MF, Huebner WP, Peters BT. The effects of target distance on eye and head movement during locomotion. *Ann NY Acad Sci.* 1992;656:699–707.

3 Pozzo T, Berthoz A, Lefort L. Head kinematics during various motor tasks in humans. *Prog Brain Res.* 1989;80:377–383.

4 Berthoz A, Pozzo T. Intermittent head stabilization during postural and locomotory tasks in humans. In: Amblard B, Berthoz A, Clarac F, eds. *Posture and Gait: Development, Adaptation, and Modulation.* Amsterdam, the Netherlands: Elsevier Science Publishers BV; 1988:189–198.

5 Winter DA. *Biomechanics and Motor Control of Human Movement.* 2nd ed. New York, NY: John Wiley & Sons Inc; 1990:93–95.

6 Assaiante C, Amblard B. Ontogenesis of head stabilization in space during locomotion in children: influence of visual cues. *Exp Brain Res.* 1993;93:499–515.

7 Gurfinkel VS, Lipshits MI, Lestienne FG. Anticipatory neck muscle activity associated with rapid arm movements. *Neurosci Lett.* 1988;94:104–108.

8 Allum JHJ, Keshner EA, Honegger F, Pfaltz CR. Organization of leg-trunk-head equilibrium movements in normals and patients with peripheral vestibular deficits. *Prog Brain Res.* 1988;76:277–290.

9 Whipple R, Wolfson L, Derby C, et al. Altered sensory function and balance in older persons. *J Gerontol.* 1993;48:71–76.

10 Woollacott MH. Age-related changes in posture and movement. *J Gerontol.* 1993;48:56–60.

11 Brocklehurst JC, Robertson D, James-Groom P. Clinical correlates of sway in old age sensory modalities. *Age Ageing.* 1982;11:1–10.

12 Lord SR, Clark RD, Webster IW. Postural stability and associated physiological factors in a population of aged persons. *J Gerontol Med Sci.* 1991;46:M69–M76.

13 Lord SR, Webster IW. Visual field dependence in elderly fallers and non-fallers. *Int J Aging Hum Dev.* 1990;31:267–277.

14 Paige GD. Senescence of human visual-vestibular interactions, 1: vestibulo-ocular reflex and adaptive plasticity with aging. *J Vestib Res.* 1992;2:133–151.

15 King OS, Seidman SH, Leigh RJ. Control of head stability and gaze during locomotion in normal subjects and patients with deficient vestibular function. In: Berthoz A, Graf W, Vidal PP, eds. *The Head-Neck Sensory Motor System.* New York, NY: Oxford University Press Inc; 1992:568–570.

16 Hirasaki E, Kubo T, Nozawa S, et al. Analysis of head and body movements of elderly people during locomotion. *Acta Otolaryngol (Stockh).* 1993;501:25–30.

17 Takahashi M. Head stability and gaze during vertical whole-body oscillations. *Ann Otol Rhinol Laryngol.* 1990;99:883–888.

18 Murata T, Kitahara M. Acceleration registrography of head movement during alternating inclination of the support platform. *Acta Otolaryngol (Stockh).* 1994;510:33–37.

19 Shupert CL, Black FO, Horak FB, Nashner LM. Coordination of the head and body in response to support surface translations in normals and patients with bilaterally reduced vestibular function. In: Amblard B, Berthoz A, Clarac F, eds. *Posture and Gait: Development, Adaptation, and Modulation.* Amsterdam, the Netherlands: Elsevier Science Publishers BV; 1988:281–289.

20 Nashner LM, Shupert CL, Horak FB. Head-trunk movement coordination in the standing posture. *Prog Brain Res.* 1988;76:243–251.

21 Grossman GE, Leigh RJ, Abel LA, et al. Frequency and velocity of rotational head perturbations during locomotion. *Exp Brain Res.* 1988;70:470–476.

22 Reschke MF, Bloomberg JJ, Harm DL, Paloski WH. Space flight and neurovestibular adaptation. *J Clin Pharmacol.* 1994;34:609–617.

23 Dichgans J, Diener HC. The contribution of vestibulo-spinal mechanisms to the maintenance of human upright posture. *Acta Otolaryngol (Stockh).* 1989;107:338–345.

24 Keshner EA, Peterson BW. Motor control strategies underlying head stabilization and voluntary head movements in humans and cats. *Prog Brain Res.* 1988;76:329–339.

25 Guitton D, Kearney RE, Wereley N, Peterson BW. Visual, vestibular, and voluntary contributions to human head stabilization. *Exp Brain Res.* 1986;64:59–69.

26 Woollacott MH, Shumway-Cook A, Nashner LM. Aging and posture control: changes in sensory organization and muscular coordination. *Intl J Aging Hum Dev.* 1986;23:97–119.

27 Wolfson L, Whipple R, Derby CA, et al. Gender differences in the balance of healthy elderly as demonstrated by dynamic posturography. *J Gerontol Med Sci.* 1994;49:M160–M167.

28 Simoneau GG, Leibowitz HW, Ulbrecht JS, et al. The effects of visual factors and head orientation on postural steadiness in women 55 to 70 years of age. *J Gerontol Med Sci.* 1992;47:M151–M158.

29 Hu M-H, Woollacott MH. Multisensory training of standing balance in older adults, I: postural stability and one-leg stance. *J Gerontol Med Sci.* 1994;49:M52–M61.

30 Blaszczyk JW, Hansen PD, Lowe DL. Postural sway and perception of the upright stance stability borders. *Perception.* 1993;22:1333–1341.

31 Schieppati M, Hugon M, Grasso M, et al. The limits of equilibrium in young and elderly normal subjects and in Parkinsonians. *Electroencephalogr Clin Neurophysiol.* 1994;93:286–298.

32 Berthoz A. Reference frames for the perception and control of movement. In: Paillard J, ed. *Brain and Space.* New York, NY: Oxford University Press Inc; 1991:81–111.

33 Paillard J. Motor and representational framing of space. In: Paillard J, ed. *Brain and Space.* New York, NY: Oxford University Press Inc; 1991:163–182.

34 Massion J. Movement, posture, and equilibrium: interaction and coordination. *Prog Neurobiol.* 1992;38:35–56.

35 Gurfinkel VS, Ivanenko YuP, Levik YuS, Babakova IA. Kinesthetic reference for human orthograde posture. *Neuroscience.* 1995;68:229–243.

36 Head H, Holmes G. Sensory disturbances from cerebral lesions. *Brain.* 1911–1912;34:102–254.

37 Hayes KC, Riach CL. Preparatory postural adjustments and postural sway in young children. In: Woollacott MH, Shumway-Cook A, eds. *Development of Posture and Gait Across the Life Span.* Columbia, SC: University of South Carolina Press; 1989:97–127.

38 Lestienne FG, Gurfinkel VS. Posture as an organizational structure based on a dual process: a formal basis to interpret changes of posture in weightlessness. In: Pompeiano O, Allum JHJ, eds. *Prog Brain Res.* 1988;76(special issue):307–313.

39 Young LR, Standish G. Influence of tactile cues on visually induced postural reactions. In: Berthoz A, Graf W, Vidal PP, eds. *The Head-Neck Sensory Motor System.* New York, NY: Oxford University Press Inc; 1992:555–559.

40 Jeka JJ, Lackner JR. Fingertip contact influences human postural control. *Exp Brain Res.* 1994;100:495–502.

41 Jeka JJ, Easton RD, Bentzen BL, Lackner JR. Haptic cues for orientation and postural control in sighted and blind individuals. *Perception and Psychophysics.* 1996;58:409–423.

42 Berthoz A. The role of gaze in the compensation of vestibular dysfunction: the gaze substitution hypothesis. In: Pompeiano O, Allum JHJ, eds. *Prog Brain Res.* 1988;76(special issue):411–420.

43 Di Fabio RP, Emasithi A. Effects of aging on adaptation of head control during exposure to sway-driven visual field displacement. *Phys Ther.* 1996;76:S22. Abstract.

44 Lackner JR. Some proprioceptive influences on the perceptual representation of body shape and orientation. *Brain.* 1988;111:281–297.

45 Fernandez C, Goldberg J. Physiology of peripheral neurons innervating otolith organs of the squirrel monkey, I: response to static tilts and to long-duration centrifugal force. *J Neurophysiol.* 1976;39:970–984.

46 Loe PR, Tompko DL, Werner G. The neural signal of angular head position in primary afferent vestibular nerve axons. *J Physiol (Lond).* 1973:230:29–50.

47 Mayne R. A systems concept of the vestibular organs. In: Kornhuber HH, ed. *Handbook of Sensory Physiology, Volume 6, Part 2: Vestibular System.* New York, NY: Springer Publishing Co Inc; 1974:493–580.

48 Fernandez C, Goldberg J. Physiology of peripheral neurons innervating otolith organs of the squirrel monkey, III: response dynamics. *J Neurophysiol.* 1976:39:996–1008.

49 Barlow JS. Inertial navigation as a basis for animal navigation. *J Theor Biol.* 1964;6:76–117.

50 Paige GD, Tomko DL. Eye movement responses to linear head motion in the squirrel monkey, I: basic characteristics. *J Neurophysiol.* 1991;65:1170–1182.

51 Collewijn H, Van Der Steen J, Ferman L, Jansen TC. Human ocular counterroll: assessment of static and dynamic properties from electromagnetic scleral coil recordings. *Exp Brain Res.* 1985;59:185–196.

52 Lichtenberg BK, Young LR, Arrott AP. Human ocular counterrolling induced by varying linear accelerations. *Exp Brain Res.* 1982;48:127–136.

53 Gresty MA, Bronstein AM. Visually controlled spatial stabilisation of the human head: compensation for the eye's limited ability to roll. *Neurosci Lett.* 1992;140:63–66.

54 Cohen B, Henn V, eds. *Representation of Three-Dimensional Space in the Vestibular, Oculomotor, and Visual Systems: A Symposium of the Bárány Society.* New York, NY: The New York Academy of Sciences; 1988.

55 Zangemeister WH, Bulgheroni MV, Pedotti A. Differential influence of vertical head posture during walking. In: Berthoz A, Graf W, Vidal PP, eds. *The Head-Neck Sensory Motor System.* New York, NY: Oxford University Press Inc; 1992:560–567.

56 Bronstein AM. Evidence for a vestibular input contribution to dynamic head stabilization in man. *Acta Otolaryngol (Stockh).* 1988;105:1–6.

57 Pozzo T, Berthoz A, Lefort L, Vitte E. Head stabilization during various locomotor tasks in humans, II: patients with bilateral peripheral vestibular deficits. *Exp Brain Res.* 1991;85:208–217.

58 Pozzo T, Berthoz A, Vitte E, Lefort L. Head stabilization during locomotion. *Acta Otolaryngol (Stockh).* 1991;481:322–327.

59 Takahashi M, Hoshikawa H, Tsujita N, Akiyama I. Effect of labyrinthine dysfunction upon head oscillation and gaze during stepping and running. *Acta Otolaryngol (Stockh).* 1988;106:348–353.

60 Taguchi K, Hirabayashi C, Kikukawa M. Clinical significance of head movement while stepping. *Acta Otolaryngol Suppl (Stockh).* 1984;406:125–128.

61 Grossman GE, Leigh RJ. Instability of gaze during locomotion in patients with deficient vestibular function. *Ann Neurol.* 1990;27:528–532.

62 Gurfinkel VS, Levik YuS, Popov KE, et al. Body scheme in the control of postural activity. In: *Stance and Motion: Third Soviet-French Roundtable Meeting on Neurobiology, 1986, Moscow and Leningrad.* New York, NY: Plenum Press; 1988:185–193.

63 Mittelstaedt H. Evidence of somatic graviception from new and classical investigations. *Acta Otolaryngol Suppl (Stockh).* 1995;520:186–187.

64 Ito T, Sanada Y. Location of receptors for righting reflexes acting upon the body in primates. *Jpn J Physiol.* 1965;15:235–242.

65 Mittelstaedt H. Somatic versus vestibular gravity reception in man. *Ann NY Acad Sci.* 1992;656:124–139.

66 Roll JP, Roll R. From eye to foot: a proprioceptive chain involved in postural control. In: Amblard B, Berthoz A, Clarac F, eds. *Posture and Gait: Development, Adaptation, and Modulation*. Amsterdam, the Netherlands: Elsevier Science Publishers BV; 1988:155–164.

67 Roll JP, Vedel JP, Roll R. Eye, head, and skeletal muscle spindle feedback in the elaboration of body references. *Prog Brain Res*. 1989;80:113–123.

68 Roll R, Velay JL, Roll JP. Eye and neck proprioceptive messages contribute to the spatial coding of retinal input in visually oriented activities. *Exp Brain Res*. 1991;85:423–431.

69 Goodwin GM, McCloskey DI, Matthews PBC. The contribution of muscle afferents to kinaesthesia shown by vibration induced illusions of movement and by the effects of paralyzing joint afferents. *Brain*. 1972;95:705–748.

70 Quoniam C, Hay L, Roll J-P, Harlay F. Age effects on reflex and postural responses to propriomuscular inputs generated by tendon vibration. *J Gerontol Biol Sci*. 1995;50:B155–B165.

71 Biguer B, Donaldson IML, Hein A, Jeannerod M. Neck muscle vibration modifies the representation of visual motion and direction in man. *Brain*. 1988;111:1405–1424.

72 Ledebt A, Bril B, Wiener-Vacher S. Trunk and head stabilization during the first months of independent walking. *Neuroreport*. 1995;6:1737–1740.

73 Peterson BW, Richmond FJ. *Control of Head Movement*. New York, NY: Oxford University Press Inc; 1988.

74 Schor RH, Kearney RE, Dieringer N. Reflex stabilization of the head. In: Peterson BW, Richmond FJ, eds. *Control of Head Movement*. Oxford, United Kingdom: Oxford University Press; 1988:141–166.

75 Horstmann GA, Dietz V. A basic control mechanism: the stabilization of the centre of gravity. *Electroencephalogr Clin Neurophysiol*. 1990;76:165–176.

76 Dietz V, Horstmann G, Berger W. Involvement of different receptors in the regulation of human posture. *Neurosci Lett*. 1988;94:82–87.

77 Dietz V, Horstmann GA, Trippel M, Gollhofer A. Human postural reflexes and gravity: an underwater simulation. *Neurosci Lett*. 1989;106:350–355.

78 Emasithi A, Di Fabio RP. Head position and orientation after exposure to altered sensory environments in different age groups. *Phys Ther*. 1996;76:S22. Abstract.

79 Di Fabio RP, Emasithi A. Aging and the influence of visual inputs on head stabilization during stance on a rotating surface. *Phys Ther*. 1996;76:S21. Abstract.

80 Sheldon JH. The effect of age on the control of sway. *Geront Clin*. 1963;5:129–138.

81 Overstall PW, Exton-Smith AN, Imms FJ, Johnson AL. Falls in the elderly related to postural imbalance. *BMJ*. 1977;1:261–264.

82 Thyssen HH, Brynskov J, Jansen EC, et al. Normal ranges in reproducibility for quantitative Romberg's test. *Acta Neurol Scand*. 1982;66:100–104.

83 Badke MB, Di Fabio RP. Effects of postural bias during support surface displacements and rapid arm movements. *Phys Ther*. 1985;65:1490–1495.

84 Diener HC, Bacher M, Guschlbauer B, Dichgans J. The coordination of posture and voluntary movement in patients with hemiparesis. *J Neurol*. 1993;240:161–167.

85 Massion J. Postural changes accompanying voluntary movement: normal and pathological aspects. *Human Neurobiology*. 1984;2:261–267.

86 Belenkii VY, Gurfinkel VS, Pal'tsev YI. Elements of control of voluntary movements. *Biofizika*. 1967;12:135–141.

87 Bouisset S, Zattara M. A sequence of postural movement precedes voluntary movement. *Neurosci Lett*. 1981;22:263–270.

88 Brown JE, Frank JS. Influence of event anticipation on postural actions accompanying voluntary movement. *Exp Brain Res*. 1987;67:645–650.

89 Cordo PJ, Nashner LM. Properties of postural adjustments associated with rapid arm movements. *J Neurophysiol*. 1982;47:287–302.

90 Friedli WG, Hallett M, Simon SR. Postural adjustments associated with rapid voluntary arm movements, I: electromyographic data. *J Neurol Neurosurg Psychiatry*. 1984;47:611–622.

91 Shumway-Cook A, McCollum G. Assessment and treatment of balance deficits. In: Montgomery PC, Connolly BH, eds. *Motor Control and Physical Therapy: Theoretical Framework and Practical Implications*. Hixson, Tenn: Chattanooga Group Inc; 1991:123–138.

92 Jones FP. Method for changing stereotyped response patterns by the inhibition of postural sets. *Psychol Rev*. 1965;72:411–425.

93 Di Fabio RP, Badke MB. Reliability of postural response as a function of muscular synergisms: effect of supraspinal lesions. *Human Movement Science*. 1989;8:447–464.

94 Di Fabio RP. Adaptation of postural stability following stroke. *Topics in Stroke Rehabilitation*. 1997;3:62–75.

95 Pal'tsev YI, El'ner AM. Preparatory and compensatory period during voluntary movement in patients with involvement of the brain of different localization. *Biofizika*. 1967;12:142–147.

96 Horak FB, Esselman P, Anderson ME, Lynch MK. The effects of movement velocity, mass displaced, and task certainty on associated postural adjustments made by normal and hemiplegic individuals. *Journal of Neurosurgery and Psychiatry*. 1984;47:1020–1028.

Appendix.
Methods Used to Study the Research Questions

Subjects
Seven subjects (six male and 1 female), ranging in age from 25 to 72 years ($\bar{X}$=42.4, SD=19), participated in this preliminary study. Five subjects were under 50 years of age ($\bar{X}$=32, SD=7), and two subjects were over 60 years of age (66 and 72 years). All subjects had no evidence of neuromuscular, orthopedic, or systemic disease. All subjects were active, living independently in the community, and did not report experiencing any falls within a year preceding the study. Each subject signed a consent form prior to participating. The protocol for this study was approved by the Committee on the Use of Human Subjects in Research at the University of Minnesota.

Control of the Sensory Environment
A modified dynamic posturography system[a] was used to manipulate the sensory environment. The sensory environment consisted of two components: a movable visual surround and a movable force platform. Servomotors tilted the foot support surface around the axis of the ankle joint (maximum tilt angle=±10°). Servomotors also tilted the visual surround forward or backward (maximum tilt angle=±10°). The magnitude and direction of platform or surround tilt were determined by the magnitude and polarity, respectively, of the "gain" selected by the tester. During the test, either the support surface or the visual surround were tilted in some proportion to anteroposterior sagittal displacement of the center of force (COF). The position of the vertical projection of the COF was calculated from the output of four vertical-thrust transducers embedded in the force platform. Precision potentiometers were mounted on the pitch rotation axis of both the visual surround and the platform to measure displacement-time history.

Two baseline conditions—stance on a fixed platform and fixed visual surround with eyes open (EO-FPS) and closed (EC-FPS)—were tested before and after the experimental conditions (see Tab. 1). The gain for the baseline conditions was 0 because neither the platform nor the surround moved in conjunction with the subjects' COF. Three experimental conditions were presented to each subject, and the investigators altered the amount of sensory input to the CNS in each of these conditions by manipulating the magnitude and polarity of the gain controlling platform or surround motion with respect to displacement of the COF (see Figs. 4 and 5). The three conditions were:

1. Surround motion (SM): Only the visual surround was moved in conjunction with displacement of the COF in the sagittal plane. For positive gains, forward displacement of the COF caused a forward tilt of the visual surround. Negative gains reversed the direction of surround tilt (see Fig. 4).
2. Eyes open–platform motion (EO-PM): Only the force platform was rotated in conjunction with the COF in the sagittal plane. For positive gains, forward displacement of the COF caused a "toes-down" rotation of the force platform. Negative gains reversed the direction of platform rotation (see Fig. 5).
3. Eyes closed–platform motion (EC-PM): Same as EO-PM but with eyes closed.

Eight experimenter-selected gains (±0.5, ±1.0, ±1.5, and ±2.0) were tested for each of three sensory conditions (see Figs. 4 and 5). Some conditions involved platform motion that was combined with surround motion, but these conditions were not analyzed.

Measurement of Head Linear Displacement and Angular Position
A 6-degree-of-freedom magnetic tracking device[b] was used to measure head position and orientation. The electromagnetic tracking device consists of a surce (transmitter) that emits a low-frequency magnetic field and a sensor that detects these magnetic fields. The device has been found to be highly reliable for measuring spatial rigid body motion,[c] and reliability was confirmed for the current application. A "bench" test was conducted by fixing the sensor approximately 1 m from the visual surround and displacing the transmitter in several known locations on a precision-drilled calibrated Plexiglas[d] plate. During the bench test, the visual surround was fully upright, tilted maximally toward the transmitter (simulating negative gain), or tilted maximally away from the transmitter (simulating positive gain).

For this study, we focused on translation and rotation of the head in the sagittal plane ("head-x" and head pitch, respectively). The linear and angular calibration measurements were found to be within 1 degree of the surround-vertical condition up to a sensor-transmitter distance of ±15 cm. The maximum error with respect to the surround-erect position was 0.18 cm for x-translation and 0.78 degrees for pitch.

Data Collection
Three DOS-based computers were interfaced for data collection. One computer controlled displacement of the sensory environment and triggered data sampling. The second computer was used to sample data simultaneously from the force platform transducers and the platform and surround-position potentiometers. The third computer was dedicated to collection of head tracking data. Force recordings and potentiometer outputs were sampled at 500 Hz, and the head tracking system was sampled at 100 Hz. All recordings were filtered with a Hanning filter[e] so that the resultant low-pass corner frequency was 20 Hz for all recordings.

Procedures
Each subject wore an adjustable plastic band firmly fitted to the head. The 6-degree-of-freedom electromagnetic sensor was mounted on the band with a plastic screw assembly. The electromagnetic transmitter was mounted on an overhead arch and fixed to a Plexiglas tube that was secured 8 cm above the subject's head. The alignment reference frame of the sensor relative to the transmitter was calibrated by digitizing the location of each external auditory canal and determining the perpendicular bisection of the imaginary "line" connecting each canal. The perpendicular bisection defined the origin of the alignment reference frame.

The subjects removed their shoes and were instructed to stand as quietly as possible on the force platform. They faced into the enclosure surrounding their field of vision (1 m deep) and were asked to maintain a standing posture with arms folded across the chest and look straight ahead. Baseline measurements were taken for three 20-second trials during EO-FPS and EC-FPS. Following the pretest baseline measures, the gain for the visual surround and the platform were altered to change the input-output relationship between the COF displacement and tilt of the physical environment (see Tab. 1, Figs. 4 and 5). A block of three trials was collected for each positive gain and was followed by a block of three trials for a negative gain of identical absolute magnitude (see Tab. 1). The presentation of blocks was randomized between subjects. Data for three trials were collected during each condition that involved displacement of the sensory environment (SM, EO-PM, and EC-PM). The duration for each trial was 20 seconds, and the intertrial interval was approximately 30 seconds to allow subjects to return to their initial starting position. Once exposure to all nonzero gain conditions was completed, the subjects were retested in EO-FPS and EC-FPS (see Tab. 1).

---

[a] EquiTest, NeuroCom International Inc, 9570 SE Lawnfield Rd, Clackamas, OR 97015.

[b] Polhemus, Div of Kaiser Aerospace Electronics Corp, 1 Hercules Dr, Colchester, VT 05446-1549.

[c] An KN, Jacobsen MC, Berglund LJ, Chao EYS. Application of a magnetic tracking device to kinesiologic studies. *J Biomech.* 1988;21:613–620.

[d] Rohm & Haas Co, Independence Mall W, Philadelphia, PA 19105.

[e] Matlab, Mathworks Inc, 24 Prime Pkwy, Natick, MA 01760.

Special Series

Light Touch Contact as a Balance Aid

Canes and crutches are commonly used mobility aids, and most studies of their use have focused on issues equating support with the resulting decrease in force required of the affected limb. Clinicians, however, often observe patients with poor balance control using light touch of surrounding objects and surfaces to stabilize themselves while standing and walking. A series of studies have shown that sensory input to the hand and arm through contact cues at the fingertip or through a cane can reduce postural sway in individuals who have no impairments and in patients without a functioning vestibular system, even when contact force levels are inadequate to provide physical support of the body. This article summarizes these results, which have implications for design considerations of rehabilitation aids. Mobility devices or rehabilitation aids that provide feedback about applied force or enhance existing resolution of applied force changes across the skin surface may lead to new rehabilitation techniques. [Jeka JJ. Light touch contact as a balance aid. *Phys Ther*. 1997;77:476–487.]

Key Words: *Cane, Fingertip, Mobility aid, Neural plasticity, Posture, Rehabilitation, Somatosensory, Vestibular.*

John J Jeka

Mobility aids such as canes and crutches are commonly used for rehabilitation from musculoskeletal or neuromuscular injuries and for balance problems with elderly individuals. A primary function of such aids is to reduce the risk of falls, because falls may lead not only to physical injury but to loss of confidence and to restrictions on mobility, which may have psychological repercussions (eg, depression). In addition, mobility aids are used to decrease loads on joints or limbs recovering from injury. The literature on mobility aids deals primarily with three general areas[1]: (1) the scientific study of variables involved during locomotion with a mobility aid, (2) their therapeutic use as rehabilitation aids, and (3) design modifications. Few studies, however, have systematically investigated these categories for the proper prescription and use of ambulatory aids.[2-4] Most studies have focused primarily on the biomechanical support provided by walking canes or crutches.[5-7] Forces applied to a cane are often measured in relation to forces applied at each foot for comparison of forces applied without cane use. Functional support provided by a cane is often equated with the resulting decrease in force required of the affected limb; the greater the support provided by the cane, the more effective its use. This belief has led to recommendations such as holding a cane in the hand contralateral to the affected limb, because the long lever arm reduces the forces across the hip joint to less than half of that of unaided locomotion.[3]

Assessing the role of the cane as a mobility aid purely in terms of absolute biomechanical forces may be underestimating its potential use in the rehabilitation of patients with balance disorders. There are many properties of cane use that have not been thoroughly investigated. Murray et al,[8] for example, demonstrated that the timing relationships between applied cane forces and the duration of stance were related to the functional use of the cane. Patients with ankle arthropathy applied peak cane force late in the stance phase of the disabled limb, suggesting that the cane was used to push forward. In contrast, patients with degenerative joint disease of the hip applied an initial peak thrust early in the stance phase, suggesting that the cane was used for restraint. Thus, an important consideration in the functional use of a cane may be the timing relationships observed between applied forces through the cane and stance forces for a particular injury or disorder that leads to poor balance.

There are also instances in which it is desirable to limit the physical support derived from a cane. Persons with lower-extremity amputations must learn to gradually shift their weight from a cane to a prosthesis to avoid residual limb irritation at the limb/socket interface.[9] Such patients often have difficulty estimating how much weight to apply to a cane to help support the affected limb. Moreover, Murray et al[8] showed that persons with above-knee amputations applied small cane forces prior to the stance phase with the prosthesis, suggesting that the cane was providing sensory information before the onset of prosthetic weight bearing.

The argument for the importance of sensory input from a balance aid is bolstered by the fact that canes are often prescribed for patients with balance disorders that stem not from an orthopedic problem but from neurological damage. For example, many patients without a functioning vestibular system have poor balance control due to the lack of sensory information about head movement,

---

JJ Jeka, PhD, is Assistant Professor, Department of Kinesiology, College of Health and Human Performance, University of Maryland at College Park, Room 2359, HHP Bldg, College Park, MD 20742-2611 (USA) (jj96@umail.umd.edu).

Dr Jeka was supported by a National Institutes of Health postdoctoral fellowship (1 F32 NS09025-02), by National Aeronautics and Space Administration grant NAG9-515, and by a Graduate Research Board grant at the University of Maryland.

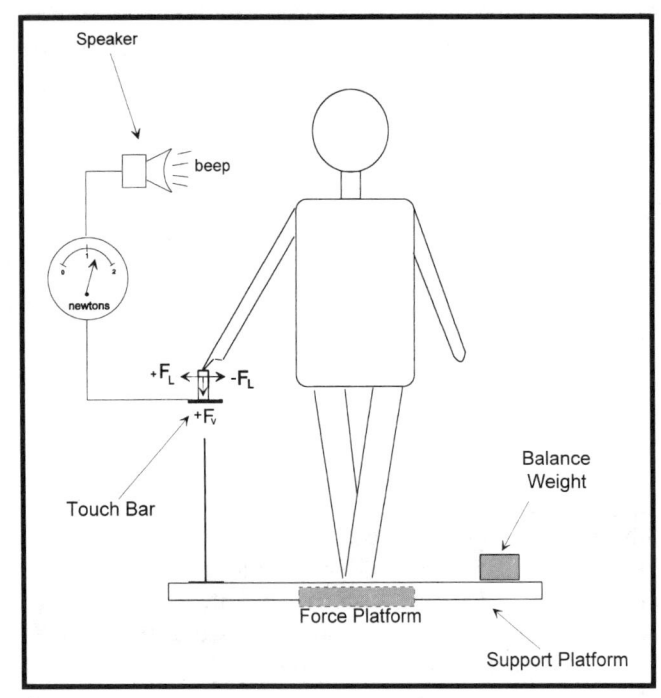

Figure 1.
A subject depicted in the heel-to-toe stance on the force platform in a touch contact condition with the tip of the right index finger on the touch bar. For the sake of illustration, the subject is shown exceeding a typical threshold force of 1 N and the alarm is sounding. In actual experiments, this occurred in less than 5% of all touch contact trials. In the force contact conditions, the auditory alarm was turned off and the subject could apply as much force as desired. In the no contact conditions, the subject's arms hung passively by the sides. F_L and F_V refer to applied contact forces in the lateral and vertical directions, respectively.

which is crucial for stable locomotion.[10-12] Patients with Parkinson's disease, whose walking patterns resemble a rigid shuffle, reported increased comfort when using a cane, even though the force applied through the cane was less than that needed for physical support of the body.[8]

The mechanical support provided by a balance aid may be the primary benefit for certain conditions (eg, hip replacement). The spontaneous adoption of different timing strategies with cane use at very low applied force levels, however, emphasizes that patients derive substantial orientation information from a hand-held cane. An underestimated source of support may be the orientation information provided from somatosensory stimulation of the hand and arm through contact of the cane with the ground or a rigid object. Recent investigations[13,14] have shown that contact cues from the fingertip provide information that leads to reduced postural sway in subjects without balance impairments and in patients with bilateral vestibular loss, even when the applied forces are physically inadequate to stabilize the body. Sighted and congenitally blind individuals may use a cane to stabilize upright stance, even at very low force levels, in the same fashion as the fingertip.[15] To provide some background on how touch and pressure cues stabilize upright stance, the results of studies on fingertip contact cane use and the control of quiet upright stance are summarized below.

Light Touch Contact Studies

Light touch contact of a fingertip to a stable surface reduced postural sway in subjects standing on one lower extremity[16] and in a heel-to-toe stance.[13,14] Figure 1 depicts a subject in the heel-to-toe stance (left lower extremity in front of right lower extremity) on a force platform touching a device used to measure the forces applied by the tip of the right index finger. The touch apparatus consisted of a horizontal metal bar attached to a metal stand, parallel with the sagittal plane of the subject. Subjects placed their right index finger on the middle of the bar while strain gauges mounted on the bar transduced the lateral (F_L) and vertical (F_V) forces applied by the fingertip. Subjects were tested with eyes open and closed in three fingertip contact conditions: (1) no contact, during which the subjects' arms hung passively by their sides, (2) touch contact, in which the subjects could apply up to 1 N ($\approx$100 g) of force on the touch apparatus before an auditory tone signaled the threshold of applied force, and (3) force contact, during which subjects could apply as much force as desired. In the light touch condition, if 1 N of force was exceeded, an auditory alarm went off, indicating that the subjects should apply less force without losing contact with the surface. The light touch task is very easy to perform. After just one practice trial to get a "feel" for the threshold force, subjects rarely set off the alarm (<5% of the light touch trials in all the experiments to date).

Figure 2 shows the combined results from five subjects.[13] Mediolateral center-of-pressure (COP_X) mean displacement* was highest in the eyes closed–no contact condition and reduced in all other conditions. *Post hoc* tests revealed that touch and force contact lowered mean COP_X displacement equivalently, with or without vision present (no touch, eyes open or closed > light touch and force touch, eyes open or closed) despite mean fingertip force levels that were over 10 times greater with force contact (4 N) than with touch contact (0.4 N).

In a model designed to study the reduction in body sway due to static and dynamic mechanical forces at the

---

* In all of the studies reviewed here, center-of-pressure displacement was used to approximate overall body sway. Center-of-pressure excursion is not equivalent to body sway. Center-of-pressure excursions tend to be larger and of higher frequency than center-of-mass movements.[17] Pilot work, however, showed that correlations between center of pressure and a single light-emitting diode located at the navel and tracked with a video camera were found to average $\rho=0.9$, with a 2.3-millisecond time lag. Such a high correlation is due primarily to the relatively small amplitude of overall body sway (<1 cm) in the present paradigm. Thus, center-of-pressure displacement is assumed to be roughly equivalent to overall body sway.

fingertip,[16] contact forces of 0.4 N predicted a 2% to 3% reduction of sway. Touch contact, however, reduced sway by 50% to 60% in all subjects. This finding suggests that fingertip forces in the touch contact conditions are inadequate to stabilize upright stance. Subjects must rely on musculature remote from the fingertip to arrest sway toward the touch bar, because touch contact forces alone are not large enough.

Temporal Relationships

When fingertip forces are providing physical support, force levels are expected to increase and decrease with body sway toward and away from the contact surface, respectively. When fingertip contact forces are limited to 1 N, the contact forces can no longer be allowed to rise and fall with body sway without exceeding the threshold force. Thus, a different temporal relationship is expected between contact forces and body sway with light touch. Figure 3 shows the time series of COP_X displacement and F_L in typical force contact (Fig. 3a) and touch contact (Fig. 3b) trials. Maximum cross-correlations and their respective time lags are also shown. Correlations between COP_X displacement and F_L were highest with force contact ($\rho \approx 0.9$), with very small time lags between the two signals (<50 milliseconds).

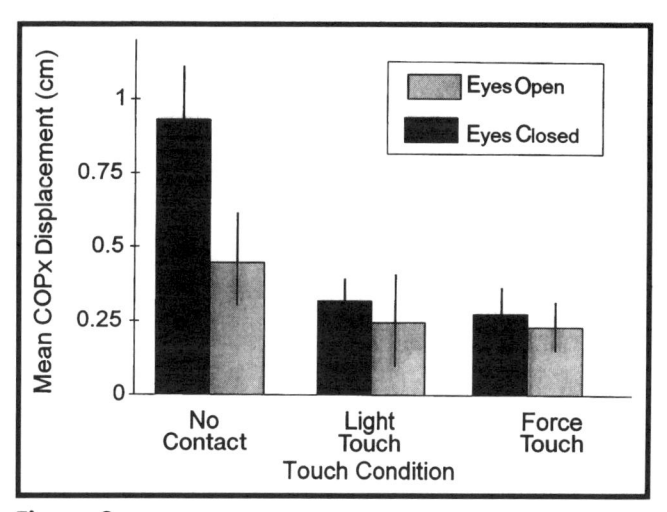

Figure 2.
Mean center-of-pressure (COP_X) displacement collapsed across subjects for each experimental condition. The COP_X displacement was highest in the no contact-eyes closed condition and lowest with any form of fingertip contact. Error bars represent standard error.

This finding means that contact forces in the force contact condition were in phase with body sway; subjects were essentially leaning on the contact surface through their finger for support. With light touch contact, COP_X-F_L correlations were lower ($\rho \approx .8$), with time lags of approximately 300 milliseconds. Figure 3b shows that the increased time lag corresponds to the F_L signal leading COP_X displacement. As subjects swayed toward the touch bar with only very light touch, contact forces initially increased, but as sway continued, F_L decreased so as not to trigger the alarm threshold. This 300-millisecond lead of the force signal was maintained throughout the trial. The key point is that the additional stabilization provided by touch contact is due to a different sensorimotor relationship than with force contact. Forces generated by the musculature remote from the fingertip (eg, lower extremities, trunk) are guided by sensory information provided by cutaneous receptors in the fingertip[18,19] and proprioceptive information about arm position.[20,21]

The same influence of light touch contact on postural control is observed in patients with bilateral loss of vestibular function. Patients with vestibular loss are thought to rely heavily on somatosensory information to indirectly derive missing information about head movement through the head-trunk linkage.[22] Consequently, an additional somatosensory reference from the fingertip may provide information about trunk movement that may enhance head-trunk coordination. In an unpublished study by Jeka and colleagues, five patients with complete bilateral vestibular loss and five age-matched subjects with normal vestibular function participated in the same paradigm as the above experiment. The subjects with vestibular loss were generally not able to maintain the tandem stance in the eyes closed–no contact condition for more than 5 seconds before falling. With light touch or force contact, however, postural sway was reduced to equivalent levels in all subjects. The same timing relationships between body sway and fingertip forces were observed in both the subjects with vestibular loss and the control subjects. Fingertip contact clearly substitutes for the sensory information that patients with vestibular loss lack to maintain upright tandem stance with eyes closed.

Leg Muscle Electromyographic Activity

In another experiment, Jeka and colleagues measured electromyographic (EMG) activity in the peroneal muscles, which are particularly important in stabilizing lateral body sway, to determine whether leg muscle activity changed with different contact cues. Two pieces of evidence suggest that light touch forces at the fingertip trigger EMG activity of the postural musculature. First, the EMG amplitude was lowest with force contact, higher with touch contact, and highest with no contact, indicating that leg muscles played a much larger role in maintaining balance with touch contact than with force contact. The increase in muscle activity with touch contact indicates that postural sway is reduced by additional muscular forces in the legs, whereas with force contact, the leg muscles play a lesser role. Forces generated by the arm musculature are a likely candidate to reduce body sway with force contact at the fingertip.

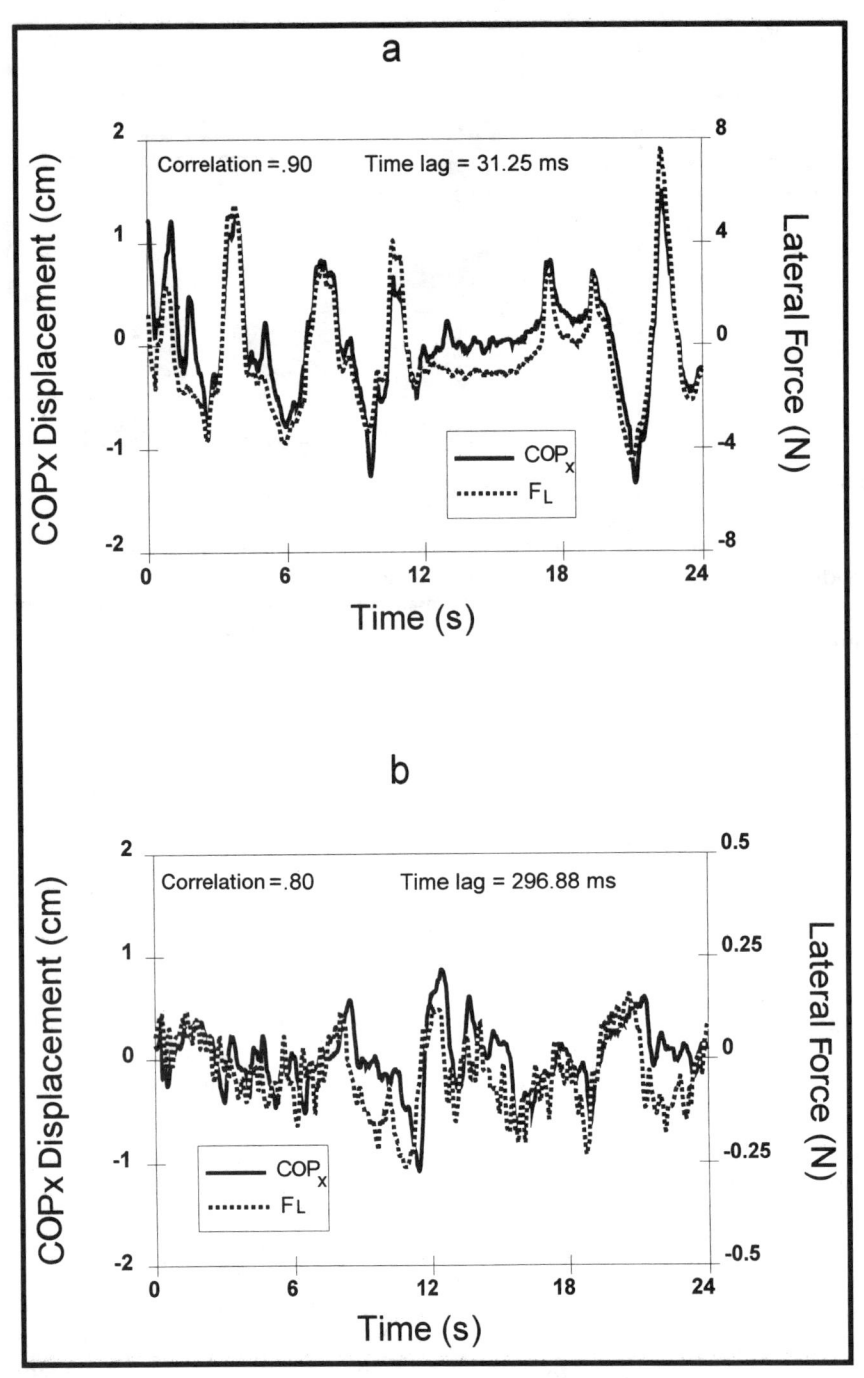

Figure 3.
Overlaid time series of center-of-pressure (COP$_X$) displacement (solid line) and lateral fingertip force (F$_L$) (dotted line) in (a) an eyes open–force contact condition and (b) an eyes open–light touch contact condition. Individual correlations and time delays for each trial are shown. A positive time delay means that F$_L$ is temporarily ahead of COP$_X$.

and decreased with leftward COP$_X$ displacement (negative slope). Right peroneal muscle EMG activity was approximately 180 degrees out of phase with left peroneal muscle EMG activity. In each condition, EMG activity led COP$_X$ displacement by about 150 milliseconds. Together with the timing relationships between COP$_X$ displacement and F$_L$ (Fig. 3), this finding means that with touch contact, changes in F$_L$ began about 150 milliseconds ahead of correlated changes in EMG activity. The observed pattern of directional changes in F$_L$ followed by leg muscle activity followed by body sway suggests that F$_L$ provided a feedforward signal of body sway. In contrast, contact force changes were in phase with COP$_X$ displacement in the force contact conditions, indicating that changes in leg muscle EMG activity were well ahead of changes in both COP$_X$ displacement and fingertip contact force. This finding suggests that fingertip contact forces in the force contact conditions were not precuing a particular muscle activity pattern but were attenuating body sway primarily with physically supportive forces.

Touch Contact With a Cane

A recent study[15] compared the use of light touch forces between individuals with congenital blindness and sighted (eyes closed) individuals. A previous study[23] had shown higher levels of sway in blind versus blindfolded sighted individuals. A possible explanation may be that visual experience is a prerequisite for establishing a precise frame of reference for spatial tasks based on nonvisual information.[24-26] Moreover, the long cane is a commonly used mobility aid for blind individuals, and its primary function is thought to be obstacle avoidance.[27,28] Somatosensory cues from a cane also may provide a spatial referent that blind individuals use to stabilize upright stance.

Figure 5 shows the experimental setup. The touch bar was mounted to the wooden platform that rests on the force platform. The tip of a lightweight adjustable metal cane rested in a tiny well mounted to the touch bar so that the cane tip could not slide horizontally. Subjects

Second, shifts in the relative timing among COP$_X$ displacement, contact force amplitude, and EMG activity were evident in the light touch versus force touch conditions. How the peroneal muscle's EMG activity behaved in each leg as the body moved in the mediolateral direction is illustrated in Figure 4. Electromyographic activity of the left peroneal muscle increased with COP$_X$ displacement to the right (positive slope)

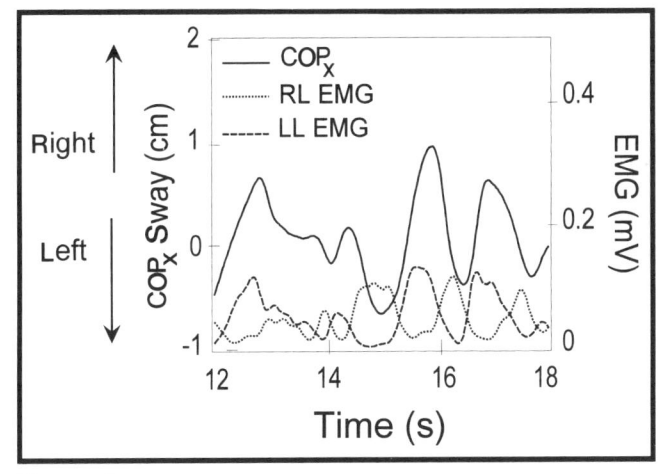

Figure 4.
Overlaid time-series segments of center-of-pressure (COP_X) displacement (solid line), right leg (RL) electromyographic (EMG) amplitude (dotted line), and left leg (LL) EMG amplitude (dashed line) from a single trial of a light touch contact condition. Electromyographic signals were full-wave rectified and band-pass filtered with a 0- to 12-Hz Blackman window.

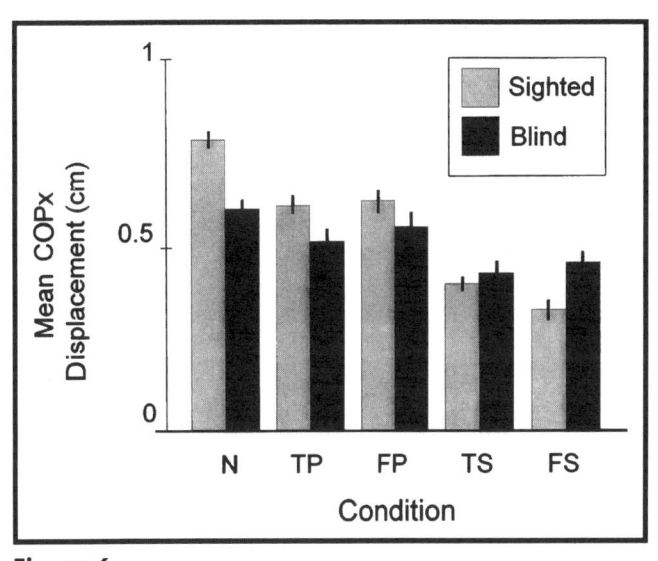

Figure 6.
Mean center-of-pressure (COP_X) displacement for sighted (eyes closed) and blind subjects in each condition. (Conditions: N=no contact, TP=touch contact–perpendicular cane, TS=touch contact–slanted cane, FP=force contact–perpendicular cane, and FS=force contact–slanted cane.) Error bars represent standard error.

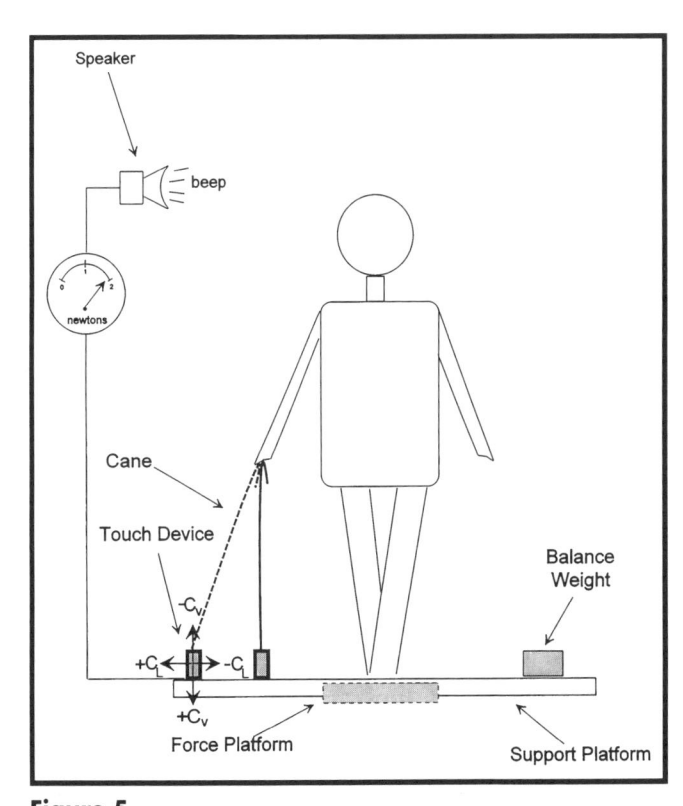

Figure 5.
A subject depicted in heel-to-toe stance on the force platform holding a cane with the tip resting on the metal bar that measures applied forces. The solid and dashed canes show the cane's orientation in the perpendicular and slanted conditions, respectively. C_L=lateral cane force, C_V=vertical cane force.

were tested with the same three contact conditions as with the fingertip (ie, no contact, touch contact, and force contact). In addition, the touch bar was anchored in two positions: 60 cm lateral to the subject so that the cane was held perpendicular to the ground or 120 cm lateral to the subject so that the cane was slanted at a 30-degree angle relative to the ground. In each condition, cane length was adjusted so that the subject's elbow was flexed at 15 degrees. The five conditions were no contact (N), touch contact–perpendicular cane (TP), touch contact–slanted cane (TS), force contact–perpendicular cane (FP), and force contact–slanted cane (FS). Figure 6 shows the mean COP_X displacement results collapsed across five subjects with congenital blindness and five control subjects (sighted with eyes closed). Mean COP_X displacement was highest with no contact. Similar to the fingertip experiment, touch contact was as effective as force contact in reducing postural sway (compare conditions TP and FP or conditions TS and FS). Moreover, postural sway was reduced most effectively with a slanted cane (conditions TS and FS), indicating that cane angle is an important consideration in its stabilizing influence (see "Light Touch With a Cane" section).

Timing Relationships With a Cane

Timing relationships between COP_X displacement and lateral cane force (C_L) changed not only with the level of applied force, as in the fingertip studies, but also with cane angle. Mean COP_X-C_L correlations and time lags in Figure 7 show negative correlations with time lags close to zero with a perpendicular cane (conditions TP and FP). With a slanted cane (conditions TS and FS), however, COP_X-C_L correlations were positive, demonstrating that C_L was now in phase with COP_X displacement. Using force contact with a slanted cane resulted in time delays close to zero, whereas touch contact with a slanted cane led to longer time delays (approximately 200

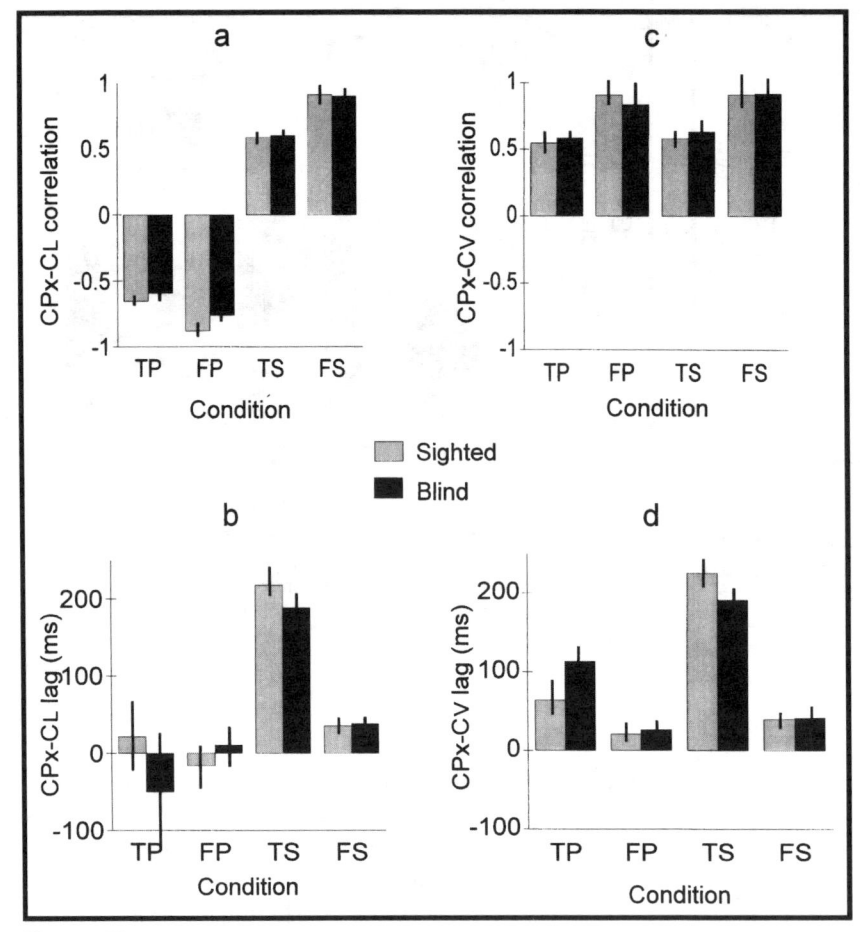

Figure 7.
Mean cross-correlation coefficients and mean time lags between center-of-pressure (COP$_X$) sway and cane forces (lateral=C$_L$, vertical=C$_V$) in each condition. (a) Mean COP$_X$-C$_L$ cross-correlation coefficients, (b) mean COP$_X$-C$_L$ time lags, (c) mean COP$_X$-C$_V$ cross-correlation coefficients, and (d) mean COP$_X$-C$_V$ time lags. (Conditions: TP=touch contact–perpendicular cane, TS=touch contact–slanted cane, FP=force contact–perpendicular cane, and FS=force contact–slanted cane.) Error bars represent standard error. A positive time lag means that C$_L$ is temporarily ahead of COP$_X$.

milliseconds), reflecting timing relationships very similar to those of the fingertip contact experiments (Fig. 3). Correlations between COP$_X$ displacement and vertical cane forces were positive and showed no differences due to cane angle. These results suggest that both vertical and lateral applied cane forces are involved in stabilizing postural sway and that stabilization is most effective when both directions of force are positively correlated to body sway.

How Does Light Touch Contact Reduce Body Sway?

These experiments have demonstrated that somatosensory contact cues at the fingertip and hand reduce postural sway in individuals without balance impairments, in persons with bilateral vestibular loss, and in individuals with congenital blindness. How do these "touch cues" serve as a source of sensory information about body orientation? Because muscular activity is greater in the peroneal muscles with light touch contact than with force contact suggests that light touch is triggering postural muscles to correct sway. The same peroneal muscles, however, are even more active without any contact. Why do we observe less sway with touch contact if muscle activity is higher with no contact? There are two possible explanations. One explanation is that additional postural musculature may be triggered with touch contact that is not active with no contact. The reference information provided by light touch contact may allow for a completely different set of muscles (eg, of the trunk) to counteract sway than with no contact, where somatosensory cues are derived primarily from around the feet and ankles. For instance, Winter et al[29] have shown that the hip abductors and adductors are prime candidates for the control of mediolateral body sway with feet side by side. Unfortunately, important hip abductor and adductor muscles, such as the gluteus medius, are deep muscles, making their EMG activity extremely difficult to isolate.

A second possibility for the reduction of body sway with light touch contact is the additional precision provided by somatosensory cues from the fingertip. Although cutaneous receptors are distributed across the entire body surface, they are particularly dense in the fingertips and hand. Analogous to the fovea of the retina, the fingertips are referred to as the "somesthetic macula."[30] Two-point discrimination studies have shown that the fingertip can resolve differences as small as 2 mm,[31] which is approximately the mean level of sway that we observe with light touch contact (Fig. 2). Interestingly, two-point discrimination at the bottom of the foot is approximately 8 to 10 mm, which is approximately the mean level of sway observed when subjects stand without fingertip contact and eyes closed.

Rapidly adapting (RA) cutaneous fibers, which have high spatial acuity and sensitivity to local vibration, are thought to be responsible for the detection of localized movement between the skin and a surface.[19] Slowly adapting (SA) cutaneous receptors, which are primarily responsible for tactual form and roughness perception through the distribution of forces across the skin surface,[19] may provide information about body sway through skin surface deformation or through "skin stretch."[32] In order to provide information about body orientation, however, cutaneous stimulation must be combined with knowledge of ongoing arm configuration that is dependent on interrelating muscle afferent and other proprioceptive activity to motor commands.[20,21,33]

There is much evidence to suggest that muscle spindle signals interpreted in relation to motor commands are the primary source of information for the position sense representation of the body and about body orientation relative to the support surface.[21,34] The fine acuity of cutaneous stimulation at the fingertip in combination with muscle spindle stimulation may allow for more precise detection of body sway with fingertip contact than somatosensory cues derived from the feet and ankles alone. Consequently, body sway is reduced because contact cues from the fingertip can detect trunk movements far earlier than those from the feet or ankles.

Light Touch With a Cane

Light touch through a cane had many of the same features of light touch with the fingertip. Jeka and colleagues' results suggest that the pattern of somatosensory stimulation with a hand-held cane could take two forms. All of the subjects they tested held the cane in the same manner, with palms resting on top of the cane and fingers wrapped around the handle in a thumb-opposing grip. The simplest pattern of stimulation could arise from body sway with the cane held still relative to the body. A traveling wave of stimulation across the palm may be interpreted as body sway, and appropriate muscular responses could inhibit further sway. Such somatosensory stimulation would be more difficult to interpret if the cane moved relative to the body. The pattern of stimulation could then be due to movement of the cane, movement of the body, or a combination of both.

As shown in Figure 8a, the negative correlation that Jeka and colleagues observed between body sway and lateral cane force with a perpendicular cane (Fig. 7) suggests that the cane and the body moved together around their respective pivot points (ie, cane tip and feet). In contrast, Figure 8b shows how positive correlations between body sway and lateral cane force suggest that the slanted cane was held still as the body swayed in the mediolateral direction. The strict threshold force of 1 N required in the light touch condition led subjects to adopt a sensorimotor relationship with a cane similar to that observed previously with the fingertip, that is, a similar lead of applied cane forces relative to body sway of 200 to 300 milliseconds. The reduction of sway that this relationship affords may be possible only with the high somatosensory precision of which the fingertips and hands are capable.

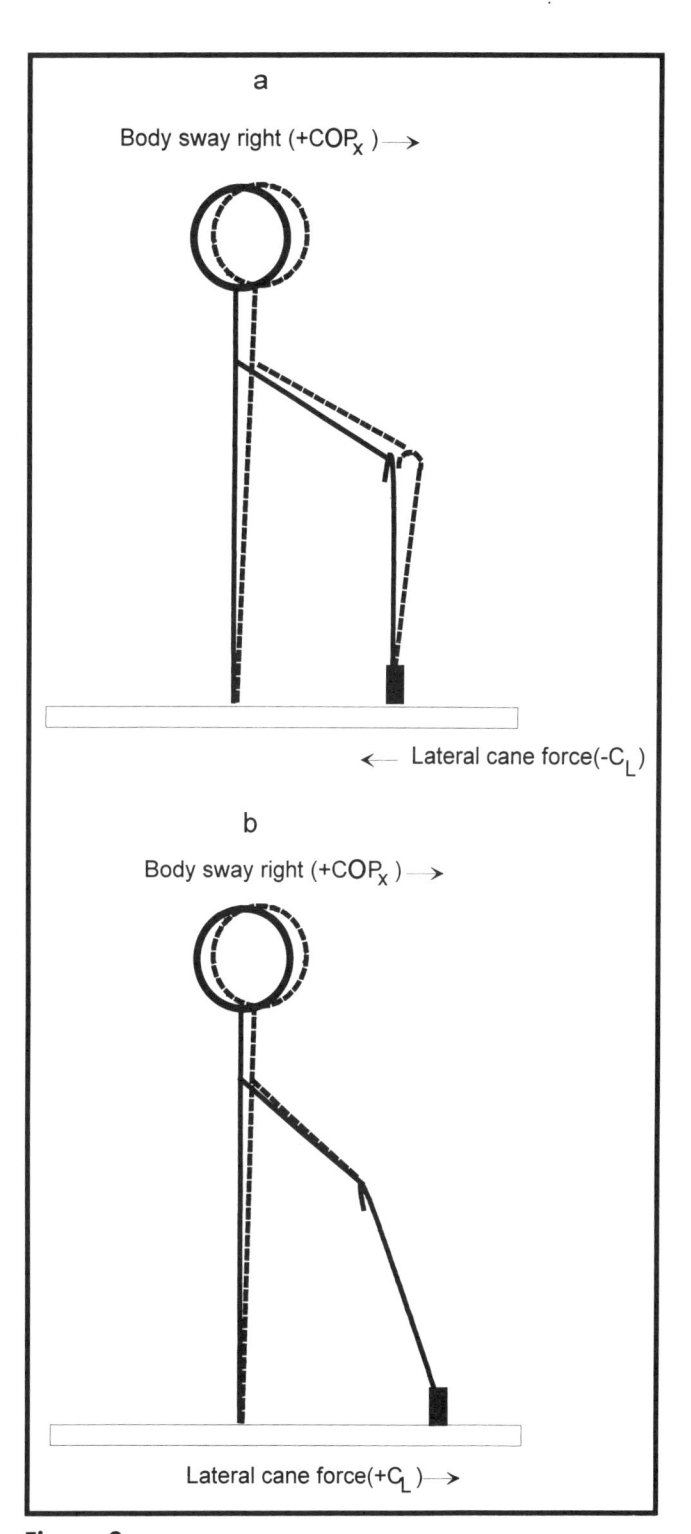

Figure 8.
Schematic depictions of a subject holding a cane viewed from behind, showing the relationship between body sway and lateral cane forces (C_L) with (a) a perpendicular cane and (b) a slanted cane. With a perpendicular cane, body sway to the right (positive center-of-pressure [COP_X] displacement) resulted in negative (leftward) lateral cane forces as the cane tip pivoted on the metal bar. With a slanted cane, lateral forces increased (rightward) with body sway to the right, implying that the cane remained stationary during body sway.

Clinical Implications

Clinicians often observe patients with balance disorders using light touch of surrounding objects and surfaces to stabilize themselves while standing and walking, but the actual use of touch contact or canes in balance control has not been studied systematically or rigorously. The findings of postural control with light touch contact may have potential applications to a large population of patients with balance and gait disorders due to neurological injury, including patients with hemiparesis, patients with Parkinson's disease, and elderly individuals. Such individuals are often capable of generating the appropriate muscular forces to maintain stable ambulation, but only if provided with sensory information that they are lacking due to neurological trauma. The additional sense of comfort that cane use provides may have little to do with physical support of the body. Two potential implications are addressed below: assistive device design and therapeutic mechanisms.

Assistive Device Design

The data on cane use with light touch contact have implications for assistive devices, where the primary design consideration is physical support for balance control.[28] Although rigidity and strength remain crucial features of any cane for instances when physical support is required, how often a cane is used for balance recovery (eg, after a "stumble") may be overestimated. Much of the time, I believe, a cane may serve the orientation function highlighted in the studies described, essentially fostering small corrections of upright stance that keep the center of mass well within stability limits and diminish the probability of a complete loss of balance. From this perspective, design features that enhance somatosensory feedback at the cane handle warrant further attention. These features may include (1) a texture of the surface at the handle that maximizes tactile resolution, (2) a shape of the handle that maximizes surface contact with the hand, and (3) indentations in the handle for the fingertips to maximize use of their fine spatial resolution.

Data indicate that the angle at which the cane contacts the ground relative to the body is a crucial influence on balance stabilization.[15] Although it is tempting to suggest that canes should be designed in a slanted manner to maximize their potential as a balance aid, a slanted shaft must be considered cautiously. Interviews of elderly cane users revealed that 30% expressed apprehension that their canes would cause them to fall as a result of tripping or a slippery tip.[2] Designers of mobility aids must recognize that the user is constantly maneuvering around obstacles that are not present in a laboratory or clinical setting. A cane with a slanted shaft increases the surrounding area that the user needs to navigate around obstacles. Thus, even if a slanted cane leads to better balance control than a vertical cane, the amount of angle may be limited by practical concerns in the real world. After extensive training, blind individuals manage to locomote freely with a cane that is extended further outward (ie, a long cane) than with a cane held vertically, but their primary goal is to perceive and avoid obstacles with the cane, even though some additional balance control may be derived. A possible compromise is to design a cane with a hinge joint near the end of the shaft that can be locked at a specific angle. This feature may afford the additional support provided by a small slanted section of the shaft while retaining the primarily vertical orientation of the shaft. Without testing these design ideas in the laboratory as well as the real world, it is possible only to speculate on their potential.

Therapeutic Mechanisms: Central and Peripheral

The inherent limitation to obtaining additional somatosensory information through the fingers or hand is that surfaces must be within reach. Obviously, this is not always practical. Patients with balance disorders often rely on light touch of a spouse for orienting information while walking through an environment without surfaces amenable to contact. These patients frequently dislike using a cane due to the image that it projects (eg, frailty). The main message from these studies of light touch is that somatosensory cues are useful for balance control up to the limits of resolving force changes across the skin surface. The fingertips have the most precise spatial resolution of any part of the body (along with the tongue) and, as a result, enhance balance control. The key for patients with balance disorders may be to artificially enhance the somatosensory information at the feet so that balance control is improved without the constraint of additional contact of surfaces with the fingertips or hand.

The potential for long-term restitution of function balance control through the enhancement of somatosensory cues at the feet may take advantage of central reorganization of cortical maps. Merzenich and Kaas[35] have shown that the body map in the somatosensory cortex of primates is capable of extensive changes following peripheral injury. Neurons in these central maps serving the damaged finger or area of the hand previous to injury reorganize to respond to adjacent areas of the skin surface. One explanation of such reorganization is that the inhibitory inputs from injured areas are eliminated, allowing previously suppressed inputs in adjacent intact regions to emerge as new receptive fields.[36,37] The time scale of reorganization is far more rapid than previously thought, on the order of hours after lesioning.[38]

Even without injury, however, a simple change of functional use can also result in rapid central reorganization.

For example, primates trained on a retrieval task requiring skilled use of individual digits showed expansion of representation in the primary motor cortex for the fingers, whereas wrist and forearm zones contracted. In a second task involving forearm movements, forearm representation expanded, whereas digit representation contracted.[39] These results argue that differences in the cortical map structure across individuals are the consequence of differences in the functional use of peripheral limbs and that these changes are reversible. Such findings of neural plasticity based on functional use are being applied to rehabilitate motor and sensory function in patients with cerebrovascular accidents of the somatosensory cortex.[40] The therapy emphasizes tools that enhance sensory appreciation during retraining of tasks involving tactile form recognition and exploration. A similar approach may be feasible to enhance somatosensory input from the feet and ankles in elderly individuals and in persons with poor balance control.

The flip side of the message from these cortical reorganization studies emphasizes that central factors can potentially worsen a sensory deficit that begins as a peripheral problem. A person with early signs of peripheral neuropathy, for example, may decrease the reliance on a peripheral limb for everyday function. Such disuse could potentially trigger cortical reorganization that may hasten further deterioration of somatosensory function in the limb. Even though the time scale of cortical reorganization with a disease such as diabetic peripheral neuropathy may be slower than that of an acute injury such as a stroke, therapies designed to intervene at the first signs of peripheral deterioration may be most prudent.

Directions for Future Research

Studies of upright stance control in humans and animals have revealed that the postural control system reconfigures with changing sensory input. Nashner and Berthoz[41] demonstrated that initial muscle activation responses to a stabilized (ie, sway-referenced) visual surround were smaller in magnitude than with normal visual feedback. With successive trials, however, muscle activity regained levels equivalent to those with normal visual feedback, indicating that somatosensory and vestibular information were reweighted once subjects deemed visual information to be unreliable. Such reweighting is often characterized in terms of system gain.

Maioli and Poppele[42] studied the changes in functional limb length and limb orientation of standing cats to varying frequencies of tilted support-surface translations. They found that the ratio of the percentage of change in limb length to table tilt position remained constant (gain of about 1, in phase) to varying frequencies of support-surface translations. The authors suggested that input from an internal model of body orientation and dynamics adapts to the system's functional goals by selectively increasing gain.

Recent evidence has also shown adaptive increases in gain to a moving visual stimulus. Dijkstra et al[43] demonstrated that postural sway closely matched the amplitude of the visual motion even as distance to the visual display was varied. Quantitative modeling revealed that not only coupling strength to visual input but also the autonomous nonvisual component of the postural control system changed.[44] Using similar techniques, potential adaptive effects were observed when subjects used light touch contact of a moving surface,[45,46] illustrating that somatosensory information can drive postural sway similarly to full-field visual stimulation.

These studies suggest that the organizational scheme for upright posture is clearly not a fixed control system on which sensory information is imposed. Instead, the change in the underlying control system is not only based on a change in sensory information but also includes a change in the control system properties that are independent of the sensory stimuli.[47] Put most simply, these studies indicate that the sensitivity to a sensory stimulus can be selectively increased. The underlying mechanisms of adaptation in postural control are not well understood, particularly in patient populations and elderly individuals. For example, studies have shown that elderly individuals use inflexible postural control "strategies" that suggest a relatively fixed (nonadaptive) control system.[48] Can the inherently adaptive capability of the postural control system be used to develop better therapies? Can we rehabilitate individuals by artificially enhancing, for example, the sensitivity to somatosensation when vestibular information has been lost? Future studies should address this question if new rehabilitative techniques are to be developed.

Studies of light touch contact with a cane beg the question of whether these findings are applicable to dynamic balance activities such as cane use during ambulation. Some studies[5-8] have implemented force-sensitive canes to assess their aid to locomotion, but these studies recorded only the vertical direction of cane force and focused primarily on mean absolute levels of cane force. The results of the study by Murray et al[8] described earlier suggest that there is much more to using a cane than simple mechanical support, particularly across different patient populations. Their results, however, are primarily descriptive and provide no insight into the mechanisms or properties of cane use that lead to more stable locomotion (or more comfort as reported by the patients in their study). Therein lies a huge problem that remains to be solved. With so many interacting components, how does one characterize overall locomotor stability? The present results[13–15] (as well as those of Murray et al[8]) suggest that temporal relationships between limb/body movements and sensory input provide information that is crucial for investigations of human upright stance control. Temporal measures have been used to characterize stability of gait, such as cycle-to-cycle relative phase.[10] These measures require numerous cycles to estimate variability adequately and are often studied on a treadmill, where the relationship to overground locomotion remains speculative. Despite their difficulties, investigations of the coupling between sensory information and locomotory patterns have begun.[49]

In summary, a series of studies on postural control with light touch contact of the fingertip have demonstrated that somatosensory cues are a powerful orientation reference for improved control of upright stance. The movement of contact forces across the skin surface of remote extremities provides orientation cues about movement of the body and signals muscular activation for corrections of body sway. Small applied forces are not capable of physically moving the body, but they still provide information about body orientation relative to the surfaces on which we stand, lean, and touch. The improvement in balance control observed with a mobility aid such as a cane is often attributed to the cane acting as "third leg," with the concomitant widening of the base of support. Data suggest that in cases of a sensory deficit, improved balance control arises from the precise cues about body sway provided by somatosensory information from the fingertips and hand. The "third leg" is uniquely different from the real legs. It has the high resolution of the fingertip to detect force changes related to body sway, resulting in postural corrections well before the boundaries of upright stability are reached.

Whether individuals with balance problems actually use light touch with any regularity remains an open issue. Unfortunately, there is no evidence of patients spontaneously adopting a light touch strategy in the clinical environment. Personal communications with numerous physicians over the last few years, however, have led me to believe that light touch contact is often used for balance control. Reports of patients lightly touching their spouse's shoulder or arm during ambulation are common. The meaning of such an observation is difficult to assess because the actual force applied by the patient is never measured. One can, however, imagine situations in which it would be advantageous to use light touch contact rather than physical support of the body frame for balance control. For example, when using a railing for support while walking down a stairway, the more force that a person applies with the hand, the more frictional shear forces the person must overcome to move forward. A person may hold and release the railing with each step. With light touch contact, however, the frictional forces are so small that continuous contact is possible without inhibiting forward progress. The continuity of contact may result in a potentially safer strategy (ie, fewer falls). Even individuals without balance impairments experience advantages from light touch contact. When entering a dark room or corridor to search for a light switch, we often use light contact of furniture or objects to maintain balance when visual information is denied. Such observations remain speculative, however, until the actual use of light touch contact is studied in more detail and across a wider range of situations.

Acknowledgment

The valuable comments of Lisa DePasquale, PT, are gratefully acknowledged.

References

1 Shoup TE, Fletcher LS, Merrill BR. Biomechanics of crutch locomotion. *J Biomech*. 1974;7:11–19.

2 Dean E, Ross J. Relationships among cane fitting, function, and falls. *Phys Ther*. 1993;73:494–500.

3 Joyce BM, Kirby RL. Canes, crutches, and walkers. *Am Fam Physician*. 1991;43:535–542.

4 Milczarek JJ, Kirby RL, Harrison ER, MacLeod DA. Standard and four-footed canes: their effect on the standing balance of patients with hemiparesis. *Arch Phys Med Rehabil*. 1993;74:281–285.

5 Baxter ML, Allington RO, Koepke GH. Weight-distribution variables in the use of crutches and canes. *Phys Ther*. 1969;49:360–365.

6 Bennett L, Murray MP, Murphy EF, Sowell TT. Locomotion assistance through cane impulse. *Bull Prosthet Res*. 1979;10–31:37–47.

7 Robinson HS. Cane for measurement and recording of stress. *Arch Phys Med Rehabil*. 1969;50:457–459.

8 Murray MP, Seireg AH, Scholz RC. A survey of the time, magnitude, and orientation of forces applied to walking sticks by disabled men. *Am J Phys Med*. 1969;18:1–13.

9 Engel J, Amir A, Messer E, Caspi I. Walking cane designed to assist partial weight bearing. *Arch Phys Med Rehabil*. 1983;64:386–388.

10 Holt KG, Jeng SF, Ratcliffe R, Jamill J. Stability and the metabolic cost of human walking. In: Woollacott MH, Horak FB, eds. *Posture and Gait: Control Mechanisms*. Eugene, Ore: University of Oregon Press; 1992:392–395.

11 Pozzo T, Berthoz A, Lefort L. Head stabilization during various locomotor tasks in humans, I: normal subjects. *Exp Brain Res*. 1990;82:97–106.

12 Pozzo T, Berthoz A, Lefort L, Vitte E. Head stabilization during various locomotor tasks in humans, II: patients with bilateral peripheral vestibular deficits. *Exp Brain Res*. 1991;85:208–217.

13 Jeka JJ, Lackner JR. Fingertip contact influences human postural control. *Exp Brain Res*. 1994;100:495–502.

14 Jeka JJ, Lackner JR. The role of haptic cues from rough and slippery surfaces in human postural control. *Exp Brain Res*. 1995;103:267–276.

15 Jeka JJ, Easton RD, Bentzen BL, Lackner JR. Haptic cues for postural control in sighted and blind individuals. *Perception and Psychophysics*. 1996;58:409–423.

16 Holden M, Ventura J, Lackner JR. Stabilization of posture by precision contact of the index finger. *J Vestib Res.* 1994;4:285–301.

17 Winter DA, Patla AE, Frank JS. Assessment of balance control in humans. *Med Prog Technol.* 1990;16:31–51.

18 Johansson RS. How is grasping modified by somatosensory input? In: Humphrey DR, Freund H-J, eds. *Motor Control: Concepts and Issues.* New York, NY: John Wiley & Sons Inc; 1991:331–355.

19 Johnson KO, Hsiao SS. Neural mechanisms of tactual form and texture perception. *Annu Rev Neurosci.* 1992;15:227–250.

20 Burgess PR, Wei JY, Clark FJ, Simon J. Signaling of kinesthetic information by peripheral sensory receptors. *Annu Rev Neurosci.* 1982;5:171–187.

21 Matthews PBC. Proprioceptors and their contribution to somatosensory mapping: complex messages require complex processing. *Can J Physiol Pharmacol.* 1988;66:430–438.

22 Horak FB. Role of the vestibular system in postural control. In: Herdman SJ, ed. *Vestibular Rehabilitation.* Philadelphia, Pa: FA Davis Co; 1994:22–46.

23 Easton RD. Inherent problems of attempts to apply sonar and vibrotactile sensory aid technology to the perceptual needs of the blind. *Optom Vis Sci.* 1992;69:3–14.

24 Pick HL. Visual coding of non-visual spatial information. In: MacLeod RB, Pick HL, eds. *Perception: Essays in Honor of James J Gibson.* Ithaca, NY: Cornell University Press; 1974:153–165.

25 Rieser J, Guth D, Hill E. Mental processes mediating independent travel: implications for orientation and mobility. *Journal of Visual Impairment and Blindness.* 1982;76:213–218.

26 Rieser J, Guth D, Hill E. Sensitivity to perspective structure while walking without vision. *Perception.* 1986;15:173–188.

27 Blasch BB, Del'Aune WR. A computer profile of mobility coverage and a safety index. *Journal of Visual Impairment and Blindness.* 1992;86:249–254.

28 Farmer LW. Mobility devices. In: Welsh RL, Blasch BB, eds. *Foundations of Orientation and Mobility.* New York, NY: American Foundation for the Blind; 1980:357–412.

29 Winter DA, Prince F, Stergiou P, Powell C. Medial-lateral and anterior-posterior motor responses associated with centre of pressure changes in quiet standing. *Neuroscience Research Communications.* 1993;12:141–148.

30 Phillips CG. *Movements of the Hand.* Liverpool, United Kingdom: Liverpool University Press; 1986.

31 Sherrick CE, Cholewiak RW. Cutaneous sensitivity. In: Boff KR, Kaufman L, Thomas JP, eds. *Handbook of Perception and Human Performance.* New York, NY: John Wiley & Sons Inc; 1986:12–24.

32 Srinivasan MA, Whitehouse JM, LaMotte RH. Tactile detection of slip: surface microgeometry and peripheral neural codes. *J Neurophysiol.* 1990;63:1323–1332.

33 Matthews PBC. Evolving views on the internal operation and functional role of the muscle spindle. *J Physiol (Lond).* 1981;320:1–30.

34 Lackner JR. Some proprioceptive influences on the perceptual representation of body shape and orientation. *Brain.* 1988;111:281–297.

35 Merzenich MM, Kaas HH. Reorganization of mammalian somatosensory cortex following peripheral nerve injury. *Trends Neurosci.* 1982;5:434–436.

36 Dykes RW. Central consequences of peripheral nerve injuries. *Ann Plast Surg.* 1984;13:412–422.

37 Jacobs KM, Donoghue JP. Reshaping the cortical motor map by unmasking latent intracortical connections. *Science.* 1991;251:944–947.

38 Donoghue JP, Suner S, Sanes JN. Dynamic organization of primary motor cortex output to target muscles in adult rats, II: rapid reorganization following motor nerve lesions. *Exp Brain Res.* 1990;79:492–503.

39 Nudo RJ, Milliken GW, Jenkins WM, Merzenich MM. Use-dependent alterations of movement representations in primary motor cortex of adult squirrel monkeys. *J Neurosci.* 1996;16:785–807.

40 Dannenbaum RM, Dykes RW. Sensory loss in the hand after sensory stroke: therapeutic rationale. *Arch Phys Med Rehabil.* 1988;69:833–839.

41 Nashner L, Berthoz A. Visual contribution to rapid motor responses during postural control. *Brain Res.* 1978;150:403–407.

42 Maioli C, Poppele RE. Parallel processing of multisensory information concerning self-motion. *Exp Brain Res.* 1991;87:119–125.

43 Dijkstra TMH, Schöner G, Gielen CCAM. Temporal stability of the action-perception cycle for postural control in a moving visual environment. *Exp Brain Res.* 1994;97:477–486.

44 Giese MA, Dijkstra TMH, Schöner G, Gielen CCAM. Identification of the nonlinear state space dynamics of the action-perception cycle for visually induced postural sway. *Biol Cybern.* 1996;74:427–437.

45 Jeka JJ, Schöner G, Lackner JR. Entrainment of postural sway to sinusoidal haptic cues. *Society for Neuroscience Abstracts.* 1994;20:336.

46 Jeka JJ, Schöner G, Dijkstra TMH, et al. Coupling of fingertip somatosensory information to head and body sway. *Exp Brain Res.* In press.

47 Schöner G. Dynamic theory of action-perception patterns: the time-before-contact paradigm. *Human Movement Science.* 1994;13:415–439.

48 Horak FB, Mirka A, Shupert CL. The role of peripheral vestibular disorders in postural dyscontrol in the elderly. In: Woollacott MH, Shumway-Cook A, eds. *Development of Posture and Gait Across the Life Span.* Columbia, SC: University of South Carolina Press; 1989:253–279.

49 Warren WH, Kay BA, Yilmaz EH. Visual control of posture during walking: functional specificity. *J Exp Psychol Hum Percept Perform.* 1996;22:818–838.

Special Series

The Role of Limb Movements in Maintaining Upright Stance: The "Change-in-Support" Strategy

Change-in-support strategies, involving stepping or grasping movements of the limbs, are prevalent reactions to instability and appear to play a more important functional role in maintaining upright stance than has generally been appreciated. Contrary to traditional views, change-in-support reactions are not just strategies of last resort, but are often initiated well before the center of mass is near the stability limits of the base of support. Furthermore, it appears that subjects, when given the option, will select these reactions in preference to the fixed-support "hip strategy" that has been purported to be of functional importance. The rapid speed of compensatory change-in-support reactions distinguishes them from "volitional" arm and leg movements. In addition, compensatory stepping reactions often lack the anticipatory control elements that are invariably present in non-compensatory stepping, such as gait initiation. Even when present, these anticipatory adjustments appear to have little functional value during rapid compensatory movements. Lateral destabilization complicates the control of compensatory stepping, a finding that may be particularly relevant to the problem of falls and hip fractures in elderly people. Older adults appear to have problems in controlling lateral stability when stepping to recover balance, even when responding to anteroposterior perturbation. Increased understanding and awareness of change-in-support reactions should lead to development of new diagnostic and therapeutic approaches for detecting and treating specific causes of imbalance and falling in elderly people and in patients with balance impairments. [Maki BE, McIlroy WE. The role of limb movements in maintaining upright stance: the "change-in-support" strategy. *Phys Ther.* 1997;77:488–507.]

Key Words: *Balance, Grasping, Postural control, Stepping.*

Brian E Maki

William E McIlroy

The age-related or pathologic changes within the neuromusculoskeletal system can lead to balance impairments that can have a tremendous impact on health care costs and quality of life. Hip fractures and other acute injuries that result from falls in elderly people, as well as the fear of falling, loss of independence, and other psychosocial consequences of falls, constitute a major health care problem.[1-3] Similarly, difficulty in controlling balance and movement can be a consequence of vestibular disorders or neurologic lesions due, for example, to Parkinson's disease or stroke.[4,5] Identifying causes of instability and developing improved methods for diagnosing and treating individuals with compromised balance can provide an important opportunity to reduce health care costs and improve independence and quality of life.

Maintenance of upright stance requires the center of mass (COM) of the body to be positioned over the base of support (BOS). The body is inherently unstable, however, due to the force of gravity, and additional destabilizing forces arise due to movement of the body and interaction with the environment. The ability to regulate the relationship between the COM and BOS during activities of daily life results from a combination of reactive (compensatory) and predictive (anticipatory) balance control strategies. Whereas predictive control can serve to minimize the destabilizing effect of predictable disturbances due, for example, to volitional movement, reactive control is the only recourse in the event of unexpected perturbation; hence, reactive control is likely to be of paramount importance in allowing stability to be maintained in the unpredictable circumstances of daily life.

There appear to be two distinct classes of strategies for reactive balance recovery, which we refer to as (1) "fixed-support" strategies and (2) "change-in-support" strategies. These two classes of strategies are distinguished by the absence or presence of limb movement to alter the BOS. The vast majority of studies have focused on the fixed-support strategies, which reflect the ability to control the movement of the COM over an unchanging BOS defined by the feet (and, in some instances, by the hands). In these studies, movement of the arms or legs has usually been restrained either explicitly (eg, by instruction) or implicitly (eg, by lack of space to step or handholds to grasp). In contrast, the more recent work that is the subject of this article has featured the change-in-support strategy, highlighted by movements of the lower or upper limbs to make new contact with support surfaces. Figure 1 presents examples of fixed-support and change-in-support balance recovery strategies.

Until recently, it was widely believed that the change-in-support strategies were only mechanisms of last resort (eg, reports that stepping occurs when fixed-support strategies have failed[6-9]). Change-in-support strategies actually appear to be very prevalent and can occur very rapidly after the onset of postural disturbances. Experimentally, these compensatory limb movements have been shown to be common reactions to externally applied postural perturbation, even when the distur-

---

BE Maki, PhD, PEng, is Senior Scientist, Sunnybrook Health Science Centre, and Associate Professor, University of Toronto. Address all correspondence to Dr Maki at Centre for Studies in Aging, Sunnybrook Health Science Centre, 2075 Bayview Ave, Toronto, Ontario, Canada M4N 3M5 (maki@srcl.sunnybrook.utoronto.ca).

WE McIlroy, PhD, is Scientist, Sunnybrook Health Science Centre, and Assistant Professor, University of Toronto.

This work was supported by operating grants (MT-10576 and MY-13355) from the Medical Research Council (MRC) of Canada. Dr McIlroy was supported by an MRC Fellowship.

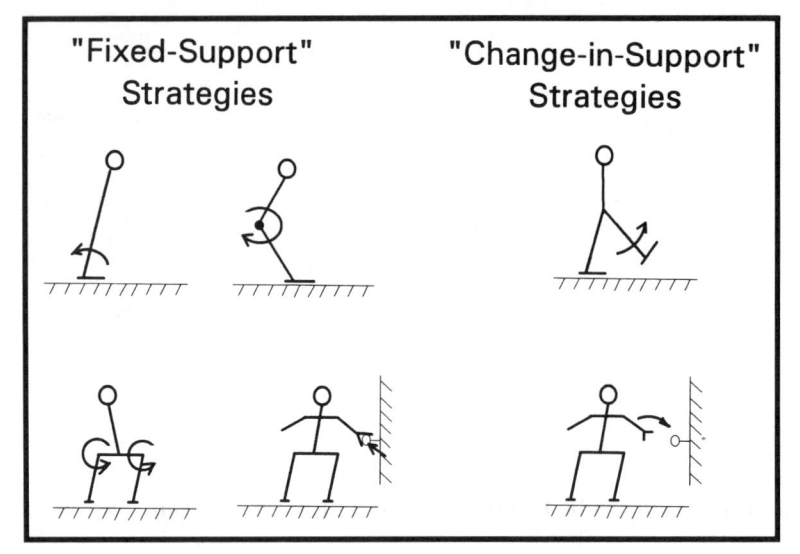

Figure 1.
Examples of fixed-support and change-in-support balance recovery strategies. Fixed-support reactions act to control the displacement of the center of mass, without alteration of the base of support. As illustrated, this may involve generating torques at the ankle or knee or exerting force on a handhold. Change-in-support reactions involve stepping or grasping movements, which serve to alter the base of support.

bances are small and stability could have been maintained without moving the arms or legs.[10–15] Furthermore, outside of the laboratory, video surveillance studies of falling incidents in geriatric health care facilities have shown that compensatory limb movements are very common reactions to loss of balance in daily life, with compensatory stepping evident in 32% to 45% of falls or near-falls and arm movements evident in 65% to 72% of these incidents.[16,17]

Although change-in-support reactions can, and do, occur even when disturbances are small, they are the only reactions that can successfully be used to maintain balance in the face of large perturbations. Fixed-support reactions may be important in providing an early defense against loss of balance; however, change-in-support reactions ultimately have, in at least two ways, the potential to make a much larger contribution to stabilization. First, in increasing the size of the BOS, the range of COM displacement that can be accommodated without loss of stability can be increased dramatically. Second, in increasing the "moment arm" between the point of action of the foot- or hand-contact force and the COM, the stabilizing moments induced by the contact force, which act to decelerate the COM, can be greatly amplified. Ability to decelerate the COM may be further enhanced by the fact that grasping reactions can serve to "anchor" the body relative to the location of the handhold.

If, as it appears, change-in-support reactions are fundamental to the control of balance and prevention of falls, then it is imperative to understand how the central nervous system (CNS) controls these reactions. Critical aspects include the spatial characteristics of the response (limb trajectory) and the timing of response initiation and execution (latency and speed), both of which must be matched to the ongoing motion of the COM and the active attempts to control this motion. Inaccurate or inappropriately timed limb movements may fail to "capture" and decelerate the COM and may even act to induce destabilizing forces and moments. In view of the potential implications for functional stability and risk of falling, it is important to understand the mechanisms by which the CNS is able to rapidly transform sensed instability into limb movements that are appropriately patterned and timed and to determine the effects of pathology, injury, and aging on the control of this process. We anticipate that such understanding will lead to the development of new diagnostic and therapeutic approaches for detecting and treating specific causes of imbalance and falling.

In the remainder of this article, we summarize the current state of knowledge with regard to the change-in-support strategies. We focus first on compensatory stepping reactions, highlighting the key characteristics: prevalence, early initiation and rapid execution, absence of functional anticipatory control, adaptive changes that can occur, and effects of lateral destabilization. This section concludes with a discussion of control mechanisms. The second section, which deals with grasping reactions, describes the similarities and differences that arise when the upper limb rather than the lower limb is used to change the base of support and examines the influence of specific task conditions (ie, sitting versus standing, light cue versus perturbation). In the third section, we examine the interactions between fixed-support and change-in-support reactions, highlighting the evidence for parallel, rather than sequential, control of the two types of reactions, the persistence of the early fixed-support "ankle strategy," and the predominance of the change-in-support reaction with respect to the fixed-support "hip strategy." In the final section, we summarize existing knowledge concerning the effects of aging and pathology on the change-in-support reactions.

Change-in-Support Movements of the Lower Limb: Stepping

Until recently, studies of step initiation have tended to focus on noncompensatory (volitional) behavior, such as gait initiation.[18–27] These responses, however, seem to show some fundamental differences when compared with the compensatory stepping reactions that are evoked by postural perturbation (see "Speed of Response" and "Anticipatory Control" sections for details).

Studies of compensatory stepping reactions are now becoming increasingly common, although almost all of these studies have examined only forward or backward responses. In several studies,[28–32] forward stepping has been evoked by suddenly releasing a cable that was supporting the subject in a forward-lean position. Forward or backward stepping has also been evoked by pulling on a cable attached to the subject's waist, by means of a motor-driven device[33] or by dropping weights attached to the cable via pulleys.[34–37] Another approach, one that we have adopted, is to perturb balance by horizontally accelerating a platform on which the subject stands (McIlroy and Maki, unpublished research).[10–13,38–46] This latter approach has the advantage of allowing the direction of perturbation to be varied in an unpredictable manner (including, in the case of multiaxis platforms, multiple planes of motion), while avoiding potential constraints on movement due to attachments to the subject. The main disadvantage of the moving-platform approach is the cost and complexity of the equipment. Some authors have also questioned the "ecologic validity" of support-surface perturbations, suggesting that the perturbations are relatively uncommon in daily life; however, the extent to which any perturbation method generalizes to control of functional stability in daily life has yet to be well established. In comparing results from different studies, readers should note that the different methods of perturbation may well evoke different patterns of joint motion and sensory drive. Results may be further affected by differences in the unpredictability of the task conditions (ie, perturbation waveform, magnitude, direction, timing) and the specific instructions given to the subject (ie, whether the subject is instructed to step, to try not to step, or is "unconstrained" by any specific instructions).

The measurement approaches that are typically used to study compensatory stepping involve perturbation of static stance. We propose that these "static" tests are relevant to functional stability in daily life for two reasons. First, a sizable proportion of falls (40%–50%) actually occur during quasi-static movements and activities.[47,48] Second, the "static" test results may also provide information that is relevant to the many falls that occur during gait,[47,49–53] because step adjustments during gait and step initiation from stance share a number of fundamental control subtasks (eg, appropriate placement of the swing foot, stabilization of the COM during swing). The multiaxis moving platform allows the control of these motor subtasks to be assessed safely, under perturbation conditions that are tightly controlled yet unpredictable to the subject, while avoiding many of the methodological difficulties of gait-perturbation studies.

Speed of Response

One of the key features that appears to distinguish compensatory stepping from noncompensatory behavior is the rapid speed of the response to instability. This difference occurs when behavior is unconstrained, but it is also evident when the perturbation-evoked response is clearly volitional.[12,39,44] In one of our studies,[39] subjects were given prior instructions to step as rapidly as possible in response to either visual cueing (as in gait initiation studies) or onset of platform motion. The results showed, for both forward and backward stepping, that instability, due to platform motion, elicits a much more rapid response, marked by a twofold (450-millisecond) reduction in the duration, as well as a 100-millisecond reduction in latency. In a similar study, Burleigh et al[44] also found very rapid response initiation (150 milliseconds from perturbation onset to start of lateral "weight shift"), with a 50-millisecond delay occurring when a proprioceptive cue was used, instead of platform motion, to elicit a rapid forward step. Although the perturbations used in these studies may passively induce a more rapid motion of the body in the anteroposterior direction, it is important to recognize that the more rapid initiation and execution of swing-leg unloading, which involves *lateral* weight transfer, must be the result of a more rapid active response.

The timing of the perturbation-evoked stepping response appears to be equally, if not more, rapid in early trials, in which subjects are free to respond "naturally" (no specific instructions), as compared with trials in which subjects are instructed to step as quickly as possible.[12,13] Response initiation is also very rapid, in most subjects, even when they are instructed to try not to step, although some subjects are able to delay the onset of swing-leg unloading under this task condition.[12] Delay of response initiation tends to occur more commonly during forward, rather than backward, stepping and appears to be associated with the ability to balance "on the toes." Even when response onset is delayed, however, the speed at which the swing leg is unloaded and moved tends to be extremely fast during compensatory stepping.[41] Data illustrating the effects of the different task conditions on the speed of the stepping response are summarized in the Table, and representative responses are shown in Figure 2.

Anticipatory Control

A second, fundamental way in which compensatory and noncompensatory stepping behaviors differ pertains to the presence or absence of an "anticipatory postural adjustment" (APA) prior to the lifting of the swing leg. For unperturbed stance, movements that involve raising

Table.
Temporal Characteristics of Compensatory and Noncompensatory Stepping Responses: Mean±Standard Deviation (Range)

Measure[a]	Task Condition[b]			
	Light-Cued (Instructed to Step as Rapidly as Possible)	Compensatory Response to Perturbation		
		Instructed to Step as Rapidly as Possible	Instructed to Try Not to Step	No Specific Instructions (Unconstrained)
Forward steps	n=26	n=20	n=18	n=23
Percentage of trials with APA	100	70	50	61
Step onset (ms)	360±106 (250–625)	216±40 (170–325)	345±135 (155–740)	232±41 (165–320)
Foot-off (ms)	778±121 (580–1,160)	376±48 (305–475)	585±130 (405–835)	409±77 (325–610)
Foot-contact (ms)	994±138 (720–1,475)	519±63 (395–620)	708±89 (515–860)	546±116 (395–830)
Preparatory duration (ms)	418±89 (250–645)	159±46 (70–265)	240±117 (85–455)	177±76 (75–390)
Swing duration (ms)	208±54 (90–315)	141±34 (60–190)	165±53 (100–260)	141±69 (30–240)
Backward steps	n=26	n=21	n=22	n=25
Percentage of trials with APA	100	81	41	48
Step onset (ms)	359±118 (215–725)	203±29 (155–250)	305±92 (220–590)	220±47 (165–365)
Foot-off (ms)	714±140 (515–1,110)	361±70 (270–495)	499±204 (340–1,200)	368±85 (265–555)
Foot-contact (ms)	931±172 (705–1,460)	524±77 (375–650)	643±230 (450–1,470)	501±105 (385–740)
Preparatory duration (ms)	356±74 (250–555)	159±66 (65–275)	194±154 (65–730)	149±63 (65–315)
Swing duration (ms)	217±68 (110–430)	169±47 (105–265)	145±50 (30–270)	129±42 (50–215)

[a] Onset of stepping response defined by onset of mediolateral center-of-pressure (COP) excursion (>4 mm, or approximately 1% of stance width); anticipatory postural adjustment (APA) present if the initial COP excursion was toward the swing leg; foot-off and foot-contact defined by vertical load <1% of body weight (in eight trials in which the foot did not land on the force plates, the foot-contact time was estimated from the onset of the sudden decrease in loading of the stance leg); preparatory duration=time from response onset to foot-off, swing duration=time from foot-off to foot-contact; response onset, foot-off, and foot-contact defined with respect to onset of platform acceleration (0.1 m/s^2) or light cue.

[b] The "try not to step" data were collected from 10 young adults in a study involving multiaxis platform perturbations.[41] All other data were collected from 5 young adults in protocols that were restricted to forward and backward platform translation (McIlroy and Maki, unpublished research).[42] In tasks involving instructions to step, subjects were asked to step to markings placed on the floor to ensure that the anteroposterior step length was similar to that observed, on average, in the other tasks (ie, 30–40 cm for forward steps, 20–30 cm for backward steps). In all perturbation tasks, perturbation direction was varied unpredictably (step direction was also varied unpredictably, in the light-cued trials). Perturbation magnitude was also varied unpredictably, except in the unconstrained task. The tabulated data correspond to perturbations of moderate magnitude (duration=0.6 s, acceleration=1.5 and 2.0 m/s^2, velocity=0.45 and 0.6 m/s, and displacement=0.14 and 0.18 m for forward and backward translations, respectively).

a leg invariably include a mediolateral (ML) APA. This anticipatory postural behavior appears as an initial increase in vertical loading of the swing foot (and ML displacement of the center of pressure toward the swing leg) prior to unloading and lifting of the foot (Fig. 2A). The ML APA acts to move the center of mass toward the stance limb and presumably serves to promote stability by reducing the tendency of the COM to fall toward the unsupported side during the subsequent foot movement.[18,27] This anticipatory postural behavior has been shown to occur, without exception, in studies involving leg abduction,[54] leg flexion,[55–57] and gait initiation.[18–20,23–25,27] Importantly, such anticipatory postural behavior is often absent during compensatory stepping in response to perturbation.[13,38] The absence of the anticipatory phase appears to be related to the absence of preplanning for compensatory stepping (ie, the ML APA is most likely to be absent in early trials, when the perturbation is unfamiliar, or in trials in which subjects are not given specific instructions to step).[13,33,38,42] Conversely, ML APAs occur most consistently when subjects are given prior instructions to step (Table).[38,39,44,45]

Inclusion of an anticipatory phase delays the lifting and placement of the swing foot by about 100 milliseconds during rapid compensatory stepping.[13] Such a delay could seriously jeopardize stability, which may explain why the ML APA tends to be absent when the perturbation is unfamiliar. Curiously, however, in view of this apparent "cost," the inclusion of the ML APA during rapid compensatory responses seems to provide little functional benefit. The ML APAs that occur appear to be either too small or too brief to have any impact on the COM dynamics, as evidenced by the lack of any measurable effect on the lateral displacement, velocity, or acceleration of the COM, either at foot-off or at foot-contact (Fig. 2B) (McIlroy and Maki, unpublished research). In this respect, it appears that the ML APA may be a "vestigial" feature of attempts to utilize the same motor programs associated with volitional stepping. Possibly, the anticipatory phase is truncated, and consequently rendered nonfunctional, as a result of the anteroposterior instability induced by the perturbation, which must drive a more rapid initiation of the unloading and swing phases of the step in order to safeguard stability. The idea that the time course of the reaction to instability defines the extent to which the anticipatory

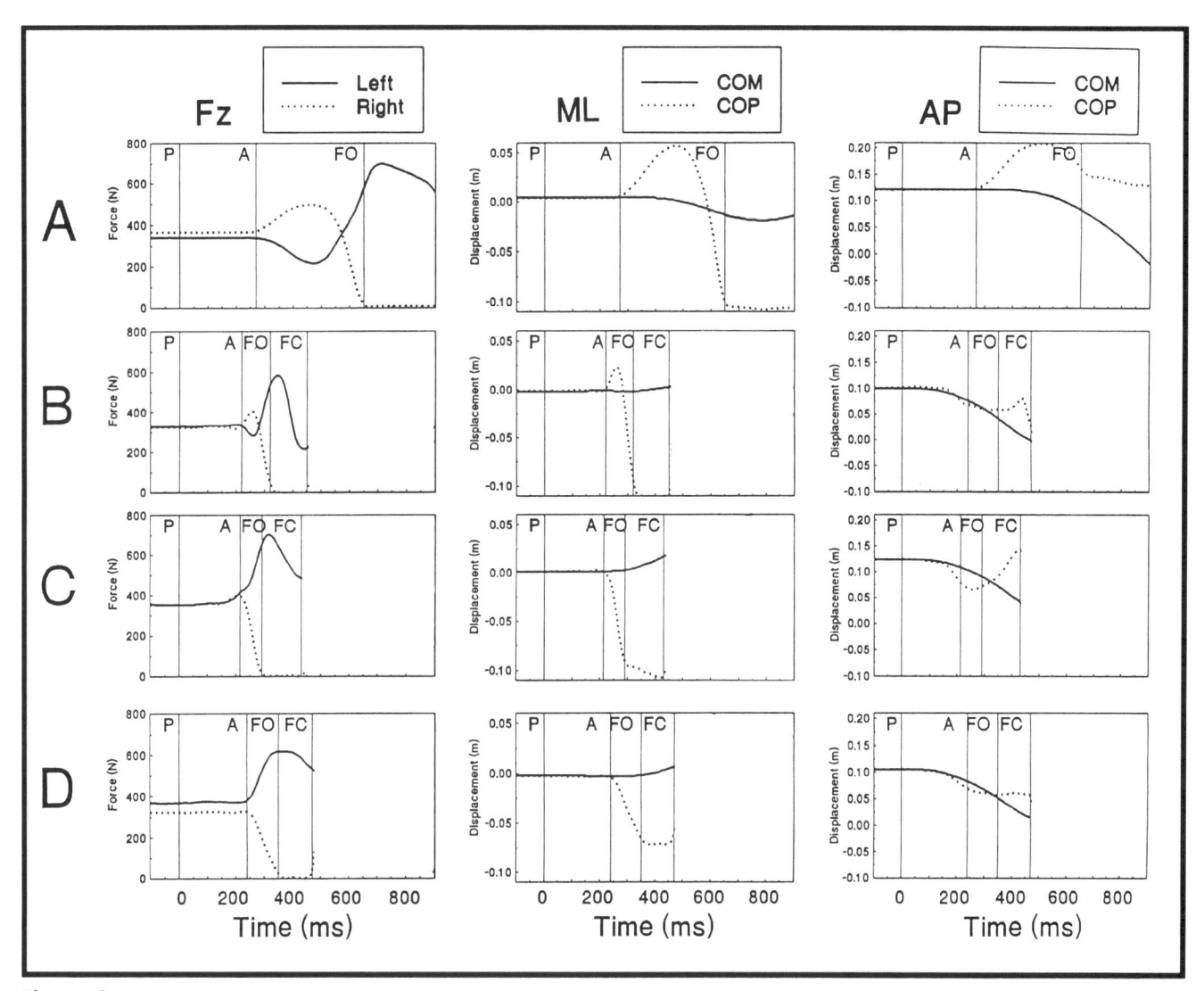

Figure 2.
Effect of task conditions on stepping. Representative backward-step responses of young adults without balance impairments are shown for (A) light-cued "volitional" stepping, (B) perturbation-cued volitional stepping, (C) unconstrained perturbation-evoked compensatory stepping, and (D) constrained perturbation-evoked compensatory stepping. In Figs. 2A and 2B, subjects were instructed to step as rapidly as possible in response to the cue (activation of a light or onset of platform motion) (McIlroy and Maki, unpublished research). Fig. 2C represents an early trial in which the subject was given no specific instructions.[42] In Fig. 2D, the subject was instructed to try not to step.[41] For each trial, the vertical ground reaction forces (Fz) and the mediolateral (ML) and anteroposterior (AP) center of mass (COM) and center of pressure (COP) are shown up to the point of foot-contact (forward AP and rightward ML displacements are positive; subjects stepped with the right lower extremity in each trial shown). Symbols P, A, FO, and FC indicate onset of perturbation (or cue), initiation of the stepping response (onset of asymmetry in Fz), foot-off, and foot-contact, respectively (in Fig. 2A, foot-contact occurred at 1,050 ms, beyond the range of the time axis). Similar moderately large platform motion was used in all perturbation trials (acceleration=1.5 m/s^2, velocity=0.5 m/s, displacement=0.14 m, duration=0.6 s). Perturbation leads to a much more rapid response, regardless of the instruction, when compared with light-cued stepping. Note the large anticipatory postural adjustment (APA) (initial increase in swing-limb Fz, initial COP displacement toward the swing limb) and the associated ML movement of the COM toward the stance limb in the light-cued task, and the absence of these features in the perturbation responses (Fig. 2B shows a very small APA but no concomitant effect on the ML COM displacement).

phase can be expressed is consistent with observations that the duration of the ML APA increases with decreasing magnitude of perturbation (McIlroy and Maki, unpublished research)[45] and that large ML APAs are seen during stepping responses to very small perturbations.[44,45] Smaller perturbations would require less rapid stepping behavior, thereby allowing an ML APA to be expressed more fully. The ML APA is more likely to be important during slower movements because the COM has greater opportunity to fall laterally as the duration of the swing phase increases.

Adaptive Changes

It appears, from our studies of unconstrained compensatory stepping reactions, that the ML APA is almost always absent when the perturbation is first presented (ie, when the perturbation is novel), but tends to appear more frequently as the subject is given an opportunity to

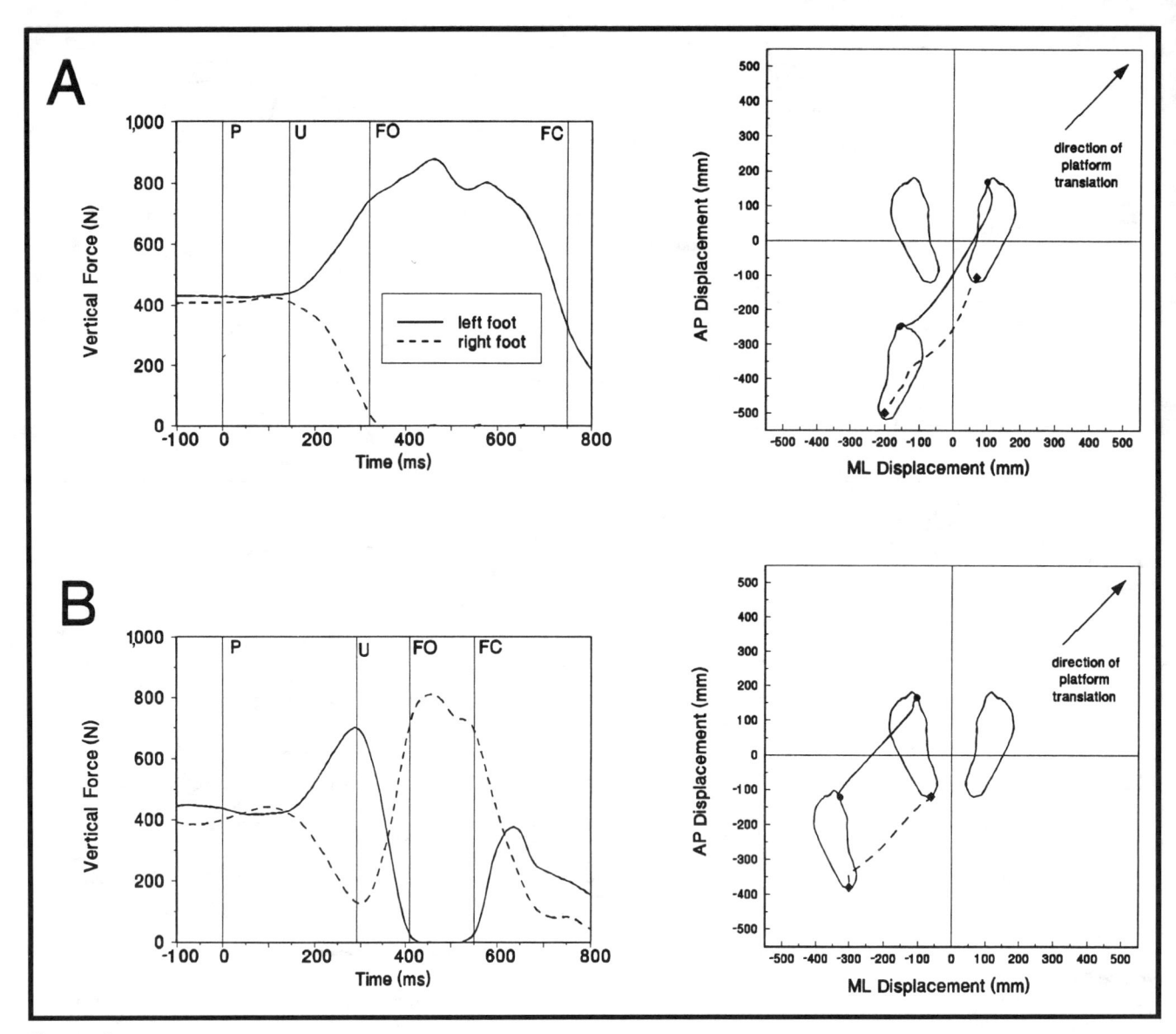

Figure 3.
Effect of lateral destabilization on compensatory stepping. In this study,[41] anteroposterior (AP), mediolateral (ML), and "oblique" perturbations of varying magnitude were presented in random order, and subjects were instructed to try not to step. Example responses from one subject are shown, illustrating the interactions between perturbation-induced loading, swing-limb selection, and swing-foot trajectory. Vertical ground reaction forces and swing-foot trajectory are shown for responses where the swing limb was (A) the perturbation-unloaded (right) leg ("cross-over step") and (B) the perturbation-loaded (left) leg ("side step"). In both trials, the platform moved forward and to the right, as indicated in the figure (acceleration= 2.6 m/s^2, velocity=0.78 m/s, displacement=0.23 m, duration=0.6 s). Symbols P, U, FO, and FC indicate onset of platform acceleration, unloading of the swing limb, foot-off, and foot-contact, respectively. Note the earlier onset of swing-limb unloading and foot-off in Fig. 3A. In Fig. 3B, unloading and foot-off are delayed until the perturbation-induced loading can be countered and reversed. The longer swing duration (FO to FC) in Fig. 3A is associated with a longer and more complex swing trajectory (the foot must cross behind the stance limb).

practice the response and to gain familiarity with the characteristics of the perturbation.[13,38] In addition, over repeated perturbation trials, subjects tend to step less frequently, and to take fewer and smaller steps when they do step, even when perturbation direction is unpredictable.[10,13] Furthermore, in a study involving multiaxis perturbations, subjects who were instructed to avoid stepping were able to reduce their frequency of stepping by 50% when perturbation direction was precued.[41] Unpracticed responses to unpredictable disturbances are likely to be most relevant to the prevention of falls because daily life rarely presents an opportunity to become familiar with the characteristics of a specific perturbation or to adapt one's response. Attempts to use clinical or experimental assessments of compensatory stepping to draw inferences about the ability of the individual to respond to unexpected perturbations in daily life could well be confounded by the adaptive changes that occur during repeated testing, and intersubject differences recorded under such conditions could well be due, in whole or in part, to differences in predictive, rather than reactive, capabilities. To minimize the potential for adaptation, we believe that test conditions should be as unpredictable as possible.

Influence of Lateral Destabilization

Almost all studies of compensatory step initiation have been limited to the forward and backward stepping that occurs in response to anteroposterior perturbation. In everyday life, perturbations can occur in an unlimited number of directions; therefore, it becomes important to characterize stepping responses that are not limited to the sagittal plane. Although relatively little attention has been given to lateral stability, the ability to compensate for lateral destabilization is particularly relevant to the problem of falling because a large proportion of falls involve lateral motion[58] and debilitating hip fractures are most likely to occur as a result of lateral falls.[59] Observations from a video surveillance study of naturally occurring falls in elderly people[16,60] showed problems in the control of laterally directed steps in a number of lateral falls.

The introduction of a lateral component to the destabilization complicates the control of stepping, due to anatomical restrictions on ML foot movement and the effects of perturbation-induced COM displacement on the unloading of the swing leg. When subjects were discouraged from preplanning to step, the predominant strategy, seen in 87% of lateral stepping responses, was to "cross over" with the foot that was unloaded by the perturbation.[41] This strategy allowed a much more rapid foot-lift in comparison with responses where the perturbation-loaded leg was swung but required a longer and more complex swing trajectory to move the foot across (either in front of or behind) the body while circumventing the stance leg (Fig. 3). In 10% of the lateral stepping responses, the need for a long trajectory was avoided by taking multiple steps, moving the perturbation-unloaded foot medially prior to a second laterally directed step with the contralateral foot. A third strategy involved "side-stepping" with the perturbation-loaded leg. Although it took much longer (200 milliseconds, on average) to unload this leg, the swing trajectory was simpler and shorter; that is, the foot was simply moved laterally (swing duration was reduced by 240 milliseconds, and step length was reduced by 9 cm). The "side-step" strategy may be dependent on preplanning. Although this strategy occurred in only 3% of constrained ("try not to step") lateral-step responses, the prevalence increased to 43% when subjects performed repeated trials in the absence of instructional constraints (Maki et al, unpublished research).

Control Mechanisms

Very little is known about how compensatory stepping reactions are controlled by the CNS. It may be that the underlying sequences of muscle activation are established by the same central pattern generators that are thought to be involved in the control of gait, whereas the initiation and amplitude scaling of the response may involve transcortical or subcortical pathways similar to those that are thought to be involved in the control of the early fixed-support postural responses. Although some authors have suggested that elements of the stepping response are "released" as predefined motor programs (based on studies of gait initiation[19-22] and "stumbling"[60-63]), sensory feedback would be expected to play a more critical role in controlling compensatory stepping, particularly when unpredictable task conditions preclude effective preplanning of an "open-loop" response. Observations that subjects are able to abort a stepping response prior to foot-lift clearly indicate that sensory information can be used to modify the response "on-line."[10-12]

One sensory source that has the potential to provide critical information for the control of stepping is the input from the soles of the feet regarding pressure. This afferent information may be particularly relevant to the control of swing-limb unloading, foot-lift, foot-contact, and weight transfer. Do and colleagues[30,31] reported that plantar pressure feedback plays an important role in controlling "volitional" stepping responses to forward perturbation (subjects instructed to step), based on the effects of variation in plantar support surface and anesthesia of the sole. Conversely, because there was negligible muscle stretch prior to response onset, Do et al[29] concluded that the early muscle activation associated with the step initiation was not triggered by muscle spindles. Do et al[29] also concluded that the response was not initiated by vestibular cues, based on testing of three patients with "vestibular syndrome"; however, observed effects of optokinetic stimulation would suggest that the interaction between the vestibular and visual systems can play an important role in initiating this type of stepping response.[32]

We have recently begun to examine the contribution of plantar pressure feedback to the control of unplanned compensatory stepping (subjects forced to step, in a proportion of trials, despite instructions to try not to step) using hypothermic anesthesia (cooling the feet in ice water) to attenuate plantar sensation in blindfolded subjects.[64] In the six subjects tested, cooling increased the incidence of stepping, as well as the incidence of multiple-step responses, in response to unpredictable multiaxis platform perturbation. Moreover, there appears to be a profound effect on control of lateral stepping. When the feet were cooled, the subjects

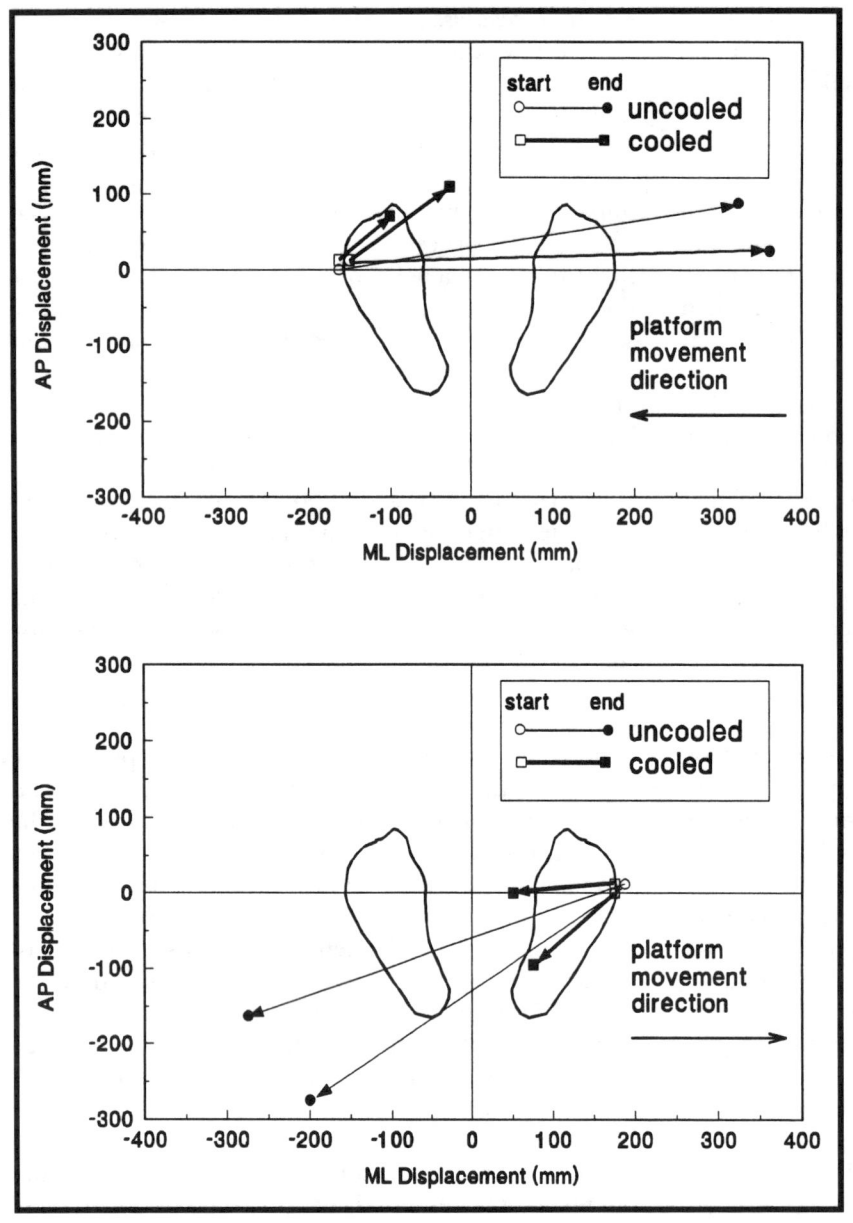

Figure 4.
Effects of attenuation of plantar sensation (due to cooling of the feet) on the placement of the initial step in response to mediolateral (ML) platform translation (acceleration=3 m/s², velocity=0.9 m/s, displacement=0.27 m, duration=0.6 s). In this study,[64] anteroposterior (AP) and ML perturbations of varying magnitude were presented in random order; subjects were blindfolded and instructed to try not to step. Initial step locations (marker on fifth metatarsal) are shown for the responses of one subject to four leftward platform translations (top panel) and four rightward translations (bottom panel). Trials where the feet were cooled are indicated by thick lines, and trials where the feet were not cooled are indicated by thin lines. Multiple small steps were taken in each cooled trial (only the first step is shown), whereas a single large "cross-over" step was used in each uncooled trial. The duration of single-limb stance was reduced by a factor of 2 in the small steps (220 ms versus 390 ms).

avoided taking large "cross-over" steps that would require a long duration of one-limb stance (Fig. 4). The implication that sensory information from the sole of the foot is critical in controlling stability during single-leg support is supported by observations that subjects are unable to balance on one leg after anesthesia of the sole (due to local injection of Xylocaine®[*]) (McIlroy et al, unpublished research).

The process by which the CNS determines the spatial and temporal step parameters is unclear, particularly because it appears that, for a given perturbation, many different combinations of step length and swing duration can achieve a stable response. We have tentatively proposed a model in which step parameters are selected to maximize the "stability margin" (ie, the distance between the COM and the boundary of the BOS), thereby maximizing the ability to decelerate the COM (Fig. 5) (Maki and Sinha, unpublished research). Studies are under way to test this model and to evaluate other possible control criteria (eg, optimizing the transfer of weight to the swing limb to facilitate subsequent stepping).

Change-in-Support Movements of the Upper Limb: Grasping

Although increasing numbers of studies are examining compensatory stepping, very few studies have addressed arm reactions resulting from instability. Arm movements can serve a protective role, to absorb impact and shield the head in the event of a fall, and can also help to stabilize the COM over a fixed BOS, through inertial effects. The focus here, however, is on grasping reactions that serve to increase external support. Control of the grasping reaction is likely to be one of the most challenging aspects of balance control, particularly when graspable surfaces are restricted in size or location. One important distinction between compensatory upper- and lower-limb reactions is the fact that the location of potential handholds can vary widely, whereas the ground (the "target" for stepping) is usually likely to remain relatively level and predictable. Because of such challenges, these arm reactions may well be more sensitive to subtle CNS changes that define an individual's ability to maintain balance.

---
[*] Astra USA Inc, 50 Otis St, Westboro, MA 01581-4500.

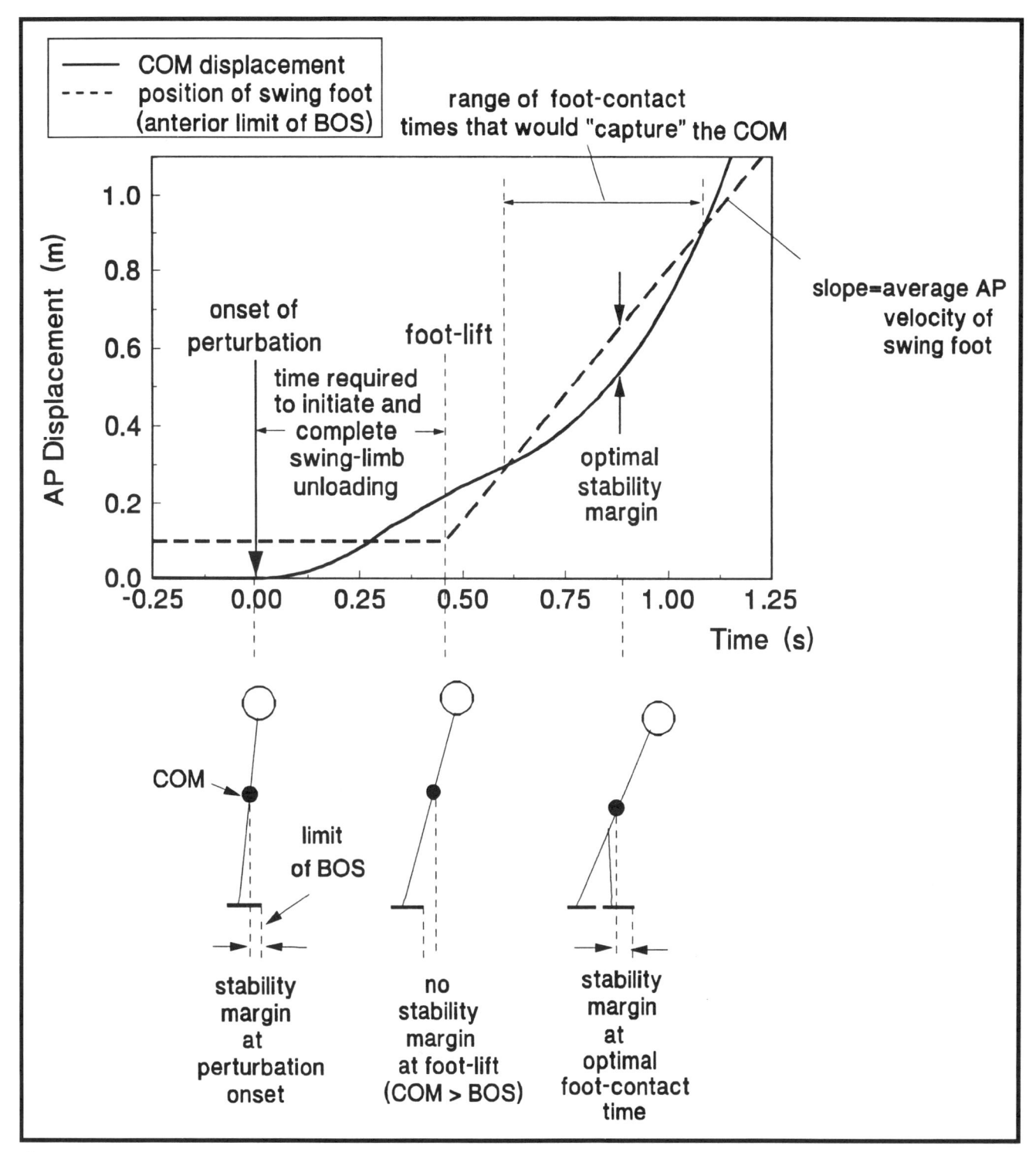

Figure 5.
Schematic representation of an optimal control model of compensatory stepping (Maki and Sinha, unpublished research). The solid line shows the anteroposterior (AP) center-of-mass (COM) displacement that would result from a large backward platform acceleration at time 0, assuming a maximal fixed-support ("ankle strategy") stabilizing response. The dashed line represents the position of the great toe of the swing foot during the forward-step response; at time of foot-contact, this point defines the anterior-most limit of the base of support (BOS). The distance between the COM and swing-foot trajectories at any given point in time (following the start of the swing phase) defines the "stability margin" that would be achieved if foot-contact occurred at that point in time. There is a finite range of foot-contact times that would allow the BOS to "capture" the COM (BOS > COM). There is also an optimal foot-contact time that maximizes the stability margin and, in doing so, allows for maximal COM deceleration.

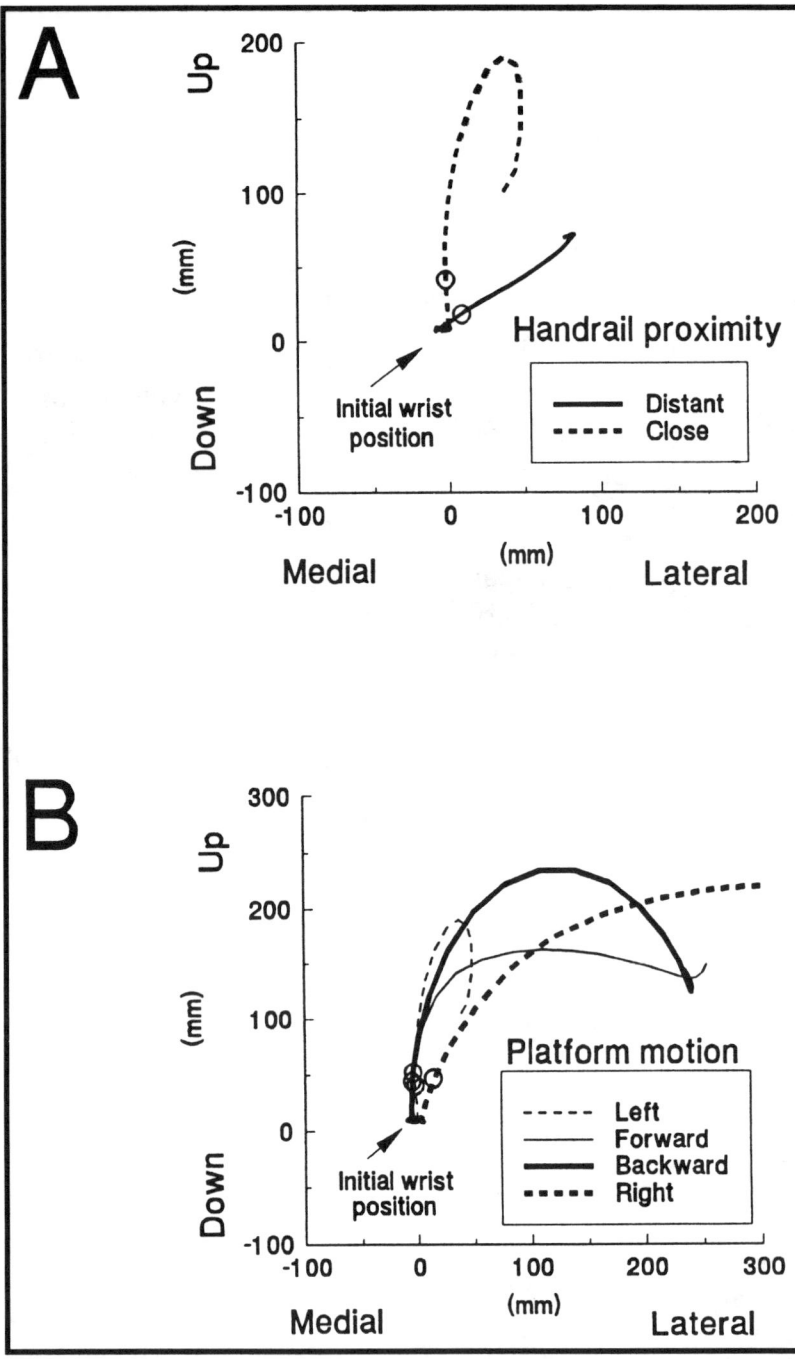

Figure 6.
Modulation of the compensatory grasping response according to (A) proximity of handrails and (B) direction of perturbation (platform translation). In this study,[14,15] anteroposterior and mediolateral perturbations of varying magnitude were presented in random order; subjects were not constrained by any specific instructions. In both panels, the first 400 ms of the wrist trajectory, relative to the shoulder, is shown in the frontal plane. Fig. 6A shows two trials where the subject grasped the rails, in response to leftward platform translation (acceleration=2.6 m/s^2, velocity=0.78 m/s, displacement=0.23 m, duration=0.6 s). Solid line=handrails distant (2 m apart), dashed line=handrails close (1 m apart). Fig. 6B shows four close-rail trials, for a single subject, where the platform moved in each of the four directions indicated (perturbation characteristics similar to those noted in Fig. 6A). The circular symbol on each trajectory indicates the point in time 150 ms after onset of perturbation. The difference in trajectory, due to change in environment or perturbation, is evident even in the earliest part of the response.

Many researchers have explored reactions of arm muscles to external loads applied to the limb itself; however, such a focus is distinctly different from balance-related arm reactions because perturbation of whole-body stability (with arms relaxed by the sides) results in complex arm responses without any prior stretch or loading of the muscles of the arms.[14,15] In addition, many investigators have studied the control of noncompensatory reaching and pointing movements of the arms, as well as the APAs associated with the execution of rapid noncompensatory arm movements. To our knowledge, we have conducted the only inquiries to date into compensatory grasping responses evoked by external perturbation of upright stance (McIlroy et al, unpublished research).[14,15]

Characteristics of Compensatory Grasping
Our initial studies[14,15] focused on arm responses to whole-body instability evoked by platform translation, both anteroposterior and ML. Handrails were located on each side of the platform, either in close proximity (1 m apart) or distant (2 m apart). Even though subjects were given no specific instructions, arm reactions were very prevalent, with activation of the shoulder muscles occurring in over 85% of trials. (Stepping occurred frequently, as well.) The prevalence of arm reactions was similarly high regardless of whether handrails were close or distant, even though subjects actually touched the rails in only 3% of distant-rail trials, in comparison with 78% of close-rail trials. Activity in the shoulder muscles began very early, 90 to 140 milliseconds after onset of perturbation, which is very similar in timing to the "automatic" (fixed-support) postural responses in the ankle muscles. Unlike the ankle muscles, however, the arm and shoulder muscles were not activated or involved in balancing prior to the perturbation nor was there any measurable motion that would have stretched or loaded the muscles prior to the onset of activation. These findings indicate that a remote sensory source was responsible for driving these responses.

The arm reaction was clearly modulated according to the characteristics of the perturbation (which were varied unpredictably), as well as of the environment. The timing and magnitude of the shoulder-muscle activation were adjusted to the perturbation magnitude, and even the earliest trajectory of the arm motion varied according to the direction of the perturbation and the location of the handrails (regardless of whether the rails were actually grasped) (Fig. 6). Furthermore, this tuning of the response was evident in the subjects' very first trial. These findings provide evidence that these reactions were not simply a generic "startle" response or the release of a stereotypical ballistic, inertial, or protective reaction. The ability of the CNS to rapidly and accurately control the trajectory of the hand to a fixed target, despite unpredictable movement of the frame of reference (ie, the shoulder), reveals the remarkable sophistication of this arm control.

Influence of Task Demands: Sitting Versus Standing

One of the potential advantages of studying arm reactions is the possibility of assessing CNS control of balance in seated subjects, which may open a number of important clinical and experimental opportunities. For example, it would be possible to test or train patients who are unable to stand (eg, patients at an early stage of recovery following a stroke) to control confounding factors such as anxiety related to fear of falling[65] and to perform measurements (eg, mapping of cortical activity) that are not as feasible in freestanding subjects. Although certain aspects of postural control are specific to whether the individual is seated or standing, we propose that the ability, or inability, of the CNS to perform the required sensorimotor transformations may well generalize across the different task conditions.

In a recent study, we compared standing and seated grasping reactions (McIlroy et al, unpublished research). Subjects either stood on a moving platform or were seated in an unstable chair that tilted slightly when the platform moved. Handrails were mounted in the same position, relative to the subjects, for each of the two tasks, and subjects were instructed to grasp the rails as rapidly as possible in response to onset of platform motion. In all trials, the arm muscles were activated very early, similar to the timing observed in our studies of unconstrained arm reactions. Moreover, the timing, pattern of muscle activity, and trajectory of these rapid grasping reactions were remarkably similar, regardless of whether subjects were standing or seated (Figs. 7A and 7B). Interestingly, the responses were also similar when the chair was translated but not allowed to tilt, suggesting that the sensation of whole-body movement is sufficient to evoke this pattern of very rapid muscle activation, regardless of the specific nature of the body motion. These findings could indicate an important role of the vestibular system in triggering the response, although we cannot rule out a possible contribution from visual or somatosensory receptors (eg, trunk pressoreceptors).

Compensatory Versus Noncompensatory Grasping

Preliminary tests have been performed to determine the differences between perturbation-cued and light-cued grasping reactions (McIlroy et al, unpublished research). In these trials, seated subjects were instructed to grasp handrails as fast as possible in response to the cue (light or platform motion). In all subjects, the timing of response to the perturbation cue was more rapid (by 130 milliseconds, on average) and less variable (mean within-subject coefficient of variation of 18% versus 32%). Furthermore, the timing and magnitude of the shoulder muscle activation were adjusted according to the perturbation magnitude and direction, which were varied unpredictably. In spite of the differences in timing and magnitude, the pattern of recruitment (relative onset of the primary arm muscles) remained the same in both compensatory and noncompensatory tasks (Fig. 7).

The modulation of the arm response according to the degree and direction of instability seems to parallel results described earlier with regard to stepping reactions. In both instances, the CNS appears to be able to respond rapidly and accurately to unpredictable perturbation. For grasping, however, there is the added complication of variation in target (handhold) location. We have found that unpredictable variation in the handhold location, prior to perturbation onset, leads to a loss of ability to direct the initial trajectory toward the handhold but does not delay response initiation (McIlroy et al, unpublished research). Based on these findings, we have proposed that (1) the compensatory grasping trajectory is preplanned by cortical neural pathways similar to those controlling noncompensatory grasping and (2) the very rapid initiation and amplitude scaling of the trajectory are controlled by transcortical or subcortical pathways similar to those that are thought to be involved in the control of the early fixed-support postural responses.

Interactions Between Fixed-Support and Change-in-Support Reactions

Sequential Versus Parallel Control

It has been suggested that change-in-support reactions, such as stepping, occur when the earlier fixed-support reactions fail to restore equilibrium[6–9] and that the stepping response will be appended to the earlier reactions.[66] Our data suggest that this is not the case. The stepping response is often initiated very early, even when subjects are instructed to try not to step (Table). For backward stepping, the asymmetry in vertical loading of the two legs, which is a biomechanical marker of the

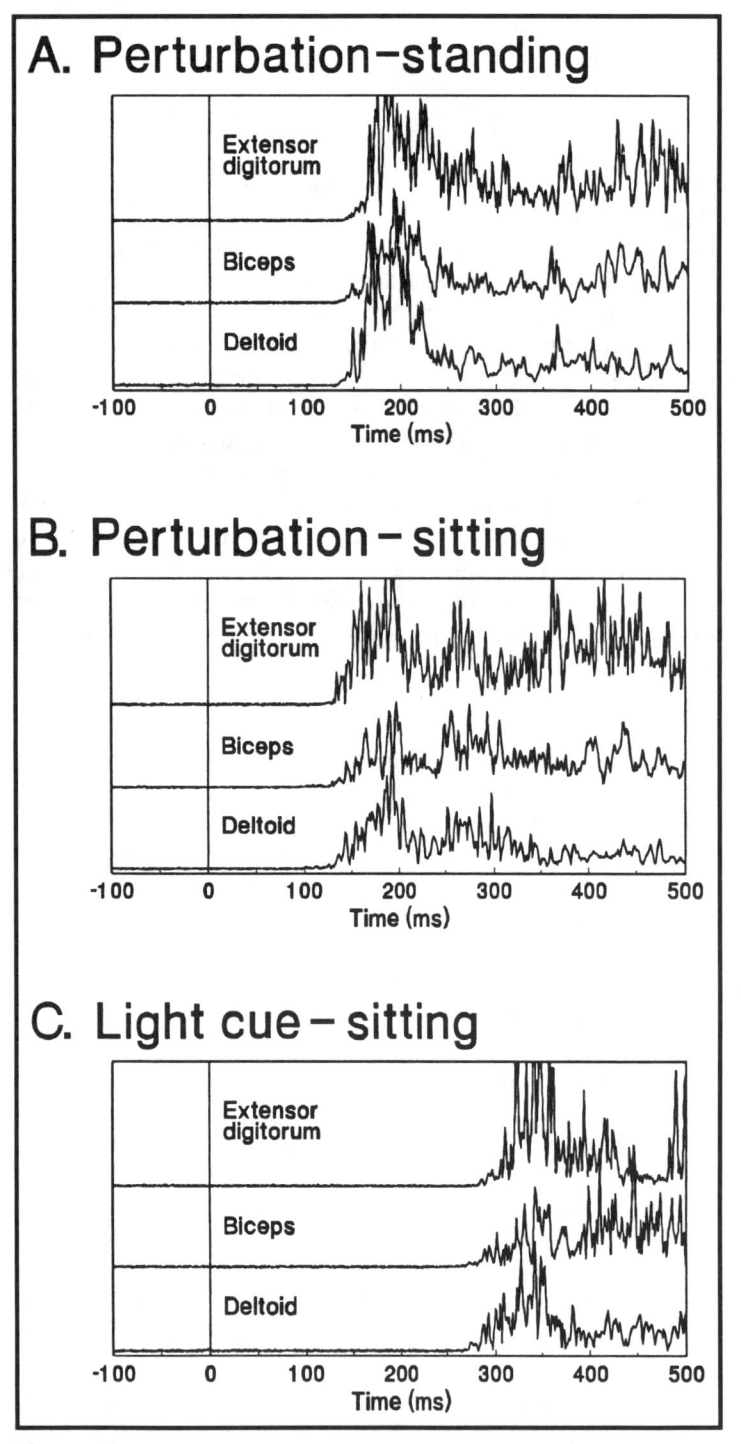

Figure 7.
Effect of task conditions on arm-muscle activation in grasping reactions (McIlroy et al, unpublished research). Rectified electromyographic profiles, averaged over five trials for one subject, are shown for the extensor digitorum, biceps, and deltoid muscles in response to forward platform translation (perturbation characteristics the same as in Fig. 2), when the subject was (A) standing or (B) seated in a chair that tilted slightly when the platform moved. The subject was instructed to grasp a handrail as rapidly as possible in response to the onset of platform motion. Fig. 7C shows the corresponding data for seated trials where the subject grasped as rapidly as possible in response to a light cue. Onset of perturbation or cue began at time 0. Note the similarity in the pattern of activation in all three tasks, but the much faster responses elicited by postural perturbation. The latter responses were equally fast regardless of whether the subject was standing or seated.

beginning of the response, was found to begin as early as 160 milliseconds after onset of platform acceleration,[12] with the underlying muscle activation likely occurring at least 50 milliseconds prior to the change in loading.[19] Given that the earliest muscle activation associated with the fixed-support reaction began at a latency of 105 milliseconds, it is clear that the step can be initiated well before the completion of the early fixed-support reaction.

Thus, in contrast to the view that the responses are sequenced, it appears that the stepping response may be initiated almost in parallel with the early fixed-support reaction. Parallel, rather than sequential, control is clearly evident in the compensatory arm reactions. As noted earlier, the activation of the shoulder muscles is coincident with the onset of the fixed-support reactions arising at the ankles.[14] Presumably, the CNS initiates the change-in-support response early to safeguard stability. This explanation is consistent with observations, noted earlier, that stepping and grasping often occur in early trials even when the perturbation is small. Potential costs of an early change-in-support reaction (eg, "unnecessary" stepping or grasping) can apparently be avoided by aborting the reaction, prior to grasping a handhold or placing the foot.[41] Stepping reactions apparently can even be aborted prior to lifting of the foot.[10-12] In such cases, there is a lateral "weight shift" that is very similar in timing and pattern to that recorded during trials in which forward or backward stepping actually occurs. Such evidence of aborted stepping is most prevalent during early trials, where subjects have been instructed to try not to step, and there is a progressive decrease in the magnitude of the lateral "weight shift" as the subject gains familiarity with the perturbation.[10,11] Responses that appear to be similar, when viewed in the sagittal plane, may actually be seen to involve quite different postural strategies, in terms of preparation for stepping, when the lateral asymmetry is examined.

Modulation of the Fixed-Support Ankle Strategy

The demands associated with the fixed-support and change-in-support reactions can conflict. For example, the fixed-support reaction acts to arrest the motion of the COM, whereas some progression of the COM is necessary to execute a step. In addition, the muscle activation required to unload and lift the swing limb may well conflict with the activation associated with the fixed-support reaction. Given the overlap in timing that has been observed within the fixed-support and change-in-support reactions, there must be a mechanism for resolving these conflicting demands. Our studies indicate that, for anteroposterior perturbation, the early fixed-support "ankle strategy" will persist even when the compensatory stepping reaction is preplanned; however, it appears that the gain of the early response can be modulated.[40] When subjects were instructed to step in response to forward platform translation, the magnitude of the initial (50-millisecond) response in the tibialis anterior muscle was reduced by about 40%, compared with "constrained" trials in which subjects were instructed to try not to step. This difference, due to instruction, occurred regardless of whether the subjects actually stepped or did not step in the constrained trials, and it suggests a centrally mediated change in the gain of the ankle reaction due to preplanning. Burleigh and colleagues[44,45] have since reported similar findings for ankle responses to small backward platform translations. Although Burleigh and Horak[45] concluded that the ability to predict platform velocity is required to suppress the early ankle reaction, the suppression in our study occurred under conditions in which platform velocity was unpredictable.[40] Apparently, there have not yet been any studies of the possible modulation of ankle responses due to compensatory arm reactions; however, it can be noted that the early fixed-support reaction at the ankle always persists, at normal latency, despite the presence of the arm reaction.[14] The persistent and automatic nature of the early fixed-support "ankle strategy" is also supported by a study of the interactions between early responses to postural perturbation and concurrent volitional (nonstepping) body movement.[67]

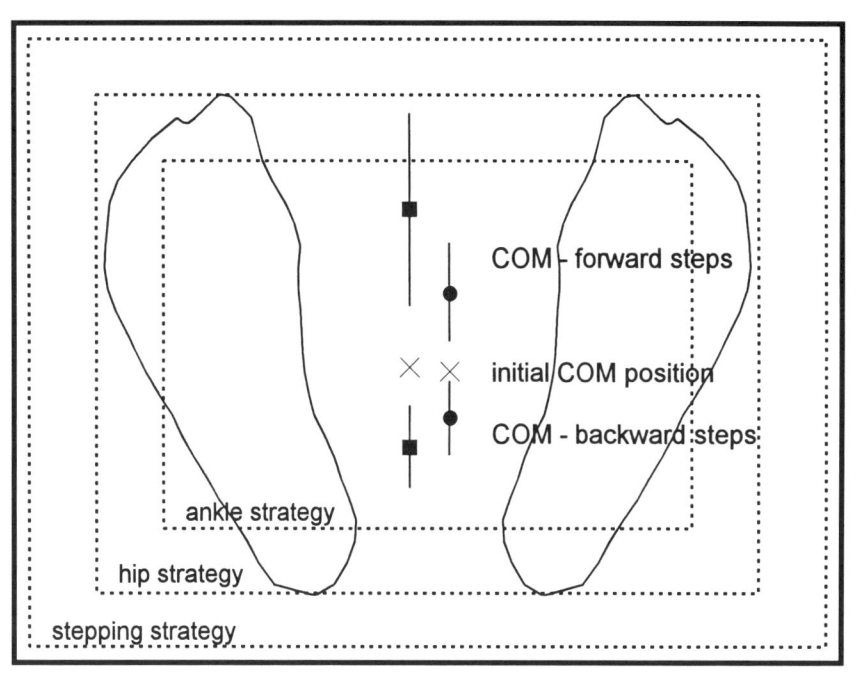

Subordination of the Fixed-Support Hip Strategy

The fixed-support "hip strategy" has, in recent years, received much attention and has been purported to be an important functional element of the postural repertoire for dealing with perturbation in the anteroposterior plane.[6-9] Our studies of young adults do not appear to support this view, however, suggesting instead that stepping is a preferred strategy. In contrast to the "ankle strategy," which relies primarily on ankle torque to stabilize the body, the hip strategy involves the use of the hip flexors or extensors to generate shear forces at the feet that act to decelerate the COM. (It is important to note that hip motion itself does not necessarily constitute a hip strategy, as classically defined.[6]) A hierarchial model has been proposed, wherein the hip strategy occurs when the stabilizing capabilities of the ankle strategy are exceeded and the stepping strategy emerges when the hip strategy is unsuccessful in keeping the COM over the BOS (Fig. 8).[6-9]

Apparently, however, the validity of this model is highly dependent on the degree to which the postural behavior is constrained. In the original experiments on which this model was based, subjects learned, over repeated trials, to execute a hip strategy in order to withstand perturbations while standing on a narrow beam.[6] We have

Figure 8.
Initiation of compensatory stepping: experimental observations versus a conceptual model of sequential control proposed by Horak and colleagues.[7,8] According to the model, transitions between ankle, hip, and stepping strategies, in response to anteroposterior perturbation, depend on "movement strategy boundaries" that can be defined in terms of the displacement of the center of mass (COM) relative to the base of support. Illustrative values for the anteroposterior boundaries are indicated by the dotted lines in the figure. The range assigned to the ankle strategy corresponds to reports that subjects without balance impairments can use this strategy to recover from up to 8° of forward sway and 4° of backward sway.[7] The boundary for step initiation corresponds to proposals that the stepping strategy emerges when the COM moves outside the base of support.[9] Superimposed on the model are measured data (mean and standard deviation) from young adults without balance impairments showing the COM displacement (normalized to foot length) at which the stepping response was actually initiated (as indicated by onset of asymmetry in vertical loading of the legs; the underlying muscle activation would have occurred at even smaller COM displacements). Square symbols=well-practiced trials where subjects were instructed to try not to step (10 subjects, total of 41 trials).[41] Circular symbols=early trials where subjects were unconstrained by specific instruction (5 subjects, total of 48 trials).[42] The "X" symbols indicate the mean COM location prior to perturbation onset. Perturbations were moderate in magnitude (forward translations same as in Fig. 2; backward translations were 33% larger). Subjects were able to maintain balance without stepping, when instructed to do so, in about 50% of trials at this perturbation level.

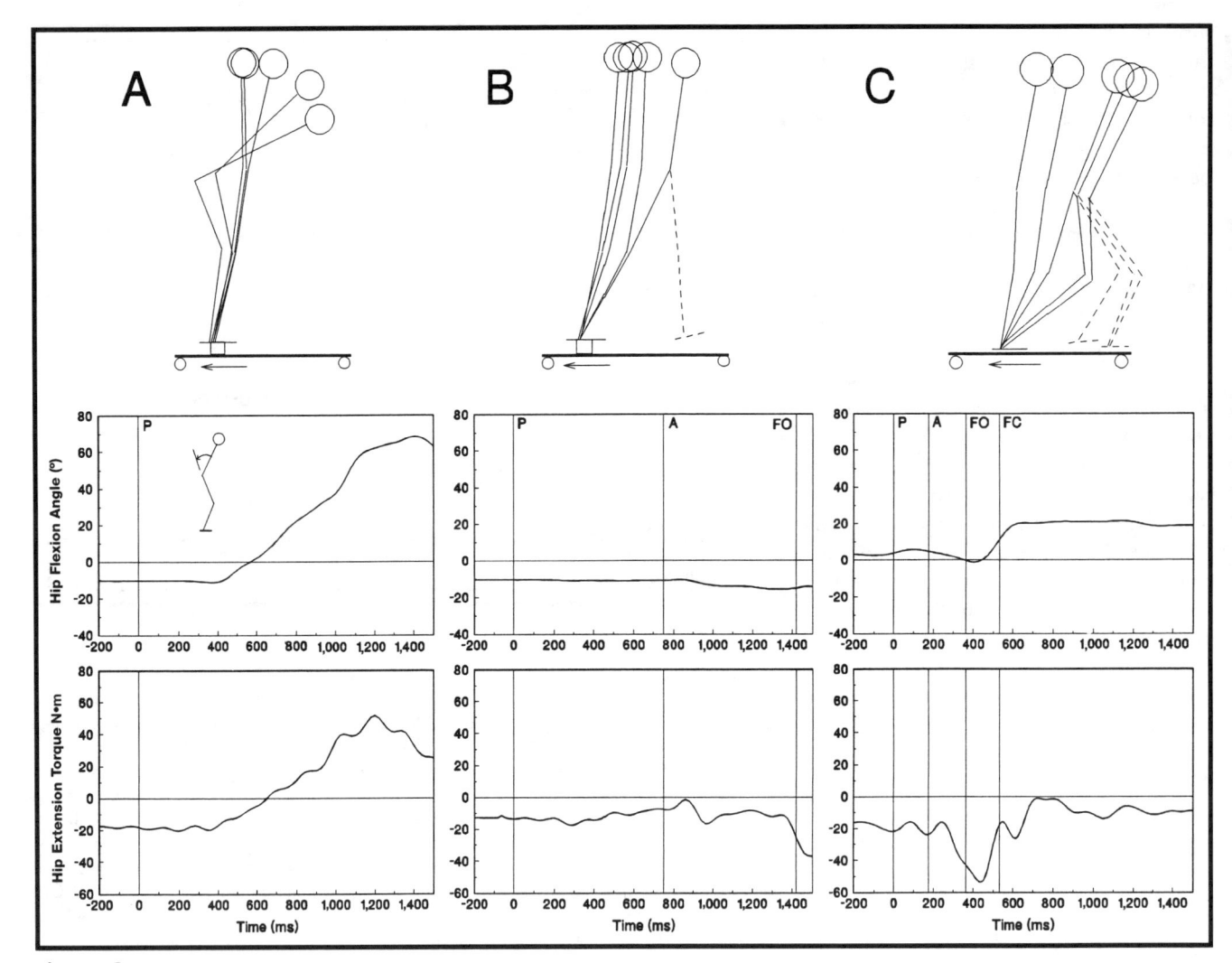

Figure 9.
Comparison of the trained fixed-support "hip strategy" (Fig. 9A) with forward stepping responses (Figs. 9B and 9C) (McIlroy and Maki, unpublished research). All responses were evoked by 600-ms backward platform translation (acceleration=0.4 m/s², velocity=0.12 m/s, displacement= 0.036 m in Figs. 9A and 9B; acceleration=3 m/s², velocity=0.9 m/s, displacement=0.27 m in Fig. 9C). Hip strategies were evoked, after approximately 7 to 10 training trials, by instructing subjects to balance, without stepping, on a narrow (10-cm) beam, according to the methodology of Horak and Nashner.[6] The stepping response shown in Fig. 9B was recorded, in the same subject, in the first training trial on the beam. The stepping response shown in Fig. 9C was recorded in a subject standing on a normal surface (no instructional constraints). The stick figures show the body posture at 333-ms intervals, starting approximately 200 ms prior to perturbation onset. Symbols P, A, FO, and FC indicate onset of platform acceleration, initiation of the stepping response (onset of left-right asymmetry in vertical limb loading), foot-off, and foot-contact, respectively. Note the large hip flexion and associated hip torque generated during the trained hip strategy and the absence of these features prior to foot-off in the stepping trials (in each panel, data are shown for the left leg, which was the stance limb for both stepping trials).

replicated this experiment and found that although it is true that the hip strategy can be learned, the natural preference is to step. In the first trial, and throughout the learning process, subjects prevented themselves from falling by stepping off the beam (McIlroy and Maki, unpublished research). Furthermore, there is no evidence, in the early "learning" trials, of substantial hip motion or hip torque that would be compatible with the classical hip strategy (Figs. 9A and 9B). Likewise, it seems doubtful that the hierarchy of responses illustrated in Figure 8 occurs under normal conditions. To date, we have seen no evidence, when subjects are allowed to respond "naturally," of substantial hip motion or torque that would be compatible with the sequencing of a classical hip strategy and step initiation (Fig. 9C). Finally, our data do not support the view that the step is initiated when the COM exceeds the limits of the BOS. As indicated in Figure 8, stepping is often initiated in response to small COM displacement, within the "zone" attributed to the ankle strategy, even when the perturbation is modest and the subject is instructed to try not to step. In early trials, when behavior is unconstrained, stepping is initiated at even smaller COM displacements.

Age- and Pathology-Related Changes

A small number of investigators have recently begun to study changes in compensatory stepping associated with aging. Studies of problems specific to visual or vestibular disorders, peripheral neuropathy, or central neurological lesions will be of equal significance in increasing our understanding of the control mechanisms and in developing new diagnostic and therapeutic approaches. Few such studies, however, have been performed to date. In one study involving three patients, there was little effect on step initiation due to vestibular deficit.[29] Another study[68] examined self- and perturbation-triggered step initiation in six patients with Parkinson's disease. Interestingly, there was further evidence of distinctions between compensatory and noncompensatory stepping, showing that dopaminergic therapy improved anticipatory force generation during self-initiated stepping but not when stepping was evoked by postural perturbation.[68] Apparently, there have not yet been any studies of age- or pathology-related changes in compensatory grasping, although we are currently beginning experiments in this area.

Effects of Aging on Incidence of Stepping

Researchers examining responses to backward pulling forces applied at the waist found that older subjects were more likely than younger subjects to take multiple backward steps in responding to the perturbation.[34,36,37] In individuals with a history of falling, there were often problems in the initiation and control of the compensatory stepping, and the stepping response was often insufficient to prevent loss of balance.[34,35] Our studies of forward and backward compensatory stepping in response to platform perturbation have also shown an increased tendency for older adults to take multiple steps.[42] On the basis of a study of backward stepping, it has been suggested that the execution of small, rapid multiple steps may represent a "conservative" strategy, in allowing increased opportunity to correct for instability.[37] It seems unlikely, however, that this strategy would apply to forward stepping responses, which tend to involve relatively large initial steps.[42]

In our study,[42] many of the multiple-step responses apparently emerged as a consequence of events that arose *after* the initiation of the first step, rather than as a strategy planned in advance. In particular, in over 30% of stepping reactions in older adults, the later steps were directed so as to recover lateral stability, even though the perturbation was in the anteroposterior direction (Fig. 10).[12] This response was rarely seen in young adults, even though the characteristics of the initial step were remarkably similar in both age groups. These findings suggest that the lateral stepping may reflect an impaired ability to control the lateral displacement of the COM during the stepping response. Interestingly, there is

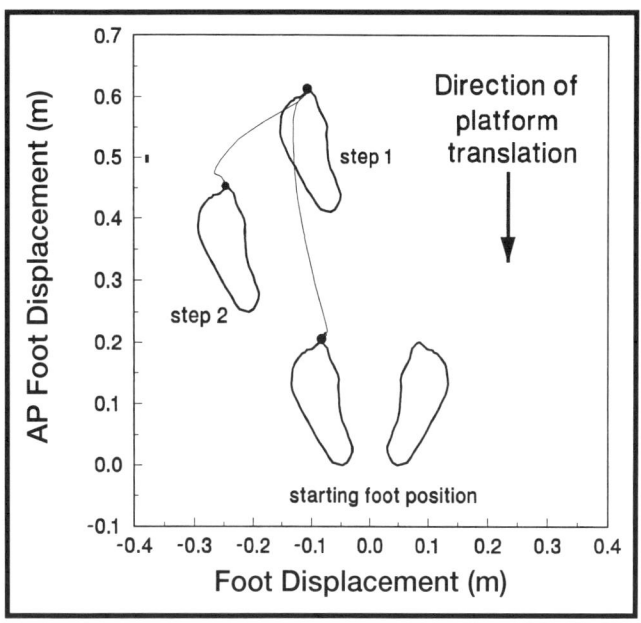

Figure 10.
Control of compensatory stepping reactions in older adults. Example data from a single trial illustrating the tendency of older adults to take a second step in the lateral direction, in responding to anteroposterior (AP) platform perturbation (this tendency was rarely seen in young adults). In this study,[42] both young and older adults were presented, at the start of their first testing session, with 10 consecutive platform-translation perturbations, 5 forward and 5 backward, in random order; there were no instructional constraints. The figure shows the response to a backward platform translation (acceleration=2.0 m/s², velocity=0.6 m/s, displacement=0.18 m, duration=0.6 s), recorded for a community-dwelling man (aged 81 years) with no recent history of falling.

recent evidence that an impaired ability to control lateral stability may distinguish elderly "fallers" from "nonfallers."[69] Recent work by Rogers[33] appears to support this view; however, in contrast to our results, Rogers found evidence of differences in the *initial* step of the response. Older subjects with a history of falling tended to include a lateral displacement in the initial step in responding to a forward pulling force applied at the waist. Attempts to compensate for lateral instability in this manner could represent a predictive strategy, which may have been facilitated by the more predictable perturbation conditions used in that study. It is also possible that such an adaptation is specific to subjects with a recent history of unsteadiness and falling; the older adults we tested were not recent fallers.

Effects of Aging on Response Initiation

In general, our results showed little evidence of age-related differences in the timing of the stepping responses, although the older subjects exhibited small delays (40 milliseconds, on average) in response initiation.[42] Our findings appear to contradict the results of Luchies and colleagues,[36,37] who reported *earlier* foot-lift (by up to 100 milliseconds) in older subjects. The discrepancy may lie in methodological differences. In our study, perturbation direction was varied unpredictably, subjects were allowed to respond in what we considered to be a "natural" manner (no instructional constraints), and we focused on the earliest trials, where the perturbations were still relatively novel, to better simulate responses evoked by unexpected disturbance in daily life. In light of evidence that aging can affect adaptive capabilities,[70] some elderly subjects in the study by Luchies and colleagues may have reached their stability limits sooner because they were less able to adapt their responses to take advantage of the more predictable features of their testing paradigm. Differences in instructional set may also account for the differences in findings. Although Luchies and colleagues did not report the instructions given to the subjects, it appears that the subjects may have been encouraged to resist stepping. In this situation, younger subjects may devote greater effort to resisting stepping and thus they may tend to delay step onset because they are less apprehensive about losing balance. The small delay in response observed in our study may reflect impaired ability to rapidly discriminate onset of instability and may be related to age-related reduction in sensitivity to peripheral sensory inputs or increased central processing and conduction time.

Effects of Aging on Anticipatory Control

Older adults appear to be less likely to include anticipatory elements in the compensatory stepping response.[33,42] Although this finding may reflect an age-related impairment in adaptive capability, we believe that it is unlikely to affect functional stability in daily life. As noted earlier, unconstrained responses to novel perturbations almost always lack an ML APA, and the ML APAs that do occur, in some experimental trials, are too small or brief to provide any functional benefit with regard to lateral stabilization. Thus, in spite of the greater prevalence of ML APAs in young adults, there was no corresponding increase in lateral stability at time of foot-contact, as reflected by the ML displacement and velocity of the COM.[42] Inclusion of the ML APA phase could actually jeopardize safety by delaying the stepping response, particularly when coupled with the age-related delay in response onset noted above. These factors might account for the reduced frequency of ML APAs in elderly persons.

Factors Contributing to Age-Related Changes

The age-related impairments in compensatory stepping described do not appear to be a consequence of impaired musculoskeletal function. Luchies and colleagues[36,37] have found that the flexion-extension joint torques, as well as the joint range of motion, required to execute rapid backward compensatory steps are well within the capabilities of "normal" older adults. In addition, we have found that the compensatory stepping movements of "normal" young and older adults are quite similar in speed of motion.[42] Because compensatory responses do not appear to require maximal muscle forces or a large range of motion, modest age-related reduction in musculoskeletal capacity may not pose a problem in generating these responses. However, readers should note that the studies to date have only examined responses up to the time of foot-contact. In addition, the possible effects of age-related decreases in hip abductor and adductor strength have not yet been examined. Weakness in these muscles could possibly contribute to the problems that older adults appear to have in controlling lateral stability during compensatory stepping. Ongoing work in our laboratory is aimed at determining the specific contributions of age-related decrements in musculoskeletal capacity, sensory function, and neural information processing to impaired control of compensatory leg and arm movements.

Summary

By removing constraints on postural behavior during experimental testing, it becomes evident that change-in-support strategies, involving compensatory stepping or grasping movements of the limbs, are very prevalent reactions to instability, even at small perturbations, and likely play a more important functional role in maintaining upright stance than has generally been appreciated in the past.

Change-in-support reactions are clearly not just strategies of last resort. Both stepping and grasping reactions can be initiated very early, well before the COM is near the stability limits of the BOS. For anteroposterior perturbations, the fixed-support ankle strategy persists despite the occurrence of change-in-support reactions, a finding that may reflect the importance of this strategy in providing an early defense against destabilization. The role of the fixed-support hip strategy, however, appears to be limited to special task conditions that preclude the option of stepping or grasping.

Compensatory stepping and grasping reactions are initiated and executed much more rapidly than the fastest noncompensatory (volitional) efforts. In addition, unplanned compensatory stepping reactions frequently lack the anticipatory control elements that invariably occur during volitional stepping. Even when anticipatory adjustments are present, they are too small or brief to have a functional impact during rapid compensatory stepping.

Lateral destabilization complicates the control of compensatory stepping, due to anatomical restrictions on lateral lower-extremity movement and the effects of perturbation-induced COM displacement on the preparatory unloading of the swing limb. Cross-over steps appear to predominate, in young adults without balance impairments, under task conditions that discourage pre-planning of the stepping response. The demands associated with this response (eg, prolonged one-limb stance), however, are likely to cause problems for individuals with balance impairments.

Sensory feedback is expected to become increasingly important when unpredictable conditions preclude pre-planning of the step or grasp. The fact that swing-limb unloading is often aborted after step initiation suggests that feedback is used to modulate the response on-line, in contrast to the view that the step is released as an immutable motor program. Evidence to date suggests that plantar pressure feedback is one of the more important sources of sensory feedback for the control of compensatory stepping.

Although older adults may be able to generate rapid compensatory stepping reactions, they are more likely to require multiple steps to recover equilibrium. Aging appears to bring particular problems in controlling lateral stability during the execution of the step, which may be of specific relevance to the problem of lateral falls and associated hip fractures. Although older adults appear to be less likely to include predictive (anticipatory) elements in the stepping response, this is unlikely to have an impact on the ability to respond to unexpected perturbation during activities of daily life.

Increased understanding of change-in-support arm and leg reactions may soon lead to development of new diagnostic and therapeutic approaches for detecting and treating specific causes of imbalance and falling. In assessing balance, clinicians need to be aware of the importance of characterizing change-in-support, as well as fixed-support, reactions and of the need to use unpredictable test conditions to prevent adaptations that are unlikely to occur in daily life. In treating balance impairments, interventions such as training programs should address specific elements of compensatory stepping or grasping reactions that are found to cause difficulty (eg, lateral weight transfer, rapid foot or arm movement, cross-over steps). The ability to assess CNS control of change-in-support reactions though tests of compensatory grasping in seated patients may present new opportunities for testing and training balance across a wider range of patients than is currently feasible.

Acknowledgments
We gratefully acknowledge the assistance of Stephen D Perry and Geoff R Fernie in the preparation of this article.

References
1 Black SE, Maki BE, Fernie GR. Aging, imbalance, and falls. In: Barber H, Sharpe J, eds. *Vestibulo-ocular Reflex, Nystagmus, and Vertigo*. New York, NY: Raven Press; 1993:317–335.

2 Baker SP, Harvey AH. Fall injuries in the elderly. In: Radebaugh TS, Hadley E, Suzman R, eds. *Symposium on Falls in the Elderly: Biologic and Behavioral Aspects*. Philadelphia, Pa: WB Saunders Co; 1985:501–512.

3 Silverton R, Tideiksaar R. Psychosocial aspects of falls. In: Tideiksaar R, ed. *Falling in Old Age: Its Prevention and Treatment*. New York, NY: Springer Publishing Co Inc; 1989:87–110.

4 Poplingher AR, Pillar T. Hip fracture for stroke patients: epidemiology and rehabilitation. *Acta Orthop Scand*. 1985;56:226–227.

5 Mion L, Gregor S, Chwirchak D, Paras W. Falls in the rehabilitation setting: incidence and characteristics. *Rehabilitation Nursing*. 1989;14:17–22.

6 Horak FB, Nashner LM. Central programming of postural movements: adaptation to altered support-surface configurations. *J Neurophysiol*. 1986;55:1369–1381.

7 Horak FB, Shupert CL, Mirka A. Components of postural dyscontrol in the elderly: a review. *Neurobiol Aging*. 1989;10:727–738.

8 Horak FB. Effects of neurological disorders on postural movement strategies in the elderly. In: Vellas B, Toupet M, Rubenstein L, et al, eds. *Falls, Balance, and Gait Disorders in the Elderly*. Paris, France: Elsevier; 1992:137–151.

9 Shumway-Cook A, Woollacott MH. *Motor Control: Theory and Practical Applications*. Baltimore, Md: Williams & Wilkins; 1995:126–131.

10 Maki BE, Whitelaw RS. Influence of expectation and arousal on centre-of-pressure responses to transient postural perturbations. *J Vestib Res*. 1993;3:25–39.

11 Maki BE, Whitelaw RS, McIlroy WE. Does frontal-plane asymmetry in compensatory postural responses represent preparation for stepping? *Neurosci Lett*. 1993;149:87–90.

12 McIlroy WE, Maki BE. Task constraints on foot movement and the incidence of compensatory stepping following perturbation of upright stance. *Brain Res*. 1993;616:30–38.

13 McIlroy WE, Maki BE. Adaptive changes to compensatory stepping responses. *Gait and Posture*. 1995;3:43–50.

14 McIlroy WE, Maki BE. Early activation of arm muscles follows external perturbations of upright stance. *Neurosci Lett*. 1995;184:177–180.

15 McIlroy WE, Maki BE. Compensatory arm movements evoked by transient perturbations of upright stance. In: Taguchi K, Igarashi M, Mori S, eds. *Vestibular and Neural Front*. Amsterdam, the Netherlands: Elsevier Science Publishers BV; 1994:489–492.

16 Holliday PJ, Fernie GR, Gryfe CI, Griggs GT. Video recording of spontaneous falls of the elderly. In: Gray BE, ed. *Slips, Stumbles, and Falls: Pedestrian Footwear and Surfaces (ASTM STP 1103)*. Philadelphia, Pa: American Society for Testing and Materials; 1990:7–16.

17 Connell BR. *Environmental and Behavioral Factors in Falls Among the Elderly*. Atlanta, Ga: US Department of Veterans Affairs Rehabilitation Research and Development Service; 1996. Merit Review Project E-539-R.

18 Breniere Y, Do MC, Bouisset S. Are dynamic phenomena prior to stepping essential to walking? *Journal of Motor Behavior*. 1987;19:62–76.

19 Brunt D, Lafferty MJ, McKeon A, et al. Invariant characteristics of gait initiation. *Am J Phys Med Rehabil*. 1991;3:206–212.

20 Herman R, Cook T, Cozzens B, Freedman W. Control of postural reactions in man: the initiation of gait. In: Stein RB, Pearson KB, Smith RS, Redford JB, eds. *Control of Posture and Locomotion*. New York, NY: Plenum Press; 1973:363–388.

21 Elble RJ, Moody C, Leffler K, Sinha R. The initiation of normal walking. *Mov Disord*. 1994;9:139–146.

22. Crenna P, Frigo C. A motor programme for the initiation of forward-oriented movements in humans. *J Physiol (Lond)*. 1991;437:635–653.

23. Carlsoo S. The initiation of walking. *Acta Anat*. 1966;65:1–9.

24. Mann R, Hagy JL, White V, Liddell D. The initiation of gait. *J Bone Joint Surg [Am]*. 1979;12:232–239.

25. Nissan M, Whittle MW. Initiation of gait in normal subjects: a preliminary study. *Biomed Eng*. 1990;12:165–171.

26. Herman R, Maulucci R, Leonard E, Pyszka V. The initiation of locomotion in man. In: Grillner S, Stein PSG, Stuart D, et al, eds. *Neurobiology of Invertebrate Locomotion*. Houndmils, Great Britain: MacMillan; 1986:623–635.

27. Jian Y, Winter DA, Ishac MG, Gilchrist L. Trajectory of the body COG and COP during initiation and termination of gait. *Gait and Posture*. 1993;1:9–22.

28. Do MC, Breniere Y, Brenguier P. A biomechanical study of balance recovery during the fall forward. *J Biomech*. 1982;15:933–939.

29. Do MC, Breniere Y, Bouisset S. Compensatory reactions in forward fall: Are they initiated by stretch receptors? *Electroencephalogr Clin Neurophysiol*. 1988;69:448–452.

30. Do MC, Bussel B, Breniere Y. Influence of plantar cutaneous afferents on early compensatory reactions to forward fall. *Exp Brain Res*. 1990;79:319–324.

31. Do MC, Roby-Brami A. The influence of a reduced plantar support surface area on the compensatory reactions to a forward fall. *Exp Brain Res*. 1991;84:439–443.

32. Hoshiyama M, Watanabe S, Kaneoke Y, et al. Effect of optokinetic stimulation on human balance recovery in unexpected forward fall. *Neurosci Res*. 1993;18:121–127.

33. Rogers MW. Disorders of posture, balance, and gait in Parkinson's disease. In: Studenski SA, ed. *Gait and Balance Disorders*. Philadelphia, Pa: WB Saunders Co; 1996:825–845.

34. Wolfson LI, Whipple R, Amerman P, Kleinberg A. Stressing the postural response: a quantitative method for testing balance. *J Am Geriatr Soc*. 1986;34:845–850.

35. Chandler JM, Duncan PW, Studenski SA. Balance performance on the postural stress test: comparison of young adults, healthy elderly, and fallers. *Phys Ther*. 1990;70:410–415.

36. Luchies CW. *Fall Arrest Biomechanics: Sway and Stepping Responses in Healthy Young and Old Adults*. Ann Arbor, Mich: The University of Michigan; 1991. Doctoral dissertation.

37. Luchies CW, Alexander NB, Schultz AB, Ashton-Miller J. Stepping responses of young and old adults to postural disturbances: kinematics. *J Am Geriatr Soc*. 1994;42:506–512.

38. McIlroy WE, Maki BE. Do anticipatory postural adjustments precede compensatory stepping reactions evoked by perturbation? *Neurosci Lett*. 1993;164:199–204.

39. McIlroy WE, Maki BE. Influence of destabilization on the temporal characteristics of "volitional" stepping. *Journal of Motor Behavior*. 1996;1:28–34.

40. McIlroy WE, Maki BE. Changes in early "automatic" postural responses associated with the prior planning and execution of a compensatory step. *Brain Res*. 1993;631:203–211.

41. Maki BE, McIlroy WE, Perry SD. Influence of lateral destabilization on compensatory stepping responses. *J Biomech*. 1996;29:343–353.

42. McIlroy WE, Maki BE. Age-related changes in compensatory stepping in response to unpredictable perturbations. *J Gerontol*. 1996;51:M289–M296.

43. Romick-Allen R, Schultz AB. Biomechanics of reactions to impending falls. *J Biomech*. 1988;21:591–600.

44. Burleigh AL, Horak FB, Malouin F. Modification of postural responses and step initiation: evidence for goal-directed postural interactions. *J Neurophysiol*. 1994;72:2892–2902.

45. Burleigh AL, Horak FB. Influence of instruction, prediction, and afferent sensory information on the postural organization of step initiation. *J Neurophysiol*. 1996;75:1619–1628.

46. Rogers MW, Hain TC, Hanke TA, Janssen I. Stimulus parameters and inertial load: effects on the incidence of protective stepping responses in healthy human subjects. *Arch Phys Med Rehabil*. 1996;77:363–368.

47. Wild D, Nayak USL, Isaacs B. Description, classification, and prevention of falls in old people at home. *Rheumatol Rehabil*. 1981;20:153–159.

48. Topper AK, Maki BE, Holliday PJ. Are activity-based assessments of balance and gait in the elderly predictive of risk of falling and/or type of fall? *J Am Geriatr Soc*. 1993;41:479–487.

49. Patla A, Frank J, Winter D. Assessment of balance control in the elderly: major issues. *Physiotherapy Canada*. 1990;42:89–97.

50. Overstall PW, Exton-Smith AN, Imms FJ, Johnson AL. Falls in the elderly related to postural imbalance. *BMJ*. 1977;1:261–264.

51. Prudham D, Evans JG. Factors associated with falls in the elderly: a community study. *Age Ageing*. 1981;10:141–146.

52. Ryynanen OP, Kivela SL, Honkanen R. Times, places, and mechanisms of falls among the elderly. *Z Gerontol*. 1991;24:154–161.

53. Maki BE. Gait changes in older adults: predictors of falls or indicators of fear? *J Am Geriatr Soc*. In press.

54. Mouchnino L, Aurenty R, Massion L, Pedotti A. Coordination between equilibrium and head-trunk orientation during leg movement: a new strategy built up by training. *J Neurophysiol*. 1992;67:1587–1598.

55. Rogers MW. Influence of task dynamics on the organization of interlimb responses accompanying standing human leg flexion movements. *Brain Res*. 1992;579:353–356.

56. Rogers MW, Pai YC. Dynamic transitions in stance support accompanying leg flexion movements in man. *Exp Brain Res*. 1990;81:398–402.

57. Do MC, Nouillot P, Bouisset S. Is balance or posture at the end of a voluntary movement programmed? *Neurosci Lett*. 1991;130:9–11.

58. Maki BE, McIlroy WE. Postural control in the older adult. In: Studenski SA, ed. *Clinics in Geriatric Medicine: Gait and Balance Disorders*. Philadelphia, Pa: WB Saunders Co; 1996:635–658.

59. Cummings SR, Nevitt MC. Non-skeletal determinants of fractures: the potential importance of the mechanics of falls. *Osteoporos Int*. 1994;1:S67–S70.

60. Dietz V, Quintern J, Berger W. Stumbling reactions in man: release of a ballistic movement pattern. *Brain Res*. 1986;362:355–357.

61. Berger W, Dietz V, Quintern J. Corrective reactions to stumbling in man: neuronal co-ordination of bilateral leg muscle activity during gait. *J Physiol (Lond)*. 1984;357:109–125.

62. Dietz V, Quintern J, Boos G, Berger W. Obstruction of the swing phase during gait: phase-dependent bilateral leg muscle coordination. *Brain Res*. 1986;384:166–169.

63. Dietz V, Quintern J, Sillem M. Stumbling reactions in man: significance of proprioceptive and pre-programmed mechanisms. *J Physiol (Lond)*. 1987;386:149–163.

64 Perry SD, Maki BE. The role of cutaneous mechanoreceptors in the control of compensatory stepping. In: *Proceedings of the Ninth Biennial Conference of the Canadian Society for Biomechanics.* 1996:168–169.

65 Maki BE, Holliday PJ, Topper AK. Fear of falling and postural performance in the elderly. *J Gerontol.* 1991;46:M123–M131.

66 Cordo PJ. Sensory triggering of a sequence of postural responses. *Neuroscience Abstracts.* 1991;17:1110. Abstract.

67 Nashner LM, Cordo PJ. Relation of automatic postural responses and reaction-time voluntary movements of human leg muscles. *Exp Brain Res.* 1981;43:395–405.

68 Burleigh-Jacobs A, Horak FB, Nutt JG, Obeso JA. Step initiation in Parkinson's disease: influence of levodopa and external sensory triggers. *Mov Disord.* In press.

69 Maki BE, Holliday PJ, Topper AK. A prospective study of postural balance and risk of falling in an ambulatory and independent elderly population. *J Gerontol.* 1994;49:M72–M84.

70 Stelmach G, Teasdale N, Di Fabio RP, Phillips J. Age-related decline in postural control mechanisms. *Int J Aging Hum Dev.* 1989;29:205–223.

Locomotion in Patients With Spinal Cord Injuries

Following central motor lesions, two forms of reorganization can be observed that lead to improved mobility: (1) the development of increased muscle tone and (2) the activation of spinal locomotor centers induced by specific treadmill training. Tension development is different from normal during spastic gait and appears to be independent of exaggerated monosynaptic stretch reflexes. Exaggerated stretch reflexes are associated with an absence or reduction of functionally essential polysynaptic reflexes. Based on observations of the locomotor capacity of the spinal cat, recent studies have indicated that spinal locomotor centers can be activated and trained in patients with complete or incomplete paraplegia when the body is partially unloaded. The level of electromyographic activity in the gastrocnemius muscle, however, is considerably lower in patients with central motor lesions than in persons without neurological impairments. During the course of a daily locomotor training program, the amplitude of gastrocnemius muscle electromyographic activity increases during the stance phase and inappropriate tibialis anterior muscle activity decreases. Such training programs can improve the ability of patients with incomplete paraplegia to walk on stationary surfaces. This article reviews the pathophysiology and functional importance of increased muscle tone and the effects of treadmill training on the locomotor pattern underlying new attempts to improve the mobility of patients with paraplegia. [Dietz V, Wirz M, Jensen L. Locomotion in patients with spinal cord injuries. *Phys Ther.* 1997;77:508–516.]

Key Words: *Incomplete/complete paraplegia, Increased muscle tone, Monosynaptic/polysynaptic reflexes, Spinal locomotor centers, Training effects.*

Volker Dietz

Markus Wirz

Lars Jensen

To control posture and gait, the central nervous system selectively utilizes afferent information from a variety of sources, which then interact with central programs to adjust the movement to the actual requirements. Although a predominant working range exists for each receptor system, considerable overlap among systems is present. Thus, under normal conditions, stepping movements are not particularly impaired in the absence of one of the main afferent systems (ie, visual, proprioceptive, or labyrinthine).

There is general agreement that locomotor movements in mammals depend primarily on neuronal mechanisms within the spinal cord that can act in the absence of any afferent input. (See review by Grillner.[1]) Nevertheless, afferent information is essential for both bipeds and quadrupeds in order to adjust the central pattern to the external requirements.[1,2] Further refinement is achieved supraspinally, namely via the cerebellum. (See review by Armstrong.[3])

The neuronal regulation of human locomotion is similarly achieved by a complex interaction of spinal and supraspinal mechanisms.[4] The rhythmic activation of lower-extremity muscles by spinal interneuronal circuits is modulated and adapted accordingly by multisensory afferent input. Muscle activity, which results from the interaction of these different mechanisms, causes functionally modulated muscle tension by the mechanical muscle fiber properties.[5] The spinal programming as well as the reflex activity are under supraspinal control. When this supraspinal control is impaired (eg, in patients with spinal cord lesions), spasticity (hypertonicity) can develop. Spasticity produces numerous physical signs such as exaggerated reflexes, clonus, and muscle hypertonia. *Spasticity* has been defined as an increase in resistance to passive muscle stretch in a velocity-dependent manner following activation of tonic stretch reflexes.[6]

The degree of spasticity bears little relationship to the patient's disability, which is due to a movement disorder. In the past, a widely accepted premise was that exaggerated reflexes are responsible for spastic muscle hypertonia, and therefore for the movement disorder. The function of these reflexes during natural movements and the relationship between exaggerated reflexes and the movement disorder are not often considered. In patients with spinal cord lesions, a characteristic gait impairment is seen. This gait impairment can be evaluated by the recording of electrophysiological and biomechanical variables. There is some difference between spasticity of cerebral origin and spasticity of spinal origin, but the main features, such as the pattern of lower-extremity muscle activity during locomotion and the pathophysiology of increased muscle tone, are quite similar.[4]

Spastic Movement Disorder

Reflexes and Muscle Tone

Neuronal reorganization occurs following central lesions in both cats[7] and humans.[8] Novel connections (eg,

---

V Dietz, MD, is Professor, Doctor, and Chair/Head of Paraplegiology, Swiss Paraplegic Centre, University Hospital Balgrist, Forchstrasse 340, CH-8008 Zurich, Switzerland (dietz@balgrist.unizh.ch). Address all correspondence to Dr Dietz.

M Wirz, PT, is Physiotherapist, Swiss Paraplegic Centre, University Hospital Balgrist.

L Jensen, DM, is Bioengineer, Swiss Paraplegic Centre, University Hospital Balgrist.

This work was supported by the Swiss National Science Foundation (No. 31–42.899.95) and the International Research Institute for Paraplegia (P16/93).

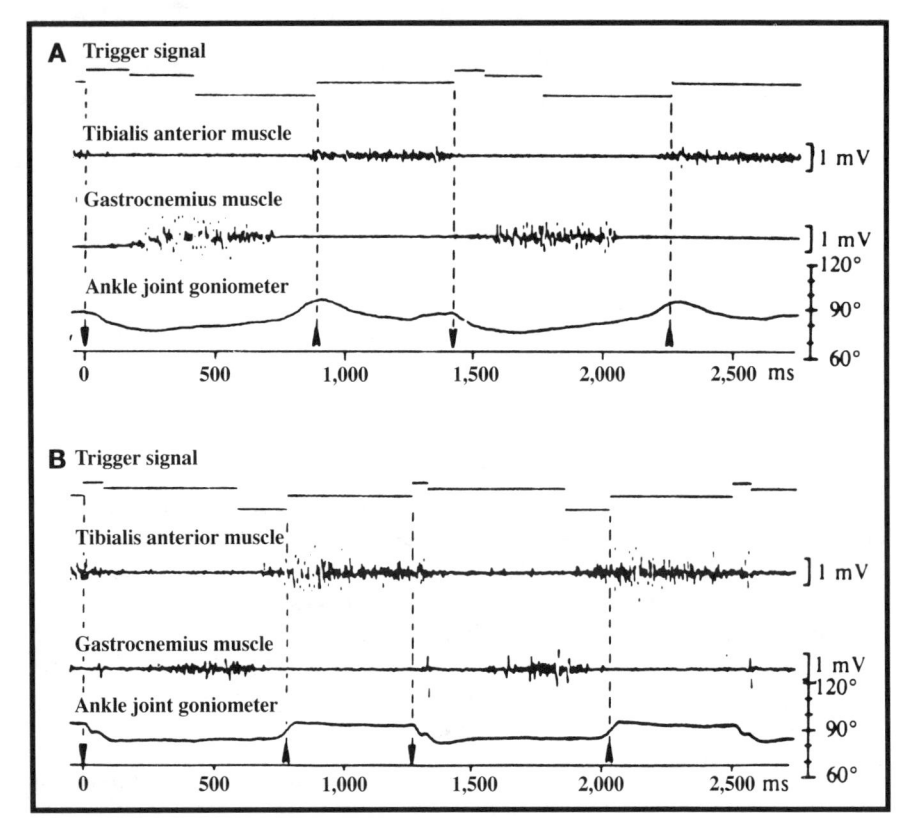

Figure 1.
Representative recordings for two step cycles during slow gait from (A) a subject without neurological impairments and (B) a patient with spastic paraparesis. From top to bottom: electrical switch signals from the heel and the ball of the foot, tibialis anterior and gastrocnemius muscle electromyographic recordings, and potentiometer signal of ankle joint. Vertical lines indicate touch-down (↑) and lift-up (↓) of the foot.[32]

sprouting, functional strengthening of existing connections, removed depression of previously inactive connections) may cause changes in the strength of inhibition. In addition, supersensitivity caused by the denervation may occur.[7] Although recent observations have indicated that spinal cord lesions do not cause sprouting of primary afferents in either cats[9] or humans,[10] changes in the reduction of presynaptic inhibition of group Ia fibers do occur,[11] which correlates with the enhanced excitability of tendon tap reflexes. In addition, reduction of presynaptic inhibition is stronger in patients with paraplegia compared with patients with hemiplegia.[12] No correlation, however, is seen between decreased presynaptic inhibition of Ia terminals and the degree of muscle tone measured by Ashworth's scale.[12] Nevertheless, treatment of spasticity is usually directed toward reducing stretch reflex activity, as it was thought that exaggerated reflexes were responsible for increased muscle tone and therefore spastic movement disorders.

The pattern of muscle activation and the development of increased muscle tone in people with spasticity, however, are basically different in the *active* motor condition compared with the clinical testing of the *passive* muscle.[13–15] During every movement, the muscle is active, and it is the movement disorder that hampers the patient. In contrast, during clinical examination of muscle tone (according to Ashworth's scale), the muscle is passive. Basically, the muscle behaves differently in response to stretch in the active and passive conditions. Extensive investigations on functional movements of lower-extremity[16,17] and arm[15,18,19] muscles have not shown any causal relationship between exaggerated reflexes and movement disorder. In adult patients with cerebral or spinal lesions, the reciprocal mode of lower-extremity muscle activation during gait is preserved in spasticity. Exaggerated stretch reflexes in persons with spasticity are associated with an absence or reduction of functionally essential polysynaptic (long-latency) reflexes.[16] Tension development during functional movements[16,20] does not depend on exaggerated stretch reflexes. The overall lower-extremity muscle activity is reduced in patients with spasticity.[16,18] For the assessment of changes in muscle electrical activity in subjects without neurological impairments, and to compare these changes with values obtained from patients with spasticity, the mean values of electromyographic (EMG) strength were determined for each group of subjects.[16,18] The sampling interval for the calculation of the mean values with standard deviations was 1/20 of one step cycle.[16,18]

Neuronal Regulation of Locomotion

During gait in patients with spasticity, the EMG activity in the calf muscles is smaller in amplitude and less well modulated compared with that of persons without neurological impairments (Fig. 1). This observation is most likely due to the impaired function of polysynaptic reflexes. Fast regulation of motoneuron discharge, which characterizes the normal muscle, is absent in patients with spasticity.[21,22] This fast regulation of motoneuron discharge corresponds to a loss of EMG modulation during gait. In patients with hemiparesis due to cerebral lesions, the strength of EMG activity in the affected lower extremity is often reduced compared with that of the unaffected lower extremity. This reduction in strength corresponds to the degree of paresis observed during both gait[16] and elbow movements.[18]

During gait in patients with spastic paresis (acquired at birth or later in life), a fundamentally different development of tension of the triceps surae muscle takes place during the stance phase.[16,17] For patients with spastic hemiparesis, tension development correlates with the modulation of EMG activity in the unaffected lower extremity (the same is true for individuals without neurological impairments), whereas tension development is correlated to the stretching period of the tonically activated (with small EMG amplitude) muscle in the spastic lower extremity (Fig. 2).[16,17] During gait, there is no visible influence of monosynaptic reflex potentials on the tension developed by the triceps surae muscle (for a description of tension recording, see Berger et al[16]). A similar discrepancy between the resistance to stretching and the level of EMG activity has been described for flexor muscles of the upper limb in patients with spasticity.[23,24]

Muscle tone during functional movements in patients with spastic paresis cannot be explained by increased activity of motoneurons, as assessed by EMG recordings. Instead, the motor units of the triceps surae muscle are transformed such that a higher-tension-to-EMG-activity relationship occurs during the stretching phase. Consequently, we believe that regulation of muscle tension takes place at a lower level of neuronal organization. Such a transformation is functionally meaningful because it enables the individual to support the body weight during gait. Fast active movements, however, become impossible.

Application of findings related to tone from studies of animals to humans must be done cautiously. An acute rigor appears in the decerebrate cat, whereas in individuals with paresis secondary to acute spinal or supraspinal lesions, muscle tone develops slowly over a period of weeks. Currently, no animal model exists to explain the development of hypertonicity in humans.

Motor Unit Transformation
Several findings support the suggestion that changes in the mechanical properties of muscle fibers occur in patients with spasticity. Contraction times of hand muscles[25] as well as of the gastrocnemius muscle[26] in patients with hemiparesis are prolonged. This is not true where there are spinal transections in cats[27] and humans.[28] Torque motor experiments applied to upper- and lower-limb muscles indicate a major, nonreflex contribution to the increased muscle tone in the antigravity muscles (ie, leg extensors and elbow flexors).[29,30] Histochemical and morphometric studies of spastic muscle have shown changes in the muscle fibers.[21,31] These changes include (1) increased levels of muscle fiber atrophy (especially of type II fibers), (2) a predominance of type I fibers in the gastrocnemius muscle 6 months after stroke, when spas-

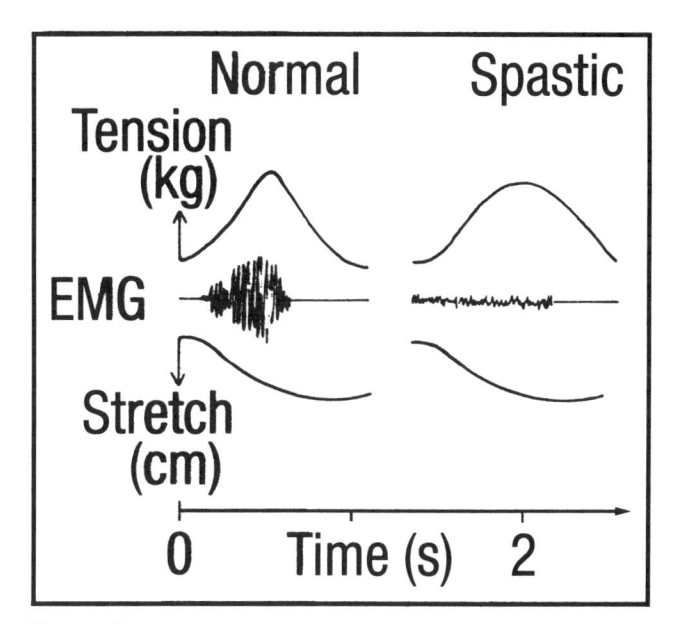

Figure 2.
Schematic illustration of tension development in a leg muscle during locomotion. (Left) Normal behavior. Increase in tension is closely correlated to muscle activation. (Right) Spastic muscle paresis. Increase in tension is closely correlated to the stretching of the slightly tonically activated muscle. This change of tension development in spastic paresis is explained by the transformation of the motor units with their muscle fibers. Changes of tension at the Achilles tendon were recorded by a buckle-type gauge. The gauge was fixed laterally near the tendon while the tendon was pressed against the force-measuring branch by a metal frame from the contralateral side. EMG=electromyographic activity.

ticity of cerebral origin has been established (however, the soleus muscle of patients with long-standing paraplegia was shown to consist of type II fibers[28]), and (3) structural changes, such as the appearance of target fibers, mainly in type I fibers.

The alteration to a simpler regulation of muscle tension could be advantageous because it enables the person with paresis due to spinal or supraspinal lesions to support the body during gait and, consequently, to achieve mobility.[32] Rapid movements, however, are no longer possible due to the absence of modulation of muscle activity. Following a severe spinal or supraspinal lesion, these transformative processes can overshoot, with unwelcome consequences (ie, painful spasms and involuntarily movements).

Patients with severe spinal or supraspinal lesions are usually much less able to perform stepping movements because the spinal locomotor centers do not provide sufficient basic activation of the leg muscles to perform functional movements such as gait. In recent years, it has been shown that specific locomotor training could enhance locomotor activity and thereby improve mobility. This approach will be discussed in the next section.

Locomotion in Patients With Paraplegia

Neuronal Capacity of Spinal Cord

For more than 30 years, functional electrical stimulation of paralyzed limb muscles was the only technique used to the improve the mobility of patients with paraplegia.[33] Despite technological developments, we believe that this method is still in at an experimental stage, and no breakthrough has occurred allowing for more extensive application of this technique.[34] The lack of a breakthrough has been due mainly to basic problems such as rapid development of muscle fatigue and adverse interactions with spinal reflexes, which cannot be overcome by technical means.[34] During the last few years, a new approach has been developed that improves the mobility of patients with paraplegia.[35–38] This improved mobility is achieved by external activation and training of spinal locomotor centers.[35–38]

In cats, recovery of locomotor function following spinal cord transection was believed to be restricted to immature animals.[39] The recovery of the locomotor patterns can be improved using regular training even in adult animals.[40] When spontaneous stepping was not stimulated, the cats lost their ability to step spontaneously.[40] During locomotor training, the animal was supported and thus only bore a part of its body weight. Locomotor movements of the hind limbs were induced by a treadmill while the forelimbs stood on a platform. With ongoing training, the body support was decreased in proportion to the animal's improving locomotor abilities. After several weeks of training, the cats were able to take more body weight and perform well-coordinated stepping movements.[35] The locomotor pattern at this stage closely resembles the pattern of the normal adult cat.[1] Thus, it can be concluded that the training represents an important factor for the recovery of locomotor function.

In humans, steplike movements are present at birth and can be initiated spontaneously or by peripheral stimuli.[41] The EMG activity underlying this newborn stepping has been shown to be centrally programmed and, as it has also been observed in children with anencephaly, it is likely that spinal mechanisms generate the EMG activity.[41] The apparent loss of locomotor movements in humans whose spinal cord was accidentally transected has been suggested to be due to a greater predominance of supraspinal over spinal neuronal mechanisms.[42] Nevertheless, there are indications that spinal interneuronal circuits exist that are involved in the generation of locomotor EMG activity in the leg muscles of humans,[3] similar to those described for cats.[35] Furthermore, involuntary steplike lower-extremity movements were recently described for a patient with an incomplete injury of the cervical spinal cord.[43]

Effect of Locomotor Training in Patients With Paraplegia

The aim of recent studies has been to determine the degree to which locomotor EMG activity and movements can be both elicited and trained in the leg muscles of patients with either complete or incomplete paraplegia.[36,37]

The induction of complex bilateral lower-extremity muscle activation combined with coordinated stepping movements in patients with incomplete and complete paraplegia was achieved by our approach of partially unloading (up to 60%) patients who were on a moving treadmill (Fig. 3).[36] To ensure consistent electrode placement over the course of training, initial electrode placement was marked by blue ink. The lower-extremity movements had to be assisted externally, especially during transitions from stance to swing, during the first phases of the training (usually 2–6 weeks, depending on the severity of paresis) in patients with incomplete paraplegia and during the whole training period (3–5 months) in patients with complete paraplegia. In comparison with subjects without neurological impairments, patients with paraplegia displayed a less dynamic mode of muscle activation (ie, it was less well modulated in amplitude) (Fig. 3). This finding may be due to the impaired function of polysynaptic spinal reflexes in patients with spinal lesions.[32] In other respects, such as the timing, the pattern of leg muscle EMG activity was similar to that seen in subjects without neurological impairments.[32] Different amplitude levels of leg extensor (the main antigravity muscle during gait) EMG activity occurred in the different subject groups, which largely exceeded the interindividual variability. The amplitude level of EMG activity was considerably smaller in patients with complete paraplegia compared with patients with incomplete paraplegia. Both patient groups had smaller EMG levels compared with those of subjects without neurological impairments (Fig. 3). Despite the reduced level of EMG activity, increased muscle tone and exaggerated reflexes were present in both patient groups. This finding supports earlier suggestions that alterations of mechanical properties of the tonically active muscle are mainly responsible for the clinical signs of spasticity.

The EMG patterns observed during locomotor training in patients with complete paraplegia may be due to rhythmic stretches of the leg muscles.[38] As shown in Figure 4, integrated EMG data for the tibialis anterior and gastrocnemius muscles were collected every 50 milliseconds over the whole step cycle and were related to the lengthening or shortening (determined by ankle and knee joint movements) of the respective muscle.[38] Leg muscle EMG activity was about equally distributed during muscle lengthening and shortening in both subjects without neurological impairments and patients

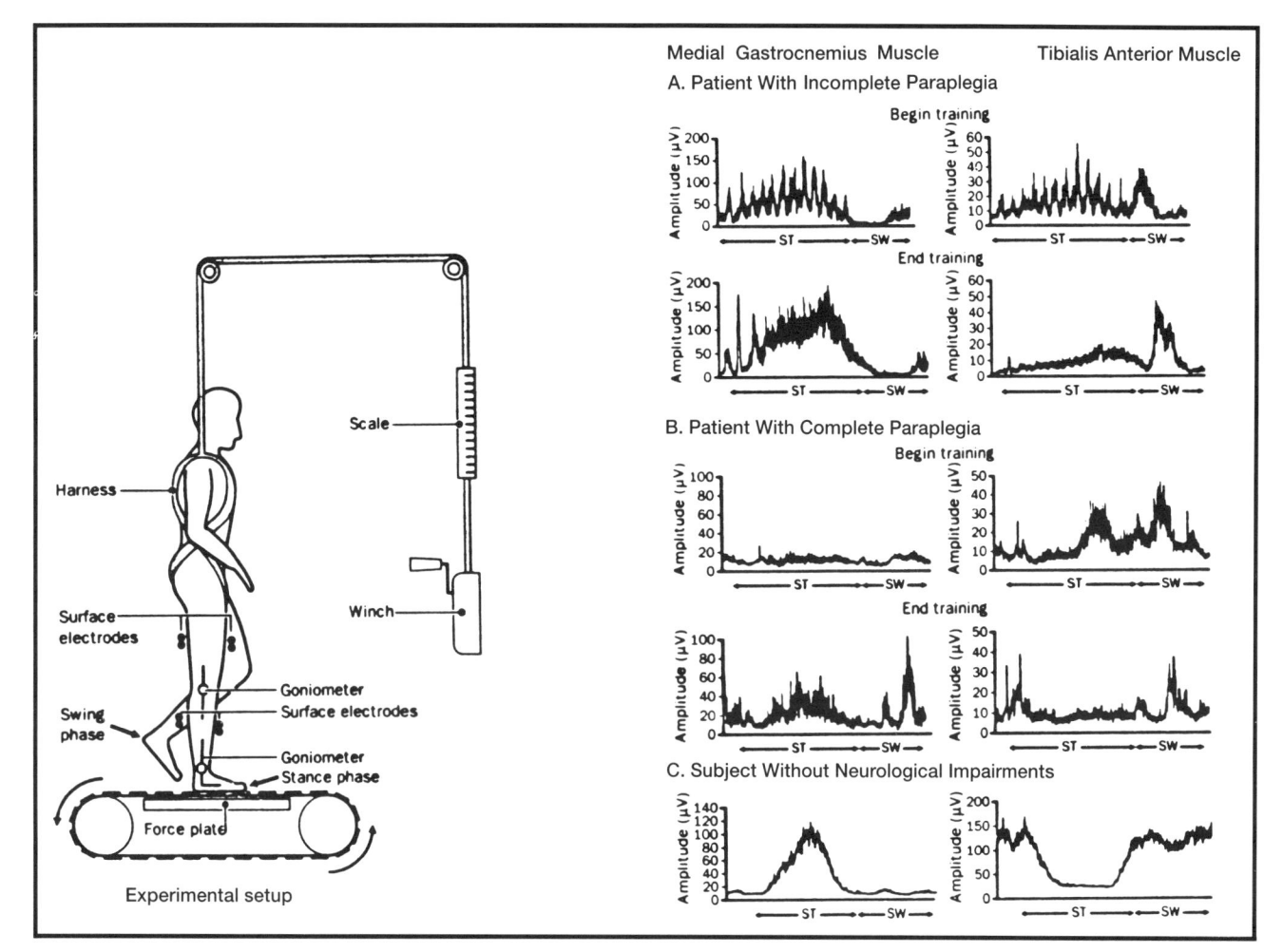

Figure 3.
Locomotor training in patients with paraplegia. (Left) Experimental setup. (Right) Rectified and averaged (n=20) electromyographic activity of lower and upper leg muscles during slow locomotion (around 1.3 km/h) for (A) a patient with incomplete paraplegia, (B) a patient with complete paraplegia, and (C) a subject without neurological impairments. For the patients, the recordings at the beginning of (above) and after (below) a locomotor training program performed daily over 5 months are displayed. The amount of unloading for the subject without neurological impairments and the patients was 50% of body load. Note different amplitude scales in the recordings. ST=stance, SW=swing phase.[36]

with complete paraplegia during locomotion. This finding indicates that stretch reflexes are unlikely to play a major role in the generation of the leg muscle EMG pattern in these patients and that the locomotor pattern is programmed at a spinal level.

During the course of a daily locomotor training program, the amplitude of gastrocnemius muscle EMG activity increased during the stance phase, whereas an inappropriate tibialis anterior muscle activation decreased.[37] These training effects were seen in both patients with incomplete and complete paraplegia (Fig. 3). The training effects were related to a greater weight-bearing function of the extensors (ie, body unloading during treadmill locomotion could be reduced). The slope of the increase of gastrocnemius muscle EMG activity was similar in patients with incomplete and complete paraplegia. This finding indicates that the isolated human spinal cord contains the capacity not only to generate a locomotor pattern, but also "to learn." Only patients with incomplete paraplegia benefited from the training program insofar as they learned to perform unsupported stepping movements on solid ground.[36,37] Patients with complete paraplegia experienced positive effects on the cardiovascular and musculoskeletal systems (ie, they had less severe spastic symptoms). In comparison with leg extensor EMG activity, only a small effect of training on leg flexor EMG amplitude was seen, which may be due to the different neuronal control of leg flexor and extensor muscles during locomotion.[44] The decreased unloading of the body (ie, successive reloading of the body) during the training may serve as a stimulus for extensor load receptors, which have been shown to be essential for leg extensor activation during locomotion in both cats[45] and humans.[46] The lower gain of extensor EMG activity (ie, the generally smaller EMG amplitude) in patients with complete paraplegia may be due to a loss of

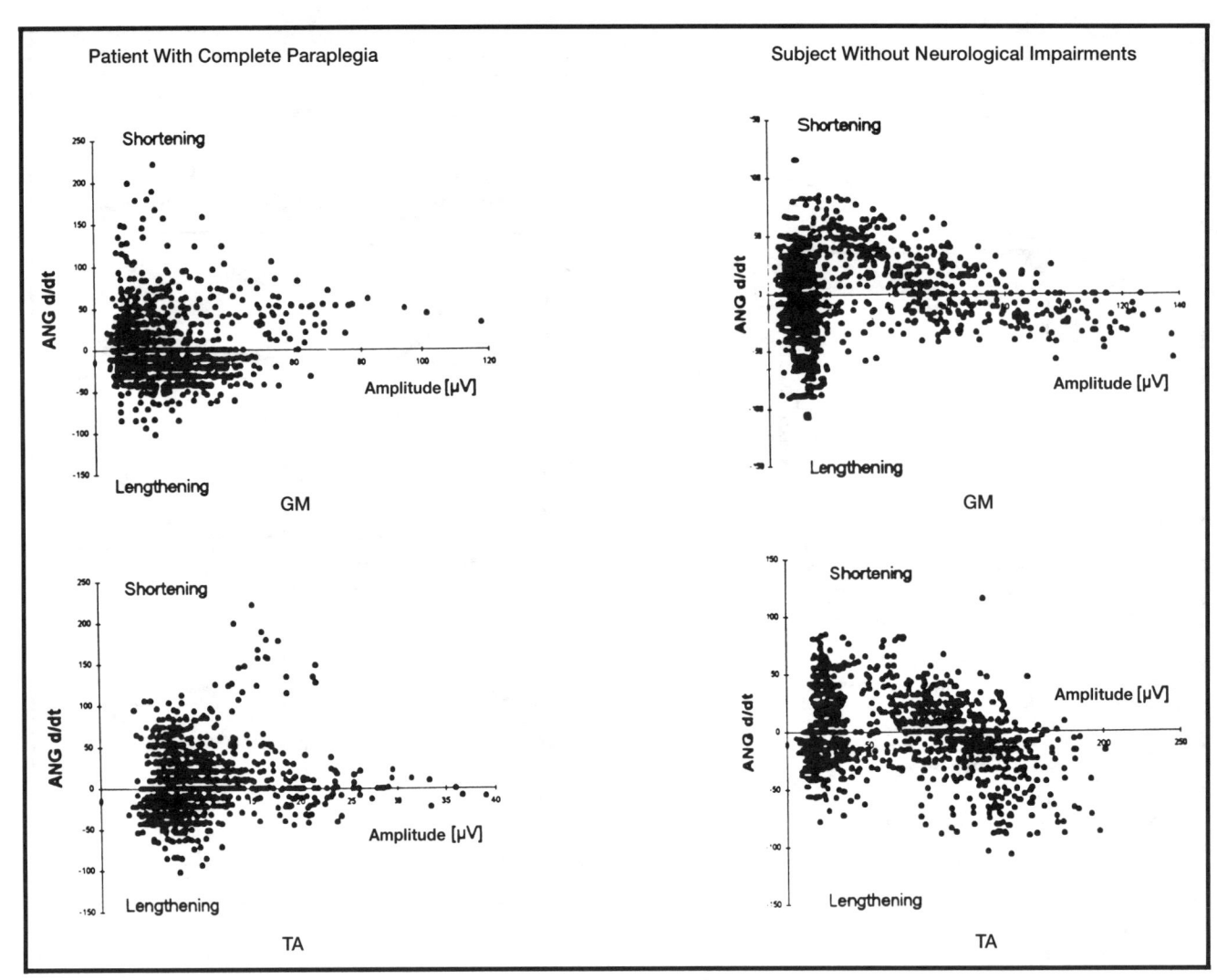

Figure 4.
Relationship between muscle lengthening and shortening (velocity at the ankle [ANG d/dt]) and electromyographic (EMG) amplitude in the medial gastrocnemius muscle (GM) and tibialis anterior muscle (TA) of a patient with complete paraplegia and a subject without neurological impairments within a step cycle (EMG amplitude measured every 100 ms). The contribution of muscle stretching to EMG activity was the key finding.

input from descending noradrenergic pathways to spinal locomotor centers.[35]

Practical Application of Locomotor Training

According to our experience over 4 years of locomotor training, the patient should be suspended by a parachute harness on the treadmill in a near-vertical body position to achieve both an axial direction of contact forces with the ground and extension of the hip during the stance phase. Depending on the severity of the spinal cord lesion, the pelvis may have to be fixed to avoid deviations in a lateral and posterior direction.

The amount of unloading should be maintained such that the maximal body load is taken over by the lower extremities but rhythmical stepping movements can still be performed. The locomotion speed should be adjusted such that an optimal rhythmicity occurs for each patient and also such that minimal assistance is required. For the assistance, an appropriate timing of stance and swing phases on either side should be achieved. Specific attention should be given to the timing of the double stance phase in order to achieve the optimal rhythmicity, which allows the patient to perform stepping movements with as little assistance as possible. The knee and hip joints should be fully extended sequentially during the stance phase to optimally support body weight. Nevertheless, hyperextension of the knees should be avoided to prevent damage of ligaments around the knee joint. The feet should pass, positioned closely together, under the vertical projection of the patient's center of gravity in order to obtain a full activation of the extensor muscles for push-off. The pelvis should be kept fixed so that loading of knee and ankle joints occurs in a physiological manner.

By unloading the body, the locomotor training can be started at an early stage of the rehabilitation program.

The locomotion training with body unloading allows the performance of rhythmical stepping movements, which can easily be assisted and controlled by the attendant physical therapists. The unloading and assistance should be adapted to the actual condition and the severity of muscle paresis of the patient. A drawback of this training approach is that in patients with complete or almost complete paraplegia, the ergonomics necessary to assist the leg movements are difficult to perform on a long-term basis (ie, over weeks to months).

Pharmacological Influences on Locomotor Activity

A recent study[37] showed no training effects in about half of the patients with complete paraplegia who underwent daily locomotor training (ie, the amplitude of leg muscle EMG activity did not increase). The a posteriori analysis led to the suggestion that this finding might be due to the action of the drugs taken by the patients. Cannabinoids[47] and prazosin (an α-1 adrenoceptor antagonist[1]) are drugs that are known to inhibit spinal neuronal activity. In contrast, Barbeau et al[48] demonstrated in spinal cats that the administration of clonidine enhances locomotor activity. Nevertheless, a contrary effect was seen in two patients following intrathecal application of a low dose (25 µg) of clonidine. This effect was also correlated with a loss of EMG activity and flaccid paresis.[37] Although a species-dependent action appears to be unlikely for this observation, there may be several explanations for the differential effects seen between cats and humans. For example, a dosage-dependent or "level of lesion"-dependent change of the drug action may explain these differential effects. The timing of drug application may also play a role because of changes of the receptor. Clonidine was applied in the acute stage following spinal cord transection in cats,[48] whereas it was given several weeks posttrauma in human patients.[37] In contrast to clonidine, the sympathomimetic drug epinephrine was shown to have a positive effect on the locomotor pattern and performance.[37] This effect was correlated with an increase of gastrocnemius muscle EMG activity during the stance phase. This finding suggests that human spinal locomotor activity can be influenced pharmacologically. Further studies are needed to determine the degree to which human spinal locomotor activity can be positively influenced by other adrenergic agonists, thereby supporting the locomotor training. Further detailed and controlled studies are needed, particularly bearing in mind that neuronal changes may occur in untreated patients during the first months following spinal cord injury.

Outlook

The analysis of neuromuscular changes following cerebral or spinal motor lesions revealed that some of these changes (eg, development of increased muscle tone) can be advantageous if they provide body support during stepping movements. This knowledge could have the consequence that these neuromuscular changes could be targeted and become incorporated into physical therapy approaches for patients.[49] However, the efficacy of such approaches is lacking, and research is needed in this area.

In severely affected patients with spinal cord injury, the strength of leg muscle activation is not sufficient to build up enough underlying muscle tone or to control limb movements for locomotion. One approach to enhance spinal locomotor activity in the patients with incomplete and complete paraplegia represents the search for substances that influence the gain of leg extensor EMG activity. Although the substances that have been investigated to date have not been convincing in their action, other substances that exhibit a stronger effect might be explored in the future. Another approach concerns the release of spinal reflexes (eg, by the electrical stimulation of cutaneous nerves[50]), thereby physiologically enhancing and controlling leg muscle EMG patterns.[51] A promising approach for the future may be to induce partial regeneration of the lesioned spinal cord tract fibers. Recent experiments with rats have indicated that after inhibition of neurite growth inhibitors, partial regeneration can occur. (See review by Schwab.[52]) Combined with appropriate locomotor training, this approach may improve functional mobility, even that of patients with almost complete paraplegia.

References

1 Grillner S. Control of locomotion in bipeds, tetrapods, and fish. In: Brookhart M, Mountcastle VB, eds. *Handbook of Physiology: The Nervous System, Volume II: Motor Control, Part 2*. Washington, DC: American Physiological Society; 1981:1179–1235.

2 Gordon CR, Fletcher WA, Melvill Jones G, Block EW. Adaptive plasticity in the control of locomotor trajectory. *Exp Brain Res*. 1995; 102:540–545.

3 Armstrong DM. The supraspinal control of mammalian locomotion. *J Physiol (Lond)*. 1988;405:1–37.

4 Dietz V. Human neuronal control of automatic functional movements: interaction between central programs and afferent input. *Physiol Rev*. 1992;73:33–69.

5 Gollhofer A, Schmidtbleicher D, Dietz V. Regulation of muscle stiffness in human locomotion. *Int J Sports Med*. 1984;5:19–22.

6 Lance JW. Symposium synopsis. In: Feldman RG, Young RR, Koella WP, eds. *Spasticity: Disordered Motor Control*. Chicago, Ill: Year Book Publishing Co Inc; 1980:485–495.

7 Mendell LM. Modifiability of spinal synapses. *Physiol Rev*. 1984;64: 260–324.

8 Carr LJ, Harrison LM, Evans AL, Stephens JA. Patterns of central motor reorganization in hemiplegic cerebral palsy. *Brain*. 1993;116: 1223–1247.

9 Nacimiento W, Mautes A, Töpper R, et al. B-50 (GAP-42) in the spinal cord caudal to hemisection: indication for lack of intraspinal sprouting in dorsal root axons. *J Neurosci Res*. 1993;35:603–617.

10 Ashby P. Discussion I. In: Emre M, Benecke R, eds. *Spasticity: The Current Status of Research and Treatment*. Carnforth, United Kingdom: Parthenon; 1989:68–69.

11 Burke D, Ashby P. Are spinal "presynaptic" inhibitory mechanisms suppressed in spasticity? *J Neurol Sci.* 1972;15:321–326.

12 Faist M, Mazevet D, Dietz V, Pierrot-Deseilligny E. A quantitative assessment of presynaptic inhibition of Ia afferents in spastics: differences in hemiplegics and paraplegics. *Brain.* 1994;117:1449–1455.

13 Thilmann AF, Fellows SJ, Garms E. Pathological stretch reflexes on the "good" side of hemiparetic patients. *J Neurol Neurosurg Psychiatry.* 1990;53:208–214.

14 Thilmann AF, Fellows SJ, Garms E. The mechanism of spastic muscle hypertonus: variation in reflex gain over the time course spasticity. *Brain.* 1991;114:233–244.

15 Ibrahim IK, Berger W, Trippel M, Dietz V. Stretch-induced electromyographic activity and torque in spastic elbow muscles. *Brain.* 1993;116:971–989.

16 Berger W, Quintern J, Dietz V. Tension development and muscle activation in the leg during gait in spastic hemiparesis: the independence of muscle hypertonia and exaggerated stretch reflexes. *J Neurol Neurosurg Psychiatry.* 1984;47:1029–1033.

17 Dietz V, Berger W. Normal and impaired regulation of muscles stiffness in gait: a new hypothesis about muscle hypertonia. *Exp Neurol.* 1983;79:680–687.

18 Dietz V, Trippel M, Berger W. Reflex activity and muscle tone during elbow movements in patients with spastic paresis. *Ann Neurol.* 1991;30:767–779.

19 Powers RK, Campbell DL, Rymer WZ. Stretch reflex dynamics in spastic elbow flexor muscles. *Ann Neurol.* 1989;25:32–42.

20 Berger W, Quintern J, Dietz V. Pathophysiology of gait in children with cerebral palsy. *Electroencephalogr Clin Neurophysiol.* 1982;53:538–548.

21 Dietz V, Ketelsen UP, Berger W, Quintern J. Motor unit involvement in spastic paresis: relationship between leg muscle activation and histochemistry. *J Neurol Sci.* 1986;75:89–103.

22 Rosenfalck A, Andreassen S. Impaired regulation of force and firing pattern of single motor units in patients with spasticity. *J Neurol Neurosurg Psychiatry.* 1980;43:907–916.

23 Powers RK, Marder-Meyer J, Rymer WZ. Quantitative relations between hypertonia and stretch reflex threshold in spastic hemiparesis. *Ann Neurol.* 1988;23:115–124.

24 Lee WA, Boughton A, Rymer WZ. Absence of stretch reflex gain enhancement in voluntarily activated spastic muscle. *Exp Neurol.* 1987;98:317–335.

25 Young JL, Mayer RF. Physiological alterations of motor units in hemiplegia. *J Neurol Sci.* 1992;54:401–412.

26 Dietz V, Berger W. Interlimb coordination of posture in patients with spastic paresis: impaired function of spinal reflexes. *Brain.* 1984;107:965–978.

27 Cope TC, Bodine SC, Fournier M, Edgerton VR. Soleus motor units in chronic spinal transected cats: physiological and morphological alterations. *J Neurophysiol.* 1986;55:1202–1220.

28 Shields RK. Fatigability, relaxation properties, and electromyographic responses of the human paralyzed soleus muscle. *J Neurophysiol.* 1995;73:1295–2205.

29 Hufschmidt A, Mauritz KH. Chronic transformation of muscle in spasticity: a peripheral contribution to increased tone. *J Neurol Neurosurg Psychiatry.* 1985;48:676–685.

30 Sinkjaer T, Toft E, Larsen K, et al. Non-reflex and reflex mediated ankle joint stiffness in multiple sclerosis patients with spasticity. *Muscle Nerve.* 1993;16:69–76.

31 Edström L. Selective changes in the size of red and white muscle fibres in upper motor lesions and parkinsonism. *J Neurol Sci.* 1970;11:537–555.

32 Dietz V, Quintern J, Berger W. Electrophysiological studies of gait in spasticity and rigidity: evidence that altered mechanical properties of muscle contribute to hypertonia. *Brain.* 1981;104:431–449.

33 Kantrowitz A. *Electronic Physiologic Aids: Report of the Maimonides Hospital.* Brooklyn, NY: Maimonides Hospital; 1960:4–5.

34 Quintern J, Minwegen P, Mauritz K-H. Control mechanisms for restoring posture and movements in paraplegics. In: Allum JHJ, Hulliger M, eds. Afferent Control of Posture and Locomotion. *Prog Brain Res.* 1989;80(special issue):489–502.

35 Barbeau H, Rossignol S. Enhancement of locomotor recovery following spinal cord injury. *Curr Opin Neurol.* 1994;7:517–524.

36 Dietz V, Colombo G, Jensen L. Locomotor activity in spinal man. *Lancet.* 1994;344:1260–1263.

37 Dietz V, Colombo G, Jensen L, Baumgartner L. Locomotor capacity of spinal cord in paraplegic patients. *Ann Neurol.* 1995;37:574–582.

38 Dietz V. Locomotor training in paraplegic patients. *Ann Neurol.* 1995;38:965.

39 Forssberg H, Grillner S, Halbertsma J. Role in spinal cord locomotion of the low spinal cat, II: interlimb coordination. *Acta Physiol Scand.* 1980;108:238–295.

40 Barbeau H, Rossignol S. Recovery of locomotion after chronic spinalization in the adult cat. *Brain Res.* 1987;412:84–95.

41 Forssberg H. A developmental model of human locomotion. In: Grillner S, Stein PSG, Stuart DG, et al, eds. *Neurobiology of Vertebrate Locomotion, Volume 45.* London, United Kingdom: Macmillan Publishers Ltd; 1986:485–501.

42 Kuhn RA. Functional capacity of the isolated human spinal cord. *Brain.* 1950;73:1–51.

43 Calancie B, Needham-Shropshine B, Jacobs P, et al. Involuntarily stepping after chronic spinal cord injury: evidence for a control rhythm generator locomotion in man. *Brain.* 1994;17:1143–1159.

44 Dietz V, Horstmann GA, Berger W. Interlimb coordination of leg-muscle activation during perturbation of stance in humans. *J Neurophysiol.* 1989;62:680–693.

45 Pearson KG, Collins DF. Reversal of the influence of group Ib-afferents from plantaris on activity in medial gastrocnemius muscle during locomotor activity. *J Neurophysiol.* 1993;70:1009–1017.

46 Dietz V, Gollhofer A, Kleiber M, Trippel M. Regulation of bipedal stance: dependency on "load" receptors. *Exp Brain Res.* 1992;89:229–231.

47 Meinck HM, Schönle PW, Conrad B. Effect of cannabinoids on spasticity and ataxia in multiple sclerosis. *J Neurol.* 1989;236:120–122.

48 Barbeau HJ, Julien C, Rossignol S. The effects of clonidine and yohimbine on locomotion and cutaneous reflexes in the adult chronic spinal cat. *Brain Res.* 1987;437:83–96.

49 O'Dwyer NJ, Ada L, Neilson PD. Spasticity and muscle contracture following stroke. *Brain.* 1996;119:1737–1749.

50 Tax AAM, van Wezel BMH, Dietz V. Bipedal reflex coordination to tactile stimulation of the sural nerve during human running. *J Neurophysiol.* 1995;73:1947–1964.

51 Jones CA, Yang JF. Reflex behaviour during walking in incomplete spinal cord injured subjects. *Exp Neurol.* 1994;128:239–248.

52 Schwab ME. Regeneration of lesioned CNS axons by neutralisation of neurite growth inhibitors: a short review. *Paraplegia.* 1991;29:294–298.

Postural Perturbations: New Insights for Treatment of Balance Disorders

This article reviews the neural control of posture as understood through studies of automatic responses to mechanical perturbations. Recent studies of responses to postural perturbations have provided a new view of how postural stability is controlled, and this view has profound implications for physical therapy practice. We discuss the implications for rehabilitation of balance disorders and demonstrate how an understanding of the specific systems underlying postural control can help to focus and enrich our therapeutic approaches. By understanding the basic systems underlying control of balance, such as strategy selection, rapid latencies, coordinated temporal spatial patterns, force control, and context-specific adaptations, therapists can focus their treatment on each patient's specific impairments. Research on postural responses to surface translations has shown that balance is not based on a fixed set of equilibrium reflexes but on a flexible, functional motor skill that can adapt with training and experience. More research is needed to determine the extent to which quantification of automatic postural responses has practical implications for predicting falls in patients with constraints in their postural control system. [Horak FB, Henry SM, Shumway-Cook A. Postural perturbations: new insights for treatment of balance disorders. *Phys Ther.* 1997;77:517–533.]

Key Words: *Balance, Electromyography, Neurology, Posture.*

Fay B Horak

Sharon M Henry

Anne Shumway-Cook

Postural control, although poorly understood, is critical for the efficient and effective performance of all goal-directed activities. A useful experimental approach to understanding neural control of posture is the disrupting of stable equilibrium and the recording of behavioral reactions to these perturbations. Magnus,[1] Rademaker,[2] and Sherrington[3] described responses to disequilibrium in infants and animals almost 100 years ago. Over the last 20 years (see reviews by Horak and Macpherson,[4] Dietz,[5] and Massion[6]), however, the application of new technology to quantify the surface forces, muscle activations, movement patterns, and joint torques that characterize postural responses involving the entire body has provided many new insights into posture and movement control. Recent studies of responses to postural perturbations have provided insight into multijoint coordination and multisensory interaction in motor control in general, and not just specific to the task of postural stability. Studies of postural responses have helped lead the way from a "reflex/hierarchical" concept of motor control to a "systems" approach, which emphasizes a goal-directed neural organization of multiple, interacting systems.[7,8]

Recent studies of responses to postural perturbations have provided new views of how postural stability is controlled. Previously, balance was viewed as resulting from a distinct set of reflex-like equilibrium responses elicited by stimuli to a particular sensory system and neural balance center.[1,2] More recently, balance has been viewed as a skill that the nervous system learns to accomplish using many systems, including passive biomechanical elements, all available sensory systems and muscles, and many different parts of the brain. We believe that balance can no longer be viewed as a totally reactive response to sensory stimuli. Instead, results from platform studies have shown that equilibrium control is quite proactive, adaptive, and centrally organized based on prior experience and intention.[9]

Changes in our basic understanding of how the central nervous system (CNS) controls postural stability have implications for physical therapy practice. Therapists are no longer limited to retraining balance by facilitating a fixed set of equilibrium reflexes. By viewing balance as a fundamental motor skill that the nervous system learns, therapists can recognize the potential for applying concepts from motor learning such as practice, feedback, experience, and education to retraining balance.

The practical importance of studying responses to external perturbations is becoming more and more apparent to physical therapists. The majority of falls among elderly persons are thought to be due to inadequate responses to perturbations. About 50% of these falls are thought to be due to sudden motion of the base of support such as slips and trips, 35% are believed to be due to external displacement of the body's center of mass (COM), and only 10% can be attributed to spontaneous falls related to physiological episodes such as dizziness, seizures, or transient ischemic attacks.[10] Maki and colleagues[11] also found that quantification of postural responses to lateral surface translations was one of the best predictors of future falls among elderly persons. Quick, coordinated responses to environmental perturbations are a very important part of effective stability during stance and gait. Therefore, we believe that laboratory quantification of postural responses may be used to predict balance in functional activities and is useful in clinical assessments of balance.

This article focuses on insights into the neural control of posture achieved through studies of automatic responses to mechanical (primarily surface) perturbations. We will summarize what perturbation studies have taught us about specific control systems that are responsible for strategy selection, rapid latency, coordinated temporal-spatial patterns, force control, and context-specific adaptation of postural responses. We will then discuss the implications for rehabilitation of balance disorders and demonstrate how a better understanding of the specific systems underlying postural control can assist in developing therapeutic approaches.

Definition of Postural Control

A postural perturbation is a sudden change in conditions that displaces the body posture away from equilibrium. These perturbations could consist of sensory perturbations, such as vestibular perturbations that result from electrical stimulation,[12] visual perturbations caused by a moving room or moving visual images,[13] or somatosensory perturbations caused by vibration of muscle.[14] The postural reactions to these sensory perturbations may be in response to perceptions of instability rather than to actual disequilibrium.[4] In contrast, mechanical perturbations actually displace the position of body segments, which may lead to displacement of the total-body COM, or disequilibrium. Small displacements of a single body segment, such as the head, can result in very

---

FB Horak, PhD, PT, is Senior Scientist and Professor, RS Dow Neurological Sciences Institute, 1120 NW 20th Ave, Portland, OR 97209-1595 (USA) (fay@nsi.lhs.org). Address all correspondence to Dr Horak.

SM Henry, PhD, PT, is Research Associate, RS Dow Neurological Sciences Institute.

Anne Shumway-Cook, PhD, PT, is Research Coordinator, Department of Physical Therapy, Northwest Hospital, Seattle, Wash.

small muscle responses throughout the body,[15] but larger displacements of the total-body COM require large enough responses to exert directionally specific forces at contact surfaces to return the body's COM to equilibrium.[16] Mechanical postural perturbations can be applied to any body part, such as a push to the trunk,[17,18] head,[15] or limbs.[19] The most common experimental approach is to perturb the support surface, which displaces the base of support under the body's COM. These support-surface perturbations are similar to a slip, trip, surface irregularity, or acceleration or deceleration of a moving surface such as a bus in which an individual is balancing.

Postural equilibrium is the condition in which all the forces acting on the body are balanced such that the COM is controlled relative to the base of support, either in a particular position or during movements. Control of balance, or equilibrium, can be reactive, that is, in response to external forces displacing the COM, or proactive, as occurs in anticipation of internally generated, destabilizing forces imposed by the body's own movements. Both external forces, including gravity and forces related to interaction with the environment, and internal forces, which are generated during all body movements, even respiration, ultimately act to destabilize the body by accelerating its COM. The role of the nervous system is to detect and predict instability and produce the appropriate muscle forces that will complement and coordinate with all the other forces acting on the body so that the COM is well controlled and balance is maintained.

No response to an external postural perturbation is totally reactive. Platform perturbation studies indicate that although automatic postural responses to external displacements of the body's COM are shaped by the sensory characteristics of the perturbation, responses also are shaped by CNS mechanisms related to expectations, attention, experience, environmental context, and intention, as well as by preprogrammed muscle activation patterns called *synergies*.[9] Thus, carefully constructed studies of automatic responses to external perturbations may reveal the relative contribution of many different central neural mechanisms in coordinating the multisegmental task of maintaining postural equilibrium.

The clinical implications of recent postural perturbation research suggest that observing how a patient responds to external perturbations provides therapists with a window into (1) how effectively the patient's sensory and motor systems respond to a particular pattern of sensory stimuli, (2) how well the patient's nervous system is prepared for and adapts to perturbations under a variety of contexts, and (3) how well the patient learns and executes a preplanned, coordinated motor pattern. Evaluation of responses to perturbations may also predict the likelihood for falls in natural environments.[20,21] We believe, however, that therapists need to recognize that responses to perturbations reveal only one aspect of the postural control system. In order to fully characterize a patient's postural control, therapists should also consider mechanisms related to control of (1) stability and antigravity muscle tone in steady-state positions such as stance and sitting, (2) sensory interpretation for spatial orientation and body alignment, and (3) equilibrium control in anticipation of and during movement, locomotion, or changes in posture. This article focuses on postural responses to external perturbations and will not address these other aspects of postural control.

Postural Responses: What Have We Learned?

Synergies and Strategies

Studies of how we control equilibrium of the multi-segmented body against gravity and environmental disturbances have led to two important motor control concepts: muscle synergy patterns and movement strategies.[22-24] Nashner[22,25] first described normal muscle synergies as stereotyped patterns of bursts of muscle activity in response to surface translations and rotations. Initially, these synergies were thought to be the result of hardwired, inflexible central pattern generators of the nervous system. Synergies were thought to be long loop extensions of the stretch reflex. Postural synergies were labeled "functional stretch reflexes" because they adapted to include activation of nonstretched muscles if required for the function of postural stability.[25] Over the last 20 years, however, the notion of muscle synergies has evolved toward a concept of "flexible" synergies, defined as centrally organized patterns of muscle activity that are responsive to initial conditions, perturbation characteristics, learning, and intention.[4,23,26] Understanding synergistic organization of multiple muscles for a common goal is useful to explain normal motor coordination, as well as disordered coordination such as occurs with brain injury.

The concept of postural strategies emerged as investigators struggled with a way to describe general sensorimotor solutions to the control of posture, including not only muscle synergies but also movement patterns, joint torques, and contact forces. Nashner and McCollum[27] predicted and Horak and Nashner[24] described two distinct postural response "strategies," an ankle strategy and a hip strategy, that people could use to maintain equilibrium in response to anterior or posterior surface translations. Horak[5,24,28,29] also predicted a "stepping strategy," which has since been well characterized.

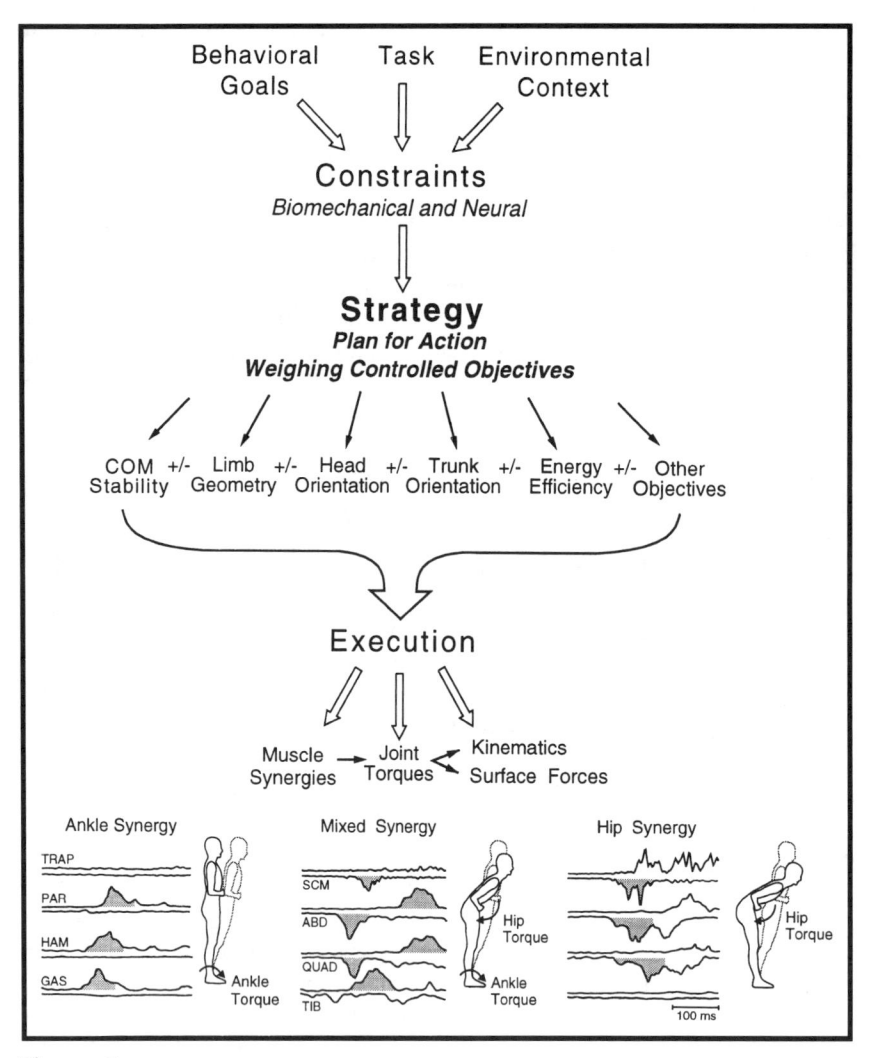

Figure 1.
A conceptual framework for the emergence of strategies that are plans for action. COM=center of mass, TRAP=trapezius muscle, SCM=sternocleidomastoid muscle, PAR=lumbar paraspinal muscles, ABD=rectus abdominis muscle, HAM=hamstring muscles, QUAD=rectus femoris muscle, GAS=gastrocnemius muscles, TIB=tibialis anterior muscle.

Horak and Nashner[24] discovered that these strategies were not hardwired like reflexes, but could gradually be learned with experience in new environmental contexts. At first, these strategies were conceived as consisting of distinct, centrally programmed patterns that were combined to provide a continuum of "mixed" strategies.[24] More recently, the continuum of postural strategies from ankle to hip is considered to be similar to the continuum of locomotor strategies in which there are transitions from walking to galloping and trotting.[22] The stepping, or stumbling, strategy could, however, represent a truly independent strategy that is usually preferred to the hip strategy when there are no surface or instructional constraints. Thus, the strategy concept has been gradually changing to allow for the functional flexibility, specificity, and motor learning apparent in postural behavior.[4]

Horak[4,7–9] now hypothesizes that strategies are emergent neural control processes providing an overall "plan for action" based on the behavioral goals, environmental context, and particular task or activity (Fig. 1). The plan for action involves prioritizing many potential controlled variables of postural control such as control of the body's COM,[6,30,33] limb geometry,[34] stabilization of the head and visual fixation,[35] alignment of the trunk in space,[12,34] energy efficiency,[36] and contact forces.[37] Thus, what the nervous system is controlling in any particular postural situation, and how this is done, can vary depending on the individual's goals, the environmental context, and the task that the person is conducting. For example, when attempting to read a hand-held book while walking, stabilization of the head and gaze to the hand with the written word may be the highest priority, whereas when attempting to balance a full glass of water while walking, stabilization of the hand and glass with respect to gravity emerges as the highest priority in order to accomplish the task.[38]

Strategies that emerge in any situation are limited by both external constraints (ie, those imposed by the environment and the particular task) and internal constraints (ie, those imposed by an individual's biomechanical system and nervous system) (Fig. 1). Inter-

These strategies can be characterized by their different muscle synergies, kinematics, and joint torques.[30] The ankle strategy uses distal-to-proximal muscle activation, the hip strategy uses early proximal hip and trunk muscle activation, and the stepping strategy uses early activation of hip abductors and ankle co-contraction.[24,29] These strategies can be differentiated by the large angular trunk acceleration of the hip strategy and by the flexible inverted-pendulum style of the ankle strategy, which includes motions at the knee and hip as well as at the ankle.[31] The ankle strategy moves the body's COM with torques primarily at the ankle and the knee.[31] The hip strategy adds hip torque to the ankle and knee torque.[31] The stepping strategy is characterized by asymmetrical loading and unloading of the legs to move the base of support under the falling COM.[24,28,32]

nal, biomechanical constraints, such as the number of limbs available, joint range of motion, and strength of muscles involved in the task, as well as internal, neural constraints, such as the extent to which attention is focused on the task, accuracy of sensory information, and force- and position-control mechanisms in the nervous system, will ultimately shape the emergent strategy.

Horak and Macpherson[4] and Horak and Shumway-Cook[32] hypothesize that postural strategies may be best differentiated by what the CNS is attempting to control. Computer models have shown that the hip strategy is optimal for quickly moving the COM, whereas the ankle strategy is optimal for maintaining a trunk vertical orientation while moving the COM.[32,36] However, these goals are not discrete and mutually exclusive. People use a whole continuum of strategies to control multiple neural objectives in the face of a variety of biomechanical and neural constraints, depending on the circumstances.

Researchers who investigate postural strategies in response to perturbations in different directions,[16,39] at different perturbation sites,[18] in different initial postural alignments,[40,41] and under different sensory conditions are searching for invariant neural objectives or "controlled variables." For example, postural strategies for recovery of stability following lateral surface perturbations may be similar to the so-called "ankle" strategy for anteroposterior perturbations. The goal of both types of strategies is to move the COM without compromising an erect trunk via loading and unloading of vertical surface force under the feet. The muscle synergies, kinematics, and joint torques used to implement the sagittal and lateral postural strategies, however, must be different to accommodate the different biomechanical constraints of sagittal-plane movement versus frontal-plane movement.[16,39,42] For example, correction for lateral perturbations involves early activation of the hip abductors rather than the ankle muscles.[39]

Thus, although a strategy may be identified by measuring kinematic, electromyographic (EMG), or force variables, these variables describe how the strategy is implemented and not, necessarily, the strategy itself (Fig. 1). A strategy is best described by what the CNS is attempting to control. Although it is often very difficult to determine what the nervous system is attempting to control, examining invariance in the way postural strategies are implemented can help researchers determine what the CNS is controlling. The implementation of many types of normal and abnormal postural strategies in response to disequilibrium have been well characterized in the literature.[15,22,24,29,43-50] This information can be very useful for improving therapists' understanding of the basis for instability and for designing effective interventions for improving balance that are specific to the underlying cause.[24,43,47,51,52]

Studies of postural strategies used by patients with sensory loss have shown that strategy selection depends not only on biomechanical constraints, but also on the sensory information available to the nervous system. Patients with complete vestibular loss are unable to utilize a hip strategy in recovery of their balance even when standing across a narrow beam where a hip strategy is required for efficient control of equilibrium.[43] In contrast, impaired somatosensory information from the lower limbs from peripheral neuropathy or ischemic leg cuffs results in an inability to use an ankle strategy effectively and reliance on a hip or stepping strategy.[43,51] This research suggests that utilization of the ankle strategy requires adequate surface somatosensory information and that utilization of the hip strategy requires adequate vestibular information. Thus, postural strategies that emerge in any situation are further constrained by the availability of sensory information inherent in the environment and perceived by the individual.

Postural Response Latencies

The earliest responses to surface perturbations are called "automatic postural responses" because postural latencies (70–180 milliseconds) are much longer than stretch reflex latencies (40–50 milliseconds), but shorter than voluntary reaction times (180–250 milliseconds).[19] Part of the delay in activating postural muscles comes from conduction delays. Muscles closer to the spinal cord, such as those of the neck or arm, are often, but not always, activated prior to muscles farther away, such as those crossing the ankles.[15,18] Results of platform perturbation studies suggest that centrally programmed synergies can delay activation of muscles more proximal to the spinal cord in order to obtain a particular functional spatiotemporal pattern. For example, in the ankle strategy, distal muscles at the ankle are activated well in advance of the trunk muscles, suggesting a central delay in activating the trunk muscles.[53]

Delays in the onset of a postural response can arise from (1) slowed sensory or motor conduction such as occurs with peripheral neuropathies,[51] (2) slowed spinal conduction such as can occur with multiple sclerosis,[54] or (3) delay in central processing such as occurs with Down syndrome,[44] cerebral palsy,[44] or aging.[45,55] Figure 2 illustrates a 45-millisecond delay in onset of ankle, knee, and hip muscle activity in response to a backward surface translation in a patient with diabetic peripheral neuropathy. Some persons compensate for delayed postural response latencies by increasing the magnitude of their responses and using more anticipatory control.[54] Apparent delays in postural responses as evaluated by body motion may not be related to an actual delay in onset of

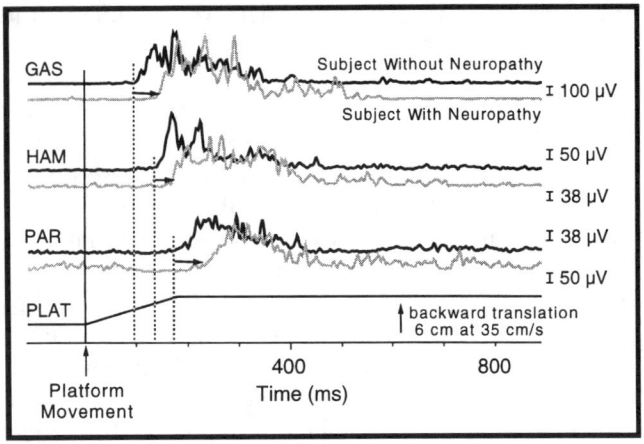

Figure 2.
Display of postural responses with impaired somatosensation for a representative subject with peripheral neuropathy (thin trace) are delayed compared with those for a subject without neuropathy (thick trace). Typical averaged electromyographic recordings from each subject activated in response to a backward platform translation of 6 cm at 35 cm/s. The three dotted vertical lines mark the burst onsets for each of the muscle groups for the subject without neuropathy. The muscle burst onsets for the subject with neuropathy are delayed. GAS=medial gastrocnemius muscle, HAM=biceps femoris muscle, PAR=paraspinal muscles, PLAT=platform. (Adapted from Inglis et al.[51])

EMG activity but to a slow rate of force production, a slow increase of muscle activity, or an abnormal spatiotemporal coordination of synergies.[47]

Spatiotemporal Coordination

Postural muscle synergies are organized in space and time to produce effective forces against support surfaces to move the body's COM and to control or prevent excessive motion at joints due to indirect, interactive torques. For example, the ankle synergy is implemented with early activation of ankle muscles to produce torques at the surface, followed by activation of knee and then hip muscles approximately 30 to 50 milliseconds later to control excessive knee and hip buckling due to the effect of ankle torques on other joints.[27,56]

Postural responses are not always initiated in the stretched muscles. For example, the first functional response to a toes-up tilt of the surface is in the shortened tibialis anterior muscle.[25] The earliest postural muscle activation may be at the neck[15] or arms,[57] instead of at the ankles, depending on the speed of perturbation and the particular context (eg, gaze instructions or presence of handrails).[57,58]

A muscle is not activated for only one direction of perturbation, but is activated over a small range of perturbation directions, with a maximum activation often in response to a diagonal direction of perturbation.[39] Figure 3A shows that activation of the left tensor fasciae latae muscle is maximal for a lateral perturbation to the right. It is also active for a range of anterolateral and posterolateral directions. When the magnitude of EMG responses to postural perturbations in 12 different directions is plotted as a polar plot, maximum muscle activation for most muscles tends to be in one of two main diagonals (Fig. 3B).[39] These results suggest that the nervous system constrains muscles to work together as synergies that are flexibly tuned to the specific biomechanical conditions, such as perturbation direction or initial stance width.

Patients with neurological impairments may show abnormal spatiotemporal coordination of automatic postural responses. Patients with stroke, head injury, or spastic cerebral palsy, as well as some elderly individuals, can show reversals in the normal distal-to-proximal temporal sequencing of postural muscle activation, resulting in excessive buckling or hyperextension of the knees and hips.[46,56,59] Abnormal spatiotemporal coordination of postural muscle responses has also been seen in patients with Parkinson's disease.[47,60] Some patients with Parkinson's disease show excessive coactivation of muscles in response to surface translations (Fig. 4).[47,60] Although patients with Parkinson's disease show normal latencies in the gastrocnemius, hamstring, and paraspinal muscles in response to forward sway, they often additionally add bursts in antagonist tibialis anterior, quadriceps femoris, and rectus abdominis muscles, which would increase stiffness but would be ineffective for direction-specific forces against the surface to preserve equilibrium. Abnormal spatiotemporal coordination of postural synergies could result from problems in creation of the synergies themselves, from interaction among simultaneous synergies, or from abnormal sensorimotor or biomechanical constraints.

Force Control

Platform perturbation studies have indicated that individuals without neurological impairments proportionally scale the magnitude of their automatic postural responses to the magnitude of their disequilibrium.[61,62] This scaling is based on both direct sensory characteristics, such as the initial speed of perturbation, and anticipatory mechanisms based on prediction of displacement characteristics, such as the estimated displacement amplitude. Figure 5A shows normal scaling of the magnitude of gastrocnemius muscle activation and the resulting surface reactive torque in response to increasing amplitudes of backward surface translations. Because automatic postural responses are initiated at 100 milliseconds, the nervous system does not have sensory information available about the amplitude of displacements of longer duration and therefore must rely on predictive mechanisms based on prior experience.[62] The role of prediction can be illustrated by comparing the scaling of postural response to predict-

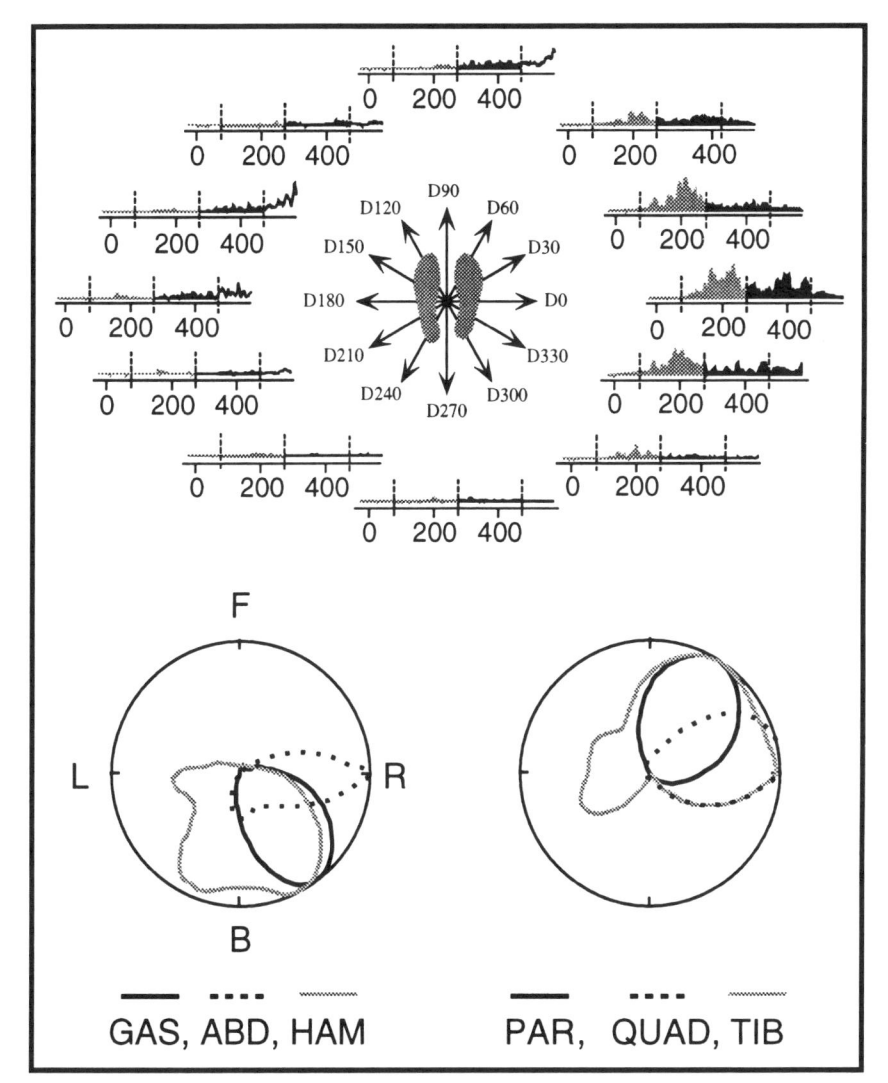

Figure 3.
The top portion of the figure shows electromyographic (EMG) activity from left tensor fasciae latae muscle that is averaged from five trials for each perturbation direction in narrow stance for one subject. The EMG integrals were calculated from individual trials using fixed windows (dotted lines) from 70 to 270 ms (early) and from 270 to 470 ms (late) after platform onset (0 ms). The bottom portion of the figure represents the six muscle amplitude changes with perturbation direction superimposed upon each other. These muscle "tuning curves" are created by normalizing the EMG integrals such that the maximum EMG amplitude reaches the circle radius. The tuning curves generally group into one of two diagonal regions. PAR=lumbar paraspinal muscles, ABD=rectus abdominis muscle, HAM=hamstring muscles, QUAD=rectus femoris muscle, GAS=gastrocnemius muscles, TIB=tibialis anterior muscle. (Adapted from Henry et al.[39])

able amplitudes and lack of scaling when the same amplitudes were unpredictable (Fig. 5C).

Many patients with neurological disorders show abnormally small (hypometric) or large (hypermetric) responses to postural displacements (Fig. 5B) despite normal latencies. For example, patients with Parkinson's disease often show hypometric postural responses related to slow buildup of EMG activation and coactivation. In contrast, patients with midline cerebellar disorders, such as anterior lobe atrophy, often show hypermetric postural responses in which each EMG burst is too large and too long, resulting in falls in the direction opposite to the direction of perturbation.[48] Patients with cerebellar dysfunction try to compensate for these hypermetric responses with large, reciprocal activation of antagonists. Despite the fact that persons with parkinsonism and cerebellar dysfunction show abnormal magnitudes of postural response, their ability to increase the magnitude of responses based on velocity feedback is intact.[60] In contrast to this ability to use sensory feedback for velocity modification, patients with cerebellar dysfunction show the unique problem of inability to adjust their postural responses based on prediction from prior experience (Fig. 5C).[60] Patients with parkinsonism adjust to predicted amplitudes when small forces are required, but they have difficulty generating the larger forces required to adjust responses to larger amplitudes (Fig. 5C). Thus, the balance problems of both persons with parkinsonism and those with cerebellar dysfunction are partly related to abnormal force control, but in very different ways, suggesting very different functional problems.

Adaptation of Postural Strategies

Context-specific adaptation. Results from platform perturbation studies have provided insight into the adaptability of the postural system. These studies have shown that automatic postural coordination is flexible and adapted to particular tasks and contexts based on the sensory information specific to each condition. The particular muscle synergies activated in response to an external perturbation depend on initial body position,[41,63] the initial support conditions,[19,64] and the location and characteristics of the sensory stimuli triggering the response.[61]

Experimental studies have shown that any group of muscles or any body segment can be used in a postural role, depending on the initial body positions and support conditions.[65] For example, responses to surface translations while maintaining bipedal versus quadrupedal stance results in a switch from using primarily ankle extensors to using primarily ventral hip flexors and co-contraction of arm muscles in both humans and cats

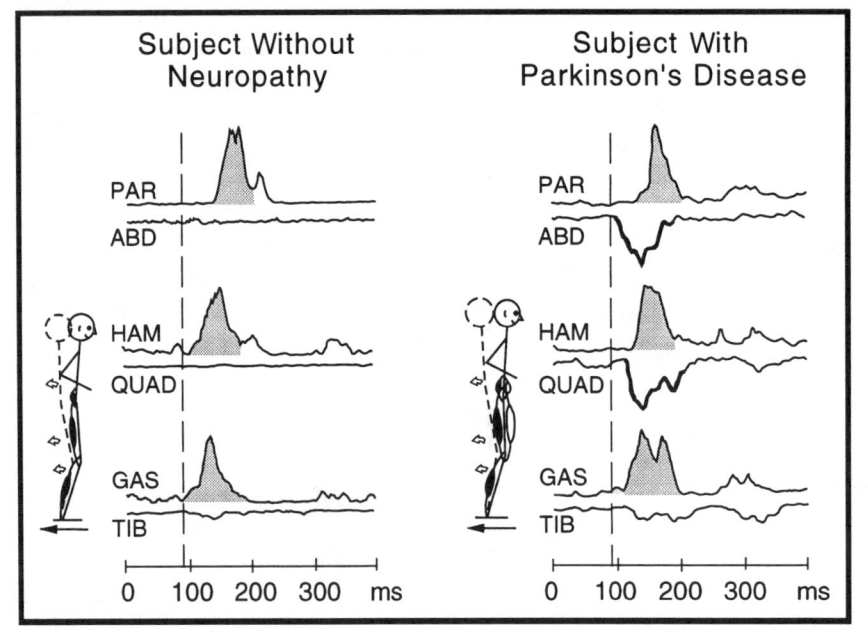

Figure 4.
Typical patterns of muscle activation in representative subject without neuropathy and subject with Parkinson's disease in response to backward surface translations. Dorsal electromyographic bursts associated with an ankle strategy are shaded, and ventral bursts associated with a hip strategy are thickened. The subject with Parkinson's disease showed normal latencies to activation of the gastrocnemius muscles (GAS), the hamstring muscles (HAM), and the paraspinal muscles (PAR), but with addition of coactivation of antagonists. Stick figures show muscles activated, and small arrows indicate direction of active correction for forward sway displacement. ABD=rectus abdominis muscle, QUAD=rectus femoris muscle, TIB=tibialis anterior muscle. (Adapted from Horak et al.[47])

(Fig. 6A).[66] Changing from a wide to a narrow stance also alters automatic postural response patterns by increasing the magnitude of responses and including more trunk activation (Fig. 6B). If individuals initially assume a leaning position prior to a perturbation, the trunk muscles rather than the ankle muscles may be activated first.[63]

When initial body positions or support conditions are changed, the same surface perturbation will result in activation of a different set of muscles on the first trial; muscles whose action is not effective in restoring equilibrium are not activated. For example, when persons support themselves by holding a handle during surface perturbations, automatic postural responses in the legs are suppressed and postural activity originates at the interface of the body and the stable surface (eg, hand, arm) (Fig. 6C).[67] Similarly, individuals who are perturbed while sitting on a stool with legs dangling use trunk, and not leg, muscle activation on the first trial.[47,68]

Practice. Perturbation studies have shown that postural strategies become more efficient and effective in response to repeated exposure to a destabilizing stimulus. When people are repeatedly exposed to a particular postural perturbation, their automatic postural responses are gradually reduced in magnitude and fewer, or different, muscles are recruited as these individuals change from a more vigorous to a less vigorous response.[62] Initial postural responses to unexpected disturbances are larger than necessary and inefficiently executed, with excessive muscle activation.[9]

Reduction in the magnitude of postural responses with repeated surface translations is shown in Figure 7A, which compares the first 10 and last 10 of 100 sequential responses. Although onset latency does not change with practice, the magnitude of responses is reduced, especially in antagonist muscles (Fig. 7B). Performance improves with less effort after practice because the time (t) it takes to reach a stable equilibrium position (sway in Fig. 7A) decreases as the torque response reduces with repetition. Although initial responses to unexpected perturbations bring the body's COM back near to its initial position, trials later in a session and over months of training show that people "pre-lean" in the direction of the predicted sway due to perturbation.[37,62] This type of "pre-leaning" can provide a mechanical advantage by increasing joint stiffness.[69]

Teaching voluntary postural responses. Voluntary responses to postural perturbations generally have a longer latency than automatically triggered postural responses.[19,49,70,71] The muscle activation patterns with voluntary sway or steps, however, may have a spatial and temporal organization that is similar to that of automatic postural responses. Although slower, these voluntary responses can be fast enough to be effective in preventing falls in patients whose automatic response latencies are delayed by sensory loss.[50] Attempts to alter automatically triggered postural responses in adults without neurological impairments by providing prior information regarding the size or direction of an impending perturbation have been unsuccessful,[72,73] although prior instruction to "resist" or "give" in response to an upcoming perturbation can alter response magnitude (Horak FA, unpublished observations).

Recent studies have shown that automatic postural responses can be suppressed by a person's intent to move, provided that the person can anticipate the characteristics of the upcoming perturbation.[70,74] When people are instructed to step, instead of remaining in

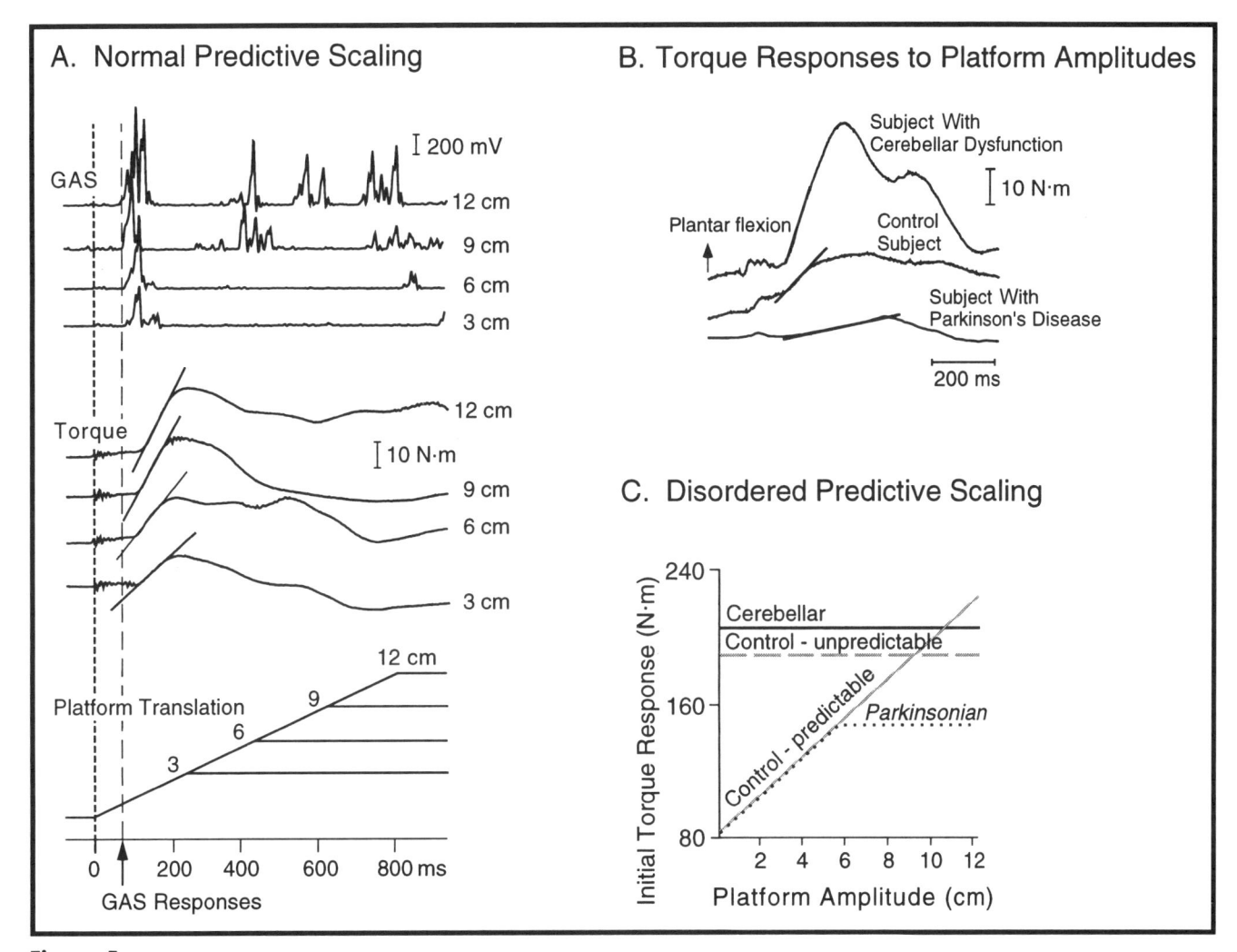

Figure 5.
(A) Initial gastrocnemius muscle (GAS) burst and resulting surface torque occur prior to completion of platform translations but are adjusted to platform amplitude when they are predictable (each amplitude is presented as a block of 5–10 like trials). (B) Effect of platform displacement amplitude (6 cm) on surface reactive torque responses in a representative subject with cerebellar dysfunction, a control subject, and a subject with Parkinson's disease. Rate of change of initial torque response (slope of regression during first 75 ms of active torque) is indicated by bold line superimposed on each torque response (average of 10 like trials). (C) Modification of postural response torque based on prediction of platform translation amplitude. Control subjects are able to modify their initial torque responses using prior experience if platform amplitude is predictable. The lack of adjustment of initial torque responses is seen when the same amplitudes were unpredictable. Persons with cerebellar dysfunction are unable to adjust their postural responses based on prediction from prior experience, whereas persons with Parkinson's disease adjust to predicted amplitudes only when small corrections forces are required. (Figs. 5A and 5C adapted from Horak[9]; Fig. 5B adapted from Horak and colleagues.[47,48])

place in response to a backward surface translation, they can suppress their automatic postural response and initiate a very rapid step. Figure 8 shows the suppression of the automatic soleus and gastrocnemius muscle activation in response to a backward surface translation with activation of the tibialis anterior muscle in order to move the COM forward in preparation for a step. The tibialis anterior muscle's EMG latency for intentional step initiation is longer than that for in-place automatic postural responses, suggesting that that voluntary, or cortical, mechanisms have substituted for the suppressed automatic postural mechanisms. This suppression of postural responses, however, is larger when individuals can predict the speed of the impending perturbation.[74] Thus, although functional, voluntary postural responses to external perturbations can be taught, patients cannot be expected to substitute fast, voluntary responses for automatic postural responses unless they are able to predict an upcoming perturbation.

Summary of Studies
Studies of automatic responses to external surface perturbations have identified quick, coordinated, multisegmental strategies responsible for maintaining equilibrium. These strategies are organized to control a variety of postural objectives and are adapted to particular conditions, behavioral goals, and environmental contexts. These strategies become more efficient with practice. Studies have also shown that patients with neurologic impairments may show many different types of

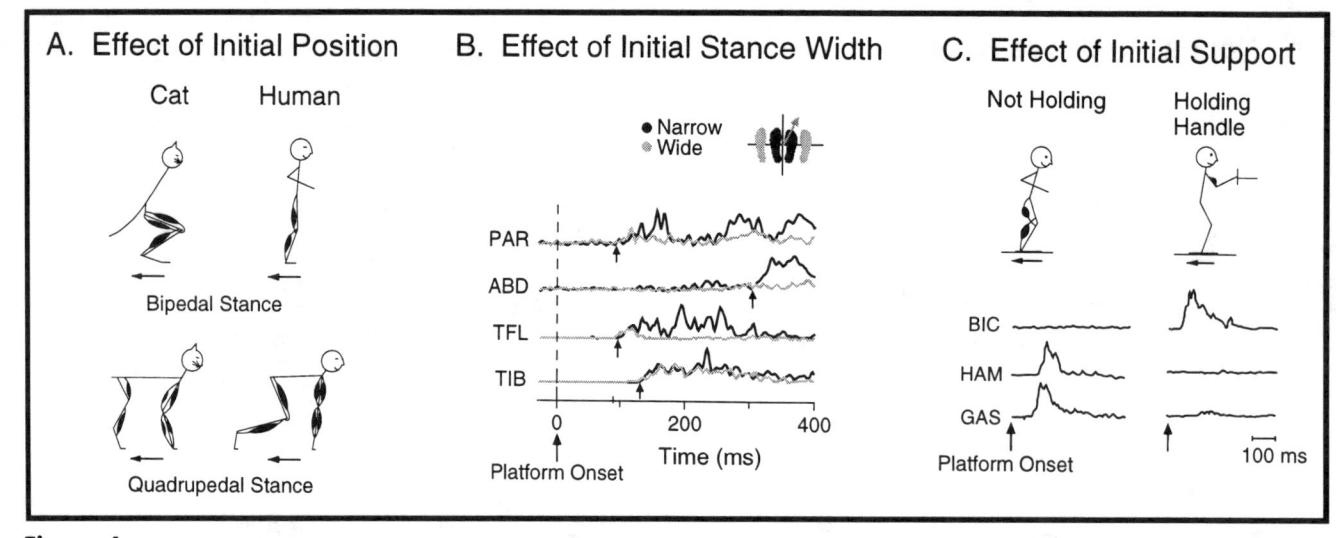

Figure 6.
(A) Cartoon shows which muscles responded to backward surface translations in bipedal and quadrupedal stance in cats and humans. (B) Average electromyographic responses from left muscles recorded during five horizontal translations that were forward and to the right in narrow (dark line) and wide (gray line) stance. Electromyographic amplitude decreases with wide stance, but latencies (arrows) do not change. (C) Muscle responses to backward surface translations during stance while not holding (on left) and while holding (on right) a handle. PAR=lumbar paraspinal muscles, ABD=rectus abdominis muscle, TFL=tensor fasciae latae muscle, TIB=tibialis anterior muscle, BIC=biceps muscle, HAM=hamstring muscles, GAS=gastrocnemius muscles. (Adapted from Henry et al,[39] Dunbar et al,[66] and Nashner.[67])

abnormalities in coordinating postural responses to disequilibrium, depending on the particular system involved and the underlying postural control impairments.

Clinical Implications of Perturbation Research

The Changing Face of Clinical Practice
Treatment success for patients with impaired balance depends on an understanding of (1) the systems controlling normal equilibrium, (2) the postural systems that are likely to be disordered by aging and pathology, and (3) a clinical framework for assessing and treating imbalance that is consistent with current research on postural control and relevant to the needs and problems of patients with impaired balance. Results from research characterizing equilibrium responses to external surface perturbations have provided insights into the contributions and interaction of the many systems that are important to normal balance. In addition, postural perturbation research has provided an approach for understanding the basis for instability during aging and in the patient with neurological pathology. This information is being used to develop a new clinical framework for assessing and treating instability, specifically by targeting the component problems that contribute to instability.[7,8,32,75]

Much has been written recently about changing theories of motor control and their effect on clinical practice.[7,8] Traditionally, balance has been conceptualized as resulting from a series of hierarchically organized reflexes and reactions.[7,8,75] This theoretical framework led to the development of assessment tools that measured the presence or absence of reflexes and interventions that focused on inhibiting primitive and pathological reflexes and facilitating the emergence of normal equilibrium reactions.[75]

Perturbation studies have shown that movement strategies for achieving balance are not the result of stereotyped reflexes, but emerge as the CNS learns to apply generalized rules for maintaining equilibrium in a variety of tasks and contexts. We suggest that balance can be viewed as a motor skill that emerges from the interaction of multiple systems that are organized to meet functional task goals and that are constrained by environmental context. Balance viewed as a motor skill suggests that, like any skill, balance can improve with practice. That is, postural motor coordination can be learned. This view of balance has led to the development of assessment tools that focus on measuring functional capacity of the patient and on quantifying underlying impairments that constrain functional performance. Therapeutic intervention is directed at changing impairments and improving functional performance, including the capacity to adapt performance to changing task and environmental demands.[8,75]

In the remaining section of this article, we discuss some of the clinical applications that have been developed in response to insights gained from postural control research. The development of new clinical approaches based on emerging research related to postural control is just beginning. Many of the new approaches discussed in the next section have yet to undergo experimental

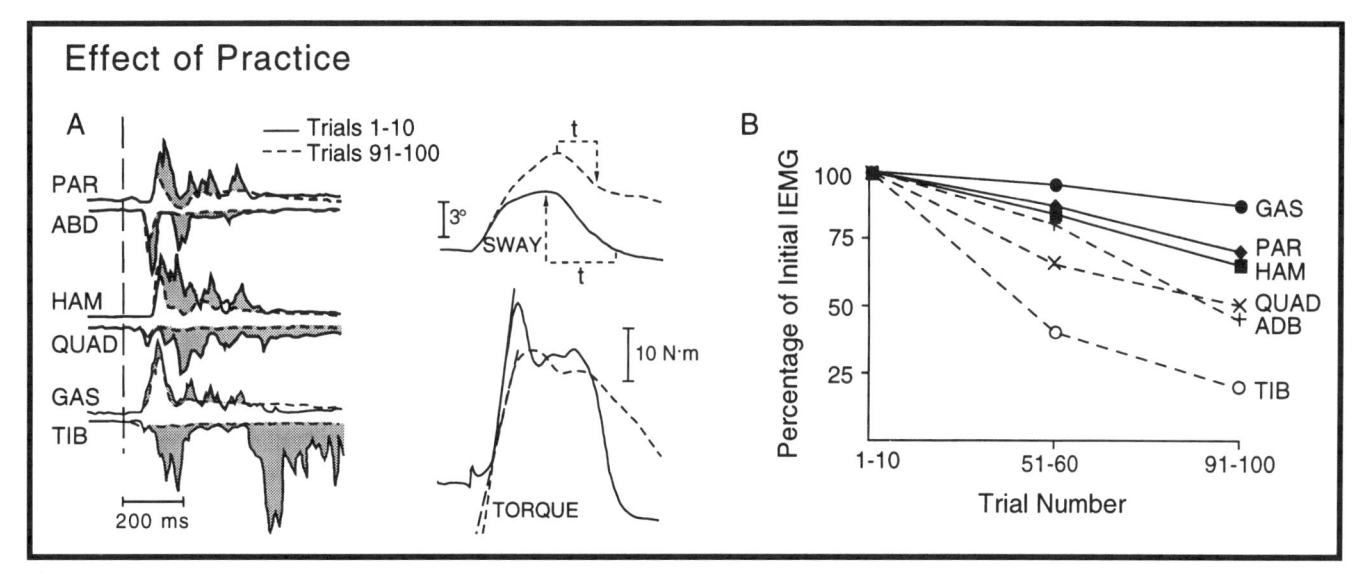

Figure 7.
Reduction of electromyographic (EMG) activity and forces with practice. (A) Reduction of EMG response, torque, and time to achieve equilibrium (t) with repetition of forward sway induced by a backward surface perturbation. Solid lines show average response of trials 1 to 10, and dashed lines show average response of trials 91 to 100. (B) Graph shows average reduction of integrated EMG (IEMG) activity (first 100 ms) in trials 51 to 60 and in trials 91 to 100 as a percentage of initial trials 1 to 10. Trial-to-trial variability was less than 10% of the average values. PAR=lumbar paraspinal muscles, ABD=rectus abdominis muscle, HAM=hamstring muscles, QUAD=rectus femoris muscle, GAS=gastrocnemius muscles, TIB=tibialis anterior muscle. (Adapted from Horak et al.[62])

validation. Nevertheless, the face of clinical practice appears to be changing in response to many factors, including recent research in postural control.

Synergies and Strategies

The selection of movement strategies that are effective in controlling the body's COM depends on numerous factors, including the biomechanical, sensory, and neuromuscular constraints within the individual, as well as on the affordances of the environment and task. Helping patients to develop effective and efficient movement strategies for postural control depends on understanding the postural system disorders that result in constraints limiting the availability and selection of movement strategies for balance.

Biomechanical constraints. Biomechanical constraints affect the development and selection of movement strategies used for balance. The development of coordinated multijoint movement strategies during balance retraining involves helping patients to develop efficient and effective ways to control their body's COM despite biomechanical constraints imposed by their musculoskeletal impairments or disabilities. For example, a musculoskeletal impairment such as limited range of motion at the ankles due to shortening of the gastrocnemius and soleus muscles may limit a patient's ability to generate forces against the surface to control the COM. Treatments aimed at lengthening these muscles may allow the person to resume use of postural movements relying on force generation at the surface. In cases in which impairments are permanent, such as may occur with an arthritic ankle, alternative postural strategies that are effective in controlling the COM must be developed. In these circumstances, use of a movement strategy that controls COM position largely through movements at the trunk, hips, and arms, or alternatively taking a step, may be appropriate.

Sensory information available. Strategy selection is also influenced by the sensory information that is available. For example, a permanent loss of sensory information may result in a restricted range of movement strategies available for postural control. In this case, patients may need to be educated to identify and avoid dangerous tasks and environments or to develop compensatory strategies using assistive devices.[76,77]

To improve balance control in patient populations where one or more senses may be impaired or not used effectively by the nervous system, therapists can develop approaches to help patients learn effective ways to organize and structure remaining senses to achieve postural control. Suggested treatment strategies designed to affect sensory systems that are important to postural control have focused both on resolution of underlying sensory impairments and on improving the organization and adaptation of sensory information for postural control.[78] For example, patients with partial vestibular loss can be taught to utilize ("tune up") the residual vestibular information that is available.[76] If the patients are unable to do this, the therapist can teach them to recognize dangerous environmental contexts and to use alternative visual and somatosensory informa-

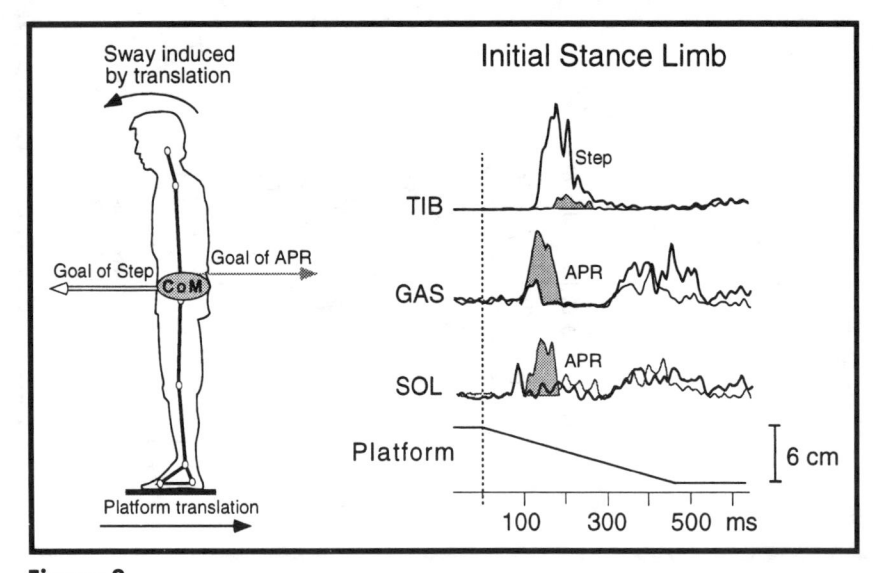

Figure 8.
Intent to step alters postural response. With intent to step, the body's center of mass (COM) moves forward with tibialis anterior muscle (TIB) activation, whereas in response to forward sway induced by a backward platform translation, the COM moves backward via the automatic postural response (APR) in the gastrocnemius muscles (GAS) and the soleus muscle (SOL) (shaded electromyographic response). With simultaneous backward platform perturbation and step initiation (open electromyographic response), the GAS and SOL postural responses are suppressed. (Adapted from Burleigh et al.[70])

tion for postural control. Initially, this type of patient should be treated barefoot on a firm surface and encouraged to attend to the sensation from the feet. Then, the information from the support surface can be made less accurate by having the patient stand on foam, which will encourage the use of vision and remaining vestibular information for orientation. Additional challenges that encourage the use of remaining vestibular information can be introduced by making the available visual information gradually more inaccurate as an orientation reference.[76,78]

Practice sessions for retraining balance can be designed to structure opportunities so that patients have a chance to become efficient in the use of given postural strategies. By initially providing a situation with accurate sensory information and progressing to more complex sensory environments, patient have an opportunity to practice while maintaining a specific level of function in increasingly difficult contexts.

Use of assistive devices. Physical therapists may choose to use assistive devices as part of their therapeutic plans. The use of a cane, for example, will alter the strategy selected based on the changes in the initial biomechanical conditions and based on the available sensory information. A study is currently underway to determine whether sensory information from light touch of the fingertip with a surface can effectively substitute for absent or impaired sensory information from the lower extremities in people with peripheral neuropathies (Horak and colleagues, unpublished research). Cutaneous information from fingertip contact with a stable surface can be more powerful than vision in stabilizing sway in stance.[79] Thus, assistive devices change both the biomechanical and sensory constraints for posture.

Improving Response Latencies
Delayed onsets of muscle responses to surface perturbations can result in increased sway and, if sufficiently delayed, an inability to regain equilibrium using an in-place movement strategy. If patients are slow in taking a step to recover balance, a fall will occur. Slowed responses can result from delays in sensory or motor conduction or from central processing problems. In most clinical settings, it is difficult to identify the problem of delayed onset latencies without force-plate and EMG recordings. Suggested treatments for shortening onset latencies include the use of sensory stimulation such as ice, sweeping, tapping, vibration, and stretching over the postural muscles themselves to increase the excitability of the motoneurons and bring them closer to firing. Other treatments designed to improve the effective recruitment of a muscle for balance include the use of electrical stimulation in conjunction with a footswitch and the use of single-channel or multichannel EMG biofeedback.[75]

Interventions aimed at improving the organization and interpretation of sensory information for postural control have been shown to have the additional effect of decreasing onset latencies of muscle responses to platform perturbations.[80,81] In a study by Hu and Woollacott,[80,81] elderly subjects practiced maintaining stance balance under altered surface and visual conditions over a period of weeks. At the end of the training period, the elderly subjects had improved their ability to stand on a compliant surfaces, and they demonstrated shortened latencies to postural responses to surface displacements.

If delayed onset latencies are due to a decreased ability to generate and sustain forces, as occurs with Parkinson's disease, interventions designed to improve force production could, in theory, affect how quickly effective movements for recovery of balance are generated. Context-specific strengthening exercises and biofeedback may also be effective treatments for improving recruitment of muscles and the rate of force development in muscles needed for postural control.

Temporal and Spatial Dyscoordination

Studies recording EMG activity in response to surface perturbations have provided considerable insight into spatial and temporal disruptions to multijoint muscle synergies essential to the recovery of balance. Although clinicians are able to observe the behavioral outcomes of dyscoordinated movements, such as buckling of the knees, excessive lateral sway, or rotation of the body, the exact nature of the dyscoordination can be determined only with the use of technology such as recording of EMG, kinematic, and kinetic patterns. This inability to identify the source of dyscoordination can hinder the development of interventions designed to improve the spatial and temporal coupling of multijoint muscle activation for balance.

Therapeutic interventions designed to improve coordination problems affecting the ability to maintain stability can begin with treatments aimed at eliminating any biomechanical constraints that may be contributing to the dyscoordination. Developing efficient and coordinated movement strategies for balance may be facilitated by having the patient practice performance of a task that requires the desired strategy. For example, working with the patient on an inclined surface such that the COM of the body is forward so the knee is less likely to buckle would allow a patient to practice the task of moving the COM without buckling of the knee.

Another potential approach to dyscoordination problems is to focus on the synergy level; that is, give patients feedback about muscle recruitment patterns. It has been well documented that to recover from instability in the backward direction, the tibialis anterior muscle fires first, followed by firing of the quadriceps femoris muscle about 30 milliseconds later.[22] In children with diplegic cerebral palsy[56] and some adults with stroke,[46] the recruitment pattern may be abnormal, with the quadriceps femoris muscle firing in advance of the tibialis anterior muscle, resulting in knee bucking. Multichannel electrical stimulation based on EMG monitoring has been used to stimulate the quadriceps femoris muscle, based on the timing of the tibialis anterior muscle activation during backward sway, to improve the distal-to-proximal temporal coordination of muscle activation to recover equilibrium.[75]

Force Control

Modifying forces appropriate to the speed and amplitude of body sway is a critical aspect of effective postural control. Generating too much force is as detrimental to the recovery of equilibrium as insufficient force generation.[48] Both hypermetric and hypometric responses result in the inability to bring the COM back to a point of stability with respect to the base of support following a perturbation.[48]

Proportional control of postural responses is based on characteristics of the perturbation. A wide variety of amplitudes and speeds of displacement, therefore, provides patients with the best opportunity to learn to modify their responses appropriately. Because predictive aspects of postural control are important to learning proportional force control, using identical perturbations that are repeated sequentially can help patients utilize prediction in formulating their postural responses. If perturbation characteristics are altered randomly, patients must rely more on reactive control.[9,62]

Numerous techniques have been developed to help patients improve the modification of forces used to predictively control postural movements. Appropriate modification of forces is needed for voluntary COM movement and for anticipatory postural adjustments when the amount of force needed to control the COM can be predicted, as well for responses to external perturbations. For voluntary postural movements, force-plate retraining systems have been designed to provide patients with visual feedback regarding movement of the center of pressure (COP) at the feet. The capacity to move the COP to designated targets placed in different quadrants on the computer monitor requires effective proactive modification of forces. This technology has been useful when retraining hypometric, as well as hypermetric, force responses (Shumway-Cook, unpublished observations). We have found that people with Parkinson's disease who demonstrate hypometric force responses respond best to a treatment progression that begins with small, slow movements of the COP and moves to large, fast movements of the COP.[61] In contrast, people with cerebellar disorders who demonstrate hypermetric force responses may need to start with large, fast movements of the COP and progress to small, slow movements of the COP.[75] The degree to which training on force-plate systems transfers to other functional tasks such as walking or responding to external perturbations has yet to be determined.[82] There is some evidence to suggest that force-plate retraining in patients with stroke does not transfer well to functional tasks such as gait.[6,81] Further research in this area is needed.

Adaptation of Postural Strategies

Context-specific adaptation. Recovery of stability requires the adaptation of effective and efficient sensorimotor strategies for postural control in the face of constraints imposed by pathology. In addition, patients must be able to adapt sensory and motor strategies to changes in task and environmental demands. We propose that the capacity to adapt is a sign of good potential for rehabilitation because it suggests the potential for change in the face of existing impairments and constraints. Research using surface perturbation paradigms indicates that under normal conditions, the strategies used to control the COM change quickly to accommodate the task and conditions.[39,66,67]

Helping people with balance disorders learn context-specific adaptation involves facilitating the development of effective strategies for controlling the COM in a wide variety of tasks and contexts. We believe that treatment should not be limited to training a single or limited set of strategies, but should include helping patients to develop strategies appropriate for each motor problem and to learn in which situations and contexts to deploy these strategies. For example, if a therapist has a patient hold on to parallel bars (or to the therapist's hands), the initial biomechanical and sensory information has changed considerably. In this context, the therapist should expect to see activation of the patient's arm muscles first during the balance response. If a patient assumes a quadrupedal position, COM is controlled primarily with hip and shoulder muscles, unlike in stance. If the patient assumes a wide stance, he or she will need to activate lower-limb muscles to a lesser degree than if standing in a very narrow stance, because the wider stance is inherently more stable.[39] By exposing patients to a multitude of environments, they are afforded the opportunity to learn how to develop context-specific strategies for solving the problems of maintaining equilibrium.

Teaching voluntary responses. People can be taught to suppress their automatic postural responses if the responses are not functional for their intended goals, especially if they can predict an upcoming perturbation.[70,74] Therapists can exploit this finding by having patients practice suppressing ineffective postural responses during functional activities. For example, patients with Parkinson's disease often have difficulty initiating postural adjustments in preparation for stepping. Therapists can assist the stepping by first moving the patient diagonally over the anticipated swing leg, then forward to the stance leg, thereby displacing the COM in preparation for a step. Initially, the patient may elicit an equilibrium response in response to the push, but with practice the therapist can teach the patient to suppress the unwanted automatic postural response and, instead, initiate a step. Such external perturbations have been shown to assist step initiation in patients with Parkinson's disease.[74]

Limitations of Postural Perturbation Research

Although studies of automatic responses to surface perturbations has increased our understanding of the underlying mechanisms involved in postural control, therapists should not limit their evaluation of balance to descriptions of responses to perturbations. Because balance control is multidimensional, involving proactive as well as reactive control, tonic as well as phasic control, and sensory as well as motor control, it is not realistic to think that any one type of postural task will be useful to analyze all of these aspects of balance control effectively. Responses to perturbation, for example, do not attempt to test the mechanisms involved in orientating the body to various sensory reference frames, steady-state stance posture, or anticipatory postural coordination with voluntary movements. Responses to perturbations of the support surface in a standing subject cannot necessarily be used to predict how the subject will adapt his or her responses to other positions, such as when sitting or kneeling. Responses to external perturbations during stance do not provide information on mechanisms needed to control balance during different tasks (eg, transferring positions), during locomotion, and while stepping over obstacles.[83] In addition, characterization of equilibrium responses to postural perturbations does not necessarily allow for the prediction of how a patient will perform functionally in activities of daily living, although it may allow for the prediction of how well the patient will respond to similar situations such as reacting to surface perturbations induced by accelerations and decelerations of a bus or subway train, a jostle in a crowd, or a pull by a pet on a leash.[84] Additional research is needed to determine the predictive value of responses to postural perturbations.

Conclusions

The ability to effectively treat patients with balance disorders will be enhanced by a clearer understanding of the problems underlying imbalance. Identifying limitations in functional performance, such as inability to stand or walk independently, does not provide information on the underlying impairments, such as prolonged latencies, poor coordination, inadequate force, or inability to adapt postural responses that may be constraining functional performance. More research is needed to develop clinical assessment tools that are effective in identifying specific problems in systems that are essential to postural control. In addition, further research is needed to determine the relative efficacy of different treatment approaches to balance disorders and the extent to which patients are able to learn effective strategies for controlling equilibrium despite the presence of underlying impairments. By understanding the basic systems underlying control of posture, therapists may be able to focus their treatments on deficits that are specific for each patient. Quantification of postural responses via new technology has the advantage of measuring changes in postural behavior that are too small to observe, of differentiating among several potential disordered systems, and of documenting progress related to rehabilitation.

References

1 Magnus R. *Body Posture (Korperstellung)*. Berlin, Federal Republic of Germany: Springer Verlag; 1924.

2 Rademaker GCJ. *Reactions Labyrinthiques et Equilibre*. Paris, France: Masson Editeur; 1935.

3 Sherrington CS. *The Integrative Action of the Nervous System*. New York, NY: Cambridge University Press; 1908:28.

4 Horak FB, Macpherson JM. Postural orientation and equilibrium. In: Smith JL, ed. *Handbook of Physiology, Section 12: Exercise: Regulation and Integration of Multiple Systems*. New York, NY: Oxford University Press Inc; 1996:255–292.

5 Dietz V. Human neuronal control of automatic functional movements: interaction between central programs and afferent input. *Physiol Rev*. 1992;72:33–69.

6 Massion J. Movement, posture, and equilibrium: interaction and coordination. *Prog Neurobiol*. 1992;38:35–56.

7 Horak FB. Motor control models underlying neurologic rehabilitation of posture in children. *Medicine and Sport Science*. 1992;36:21–30.

8 Horak FB. Assumptions underlying motor control for neurologic rehabilitation. In: Lister MJ, ed. *Contemporary Management of Motor Control Problems: Proceedings of the II Step Conference*. Alexandria, Va: Foundation for Physical Therapy Inc; 1991:11–27.

9 Horak FB. Adaptation of automatic postural responses. In: Bloedel J, Ebner TJ, Wise SP, eds. *Acquisition of Motor Behavior in Vertebrates*. Cambridge, Mass: The MIT Press; 1996:57–85.

10 Black SE, Maki BE, Fernie GR. Aging, imbalance, and falls. In: Sharpe JA, Barber HO, eds. *The Vestibulo-Ocular Reflex and Vertigo*. New York, NY: Raven Press; 1994:1–24.

11 Maki BE, Holliday PJ, Topper AK. A prospective study of postural balance and risk of falling in an ambulatory and independent elderly population. *J Gerontol*. 1994;49:M72–M84.

12 Inglis JT, Shupert CL, Hlavacka F, Horak FB. The effect of galvanic vestibular stimulation on human postural responses during support surface translations. *J Neurophysiol*. 1995;73:896–901.

13 Lee DN, Lishman JR. Visual proprioceptive control of stance. *Perception and Psychophysics*. 1975;1:87–95.

14 Pyykko I, Enbom H, Magnusson M, Schalen L. Effect of proprioceptor stimulation on postural stability in patients with peripheral or central vestibular lesion. *Acta Otolaryngol (Stockh)*. 1991;111:27–35.

15 Horak FB, Shupert CL, Dietz V, Horstmann G. Vestibular and somatosensory contributions to responses to head and body displacements in stance. *Exp Brain Res*. 1994;100:93–106.

16 Fung J, Henry SM, Horak FB. Is the force constraint strategy used by humans to maintain stance and equilibrium? *Soc Neurosci Abstr*. 1995;21:683. Abstract.

17 Brown LA, Frank JS. Are accommodations to postural perturbations affected by fear of falling? *Soc Neurosci Abstr*. 1995;21:1202. Abstract.

18 Do MC, Breniere Y, Bouisset S. Compensatory reactions in forward fall: Are they initiated by stretch receptors? *Electroencephalogr Clin Neurophysiol*. 1988;69:448–452.

19 Nashner LM, Cordo PJ. Relation of automatic postural responses and reaction-time voluntary movements of human leg muscles. *Exp Brain Res*. 1981;43:395–405.

20 Shepard NT, Schultz A, Gu MJ, et al. Postural control in young and elderly adults when stance is challenged: clinical versus laboratory measurements. *Ann Otol Rhinol Laryngol*. 1993;102:508–517.

21 Maki BE, Holliday PJ, Fernie GR. Aging and postural control: a comparison of spontaneous- and induced-sway balance tests. *J Am Geriatr Soc*. 1990;38:1–9.

22 Nashner LM. Fixed patterns of rapid postural responses among leg muscles during stance. *Exp Brain Res*. 1977;30:13–24.

23 Macpherson JM. How flexible are muscle synergies? In: Humphrey DR, Freund HJ, eds. *Motor Control: Concepts and Issues*. New York, NY: John Wiley & Sons Inc; 1991:33–47.

24 Horak FB, Nashner LM. Central programming of postural movements: adaptation to altered support surface configurations. *J Neurophysiol*. 1986;55:1369–1381.

25 Nashner LM. Adapting reflexes controlling the human posture. *Exp Brain Res*. 1976;26:59–72.

26 Lee WA. Neuromotor synergies as a basis for coordinated intentional action. *Journal of Motor Behavior*. 1984;16:135–170.

27 Nashner LM, McCollum G. The organization of human postural movements: a formal basis and experimental synthesis. *Behav Brain Sci*. 1985;8:135–172.

28 Horak FB. Clinical measurement of postural control in adults. *Phys Ther*. 1987;67:1881–1885.

29 McIlroy WE, Maki BE. Adaptive changes to compensatory stepping responses. *Gait and Posture*. 1995;3:43–50.

30 Kuo AD, Zajac FE. Human standing posture: multi-joint movement strategies based on biomechanical constraints. *Prog Brain Res*. 1993;97:349–358.

31 Runge CF, Shupert CL, Horak FB, Zajac FE. Possible contribution of an otolith signal to automatic postural strategies. *Soc Neurosci Abstr*. 1994;20:793. Abstract.

32 Horak FB, Shumway-Cook A. Clinical implications of posture control research. In: Duncan PW, ed. *Balance*. Alexandria, Va: American Physical Therapy Association; 1990:105–111.

33 Horstmann GA, Dietz V. A basic posture control mechanism: the stabilization of the centre of gravity. *Electroencephalogr Clin Neurophysiol*. 1990;76:165–176.

34 Lacquaniti F, LeTaillanter M, Lopiano L, Maioli C. The control of limb geometry in cat posture. *J Physiol (Lond)*. 1990;426:177–192.

35 Pozzo T, Levik Y, Berthoz A. Head stabilization in the frontal plane during complex equilibrium tasks in humans. In: Woollacott MH, Horak FB, eds. *Posture and Gait: Control Mechanisms, Volume 1*. Eugene, Ore: University of Oregon Books; 1992:100.

36 Kuo AD. An optimal control model for analyzing human postural balance. *IEEE Trans Biomed Eng*. 1995;42:87–101.

37 Macpherson JM. The force constraint strategy for stance is independent of prior experience. *Exp Brain Res*. 1994;101:397–405.

38 Droulez J, Berthoz A. Servo-controlled (conservative) versus topological (projective) mode of sensory motor control. In: Bles W, Brandt T, eds. *Disorders of Posture and Gait*. Amsterdam, the Netherlands: Elsevier Science Publishers BV; 1986:83–97.

39 Henry SM, Fung J, Horak FB. EMG responses to multidirectional surface translations. *Soc Neurosci Abstr*. 1995;21:683. Abstract.

40 Moore SP, Horak FB, Nashner LM. Influence of initial stance position on human postural responses. *Soc Neurosci Abstr*. 1986;12:1301. Abstract.

41 Macpherson JM, Horak FB, Dunbar DC. Stance dependence of automatic postural adjustments in humans. *Exp Brain Res*. 1989;78:557–566.

42 Henry SM, Fung J, Horak FB. Postural responses to lateral surface perturbations. *Soc Neurosci Abstr.* 1996;22:1632.

43 Horak FB, Nashner LM, Diener HC. Postural strategies associated with somatosensory and vestibular loss. *Exp Brain Res.* 1990;82:167–177.

44 Shumway-Cook A, Woollacott MH. Dynamics of postural control in the child with Down syndrome. *Phys Ther.* 1985;65:1315–1322.

45 Woollacott MH, Shumway-Cook A, Nashner LM. Aging and postural control: changes in sensory organization and muscular coordination. *Int J Aging Hum Dev.* 1986;23:97–114.

46 Di Fabio RP, Badke MB, McEvoy A, Ogden E. Kinematic properties of voluntary postural sway in patients with unilateral primary hemispheric lesions. *Brain Res.* 1990;513:248–254.

47 Horak FB, Nutt JG, Nashner LM. Postural inflexibility in parkinsonian subjects. *J Neurol Sci.* 1995;111:46–58.

48 Horak FB, Diener HC. Cerebellar control of postural scaling and central set in stance. *J Neurophysiol.* 1994;72:479–493.

49 Shupert CL, Horak FB, Black FO. Hip sway associated with vestibulopathy. *J Vestib Res.* 1994;4:231–244.

50 Horak FB, Lamarre Y, Macpherson JM, et al. Postural control in a patient with total body somatosensory loss. *Soc Neurosci Abstr.* 1996;22:1632. Abstract.

51 Inglis JT, Horak FB, Shupert CL, Jones-Rycewicz C. The importance of somatosensory information in triggering and scaling automatic postural responses in humans. *Exp Brain Res.* 1994;101:159–164.

52 Nashner LM, Woollacott MH, Tuma G. Organization of rapid responses to postural and locomotor-like perturbations of standing man. *Exp Brain Res.* 1979;36:463–476.

53 McCollum G, Horak FB, Nashner LM. Parsimony in neural calculations for postural movement. In: Bloedel J, Dichgans J, Precht W, eds. *Cerebellar Functions.* Berlin, Federal Republic of Germany: Springer-Verlag; 1984:52–66.

54 Pratt CA, Horak FB, Herndon RM. Differential effects of somatosensory and motor system deficits on postural dyscontrol in multiple sclerosis. In: Woollacott MH, Horak FB, eds. *Posture and Gait: Control Mechanisms.* Eugene, Ore: University of Oregon Press; 1992:118–121.

55 Stelmach GE, Teasdale N, Di Fabio RP, Phillips J. Age-related decline in postural control mechanisms. *Int J Aging Hum Dev.* 1989;29:205–223.

56 Nashner LM, Shumway-Cook A, Marin O. Stance posture control in select groups of children with cerebral palsy: deficits in sensory organization and muscular coordination. *Exp Brain Res.* 1983;49:393–409.

57 McIlroy WE, Maki BE. Early activation of arm muscles follows external perturbation of upright stance. *Neurosci Lett.* 1995;184:1–4.

58 Shupert CL, Black FO, Horak FB, Nashner LM. Coordination of the head and body in response to support surface translations in normals and patients with bilaterally reduced vestibular function. In: Amblard B, Berthoz A, Clarac F, eds. *Posture and Gait: Development, Adaptation, and Modulation.* Amsterdam, the Netherlands: Elsevier Science Publishers BV; 1988:281–289.

59 Woollacott MH, Shumway-Cook A. *Development of Posture and Gait Across the Lifespan.* Columbia, SC: University of South Carolina Press; 1989.

60 Horak FB, Frank J, Nutt JG. Effects of dopamine on postural control in parkinsonian subjects: scaling, set, and tone. *J Neurophysiol.* 1996;75:2380–2396.

61 Diener HC, Horak FB, Nashner LM. Influence of stimulus parameters on human postural responses. *J Neurophysiol.* 1988;59:1888–1895.

62 Horak FB, Diener HC, Nashner LM. Influence of central set on human postural responses. *J Neurophysiol.* 1989;62:841–853.

63 Horak FB, Moore SP. The effect of prior leaning on human postural responses. *Gait and Posture.* 1993;1:203–210.

64 Schieppati M, Nardone A. Free and supported stance in Parkinson's disease: the effect of posture and "postural set" on leg muscle responses to perturbation, and its relation to the severity of the disease. *Brain.* 1991;114:1227–1244.

65 Marsden CD, Merton PA, Mortan HB. Anticipatory postural responses in the human subject. *Proceedings of the Physiological Society.* 1977;275:47P–48P.

66 Dunbar DC, Horak FB, Macpherson JM, Rushmer DS. Neural control of quadrupedal and bipedal stance: implications for the evolution of erect posture. *Am J Phys Anthropol.* 1986;69:93–105.

67 Nashner LM. Adaptation of human movement to altered environments. *Trends Neurosci.* 1982;5:358–361.

68 Hirschfeld H, Forssberg H. Epigenetic development of postural responses for sitting during infancy. *Exp Brain Res.* 1994;97:528–540.

69 McIlroy WE, Maki BE. Changes in early automatic postural responses associated with the prior planning and execution of a compensatory step. *Brain Res.* 1993;631:203–211.

70 Burleigh AL, Horak FB, Malouin F. Modification of postural responses and step initiation: evidence for goal directed postural interactions. *J Neurophysiol.* 1995;72:2892–2902.

71 McIlroy WE, Maki BE. Do anticipatory postural adjustments precede compensatory stepping reactions evoked by perturbation? *Neurosci Lett.* 1993;164:199–202.

72 Diener HC, Horak FB, Stelmach G, et al. Direction and amplitude precuing has no effect on automatic posture responses. *Exp Brain Res.* 1991;84:219–223.

73 Maki BE, Whitelaw RS. Influence of expectation and arousal on center-of-pressure responses to transient postural perturbations. *J Vestib Res.* 1993;3:25–39.

74 Burleigh A, Horak FB, Nutt JG, Obeso J. Step initiation in Parkinson's disease: influence of levodopa and external sensory triggers. *Mov Disord.* In press.

75 Shumway-Cook A, Woollacott MH. *Motor Control: Theory and Practical Applications.* Baltimore, Md: Williams & Wilkins; 1995.

76 Shumway-Cook A, Horak FB. Rehabilitation strategies for patients with vestibular deficits. *Neurol Clin.* 1990;8:441–457.

77 Horak FB, Shupert CL. Role of the vestibular system in postural control. In: Herdman SJ, ed. *Vestibular Rehabilitation.* Philadelphia, Pa: FA Davis Co; 1994:22–46.

78 Shumway-Cook A, Horak FB, Yardley L, Bronstein AM. Rehabilitation of balance disorders in the patient with vestibular pathology. In: Bronstein AM, Brandt T, Woollacott MH, eds. *Clinical Aspects of Balance and Related Gait Disorders.* New York, NY: Arnold and Oxford University Press; 1996:211–235.

79 Jeka JJ, Lackner JR. Fingertip contact influences human postural control. *Exp Brain Res.* 1994;100:495–502.

80 Hu M, Woollacott MH. Multisensory training of standing balance in older adults, I: postural stability and one-leg stance balance. *J Gerontol.* 1994;49:M52–M61.

81 Hu M, Woollacott MH. Multisensory training of standing balance in older adults, II: kinematic and electromyographic postural responses. *J Gerontol.* 1994;49:M62–M71.

82 Winstein CJ, Gardner ER, McNeal DR, et al. Standing balance training: effect on balance and locomotion in hemiparetic adults. *Arch Phys Med Rehabil.* 1989;70:755–762.

83 Patla AE, Rietdyk S. Visual control of limb trajectory over obstacles during locomotion: effect of obstacle height and width. *Gait and Posture.* 1993;1:45–60.

84 Topper AK, Maki BE, Holliday PJ. Are activity-based assessments of balance and gait in the elderly predictive of risk of falling and/or type of fall? *J Am Geriatr Soc.* 1993;41:479–487.

Rehabilitation of Balance in Two Patients With Cerebellar Dysfunction

The treatment of two patients with cerebellar dysfunction is described. One patient was a 36-year-old woman with a 7-month history of dizziness and unsteadiness following surgical resection of a recurrent pilocystic astrocytoma located in the cerebellar vermis. The other patient was a 48-year-old man with cerebrotendinous xanthamatosis (CTX) and diffuse cerebellar atrophy, and a 10-year history of progressive gait and balance difficulties. Each patient was treated with a 6-week course of physical therapy that emphasized the practice of activities that challenged stability. The patient with the cerebellar tumor resection also performed eye-head coordination exercises. Each patient had weekly therapy and performed selected balance retraining exercises on a daily basis at home. Measurements taken before and after treatment for each patient included self-perception of symptoms, clinical balance tests, and stability during selected standing and gait activities; for the patient with the cerebellar tumor resection, vestibular function tests and posturography were also performed. Both patients reported improvements in symptoms and demonstrated similar improvements on several kinematic indicators of stability during gait. The patient with the cerebellar tumor resection improved on posturography following treatment, whereas the patient with CTX improved on clinical balance tests. This case report describes two individualized treatment programs and documents functional improvements in two patients with different etiologies, durations, and clinical presentations of cerebellar dysfunction. The outcomes suggest that patients with cerebellar lesions, acute or chronic, may be able to learn to improve their postural stability. [Gill-Body KM, Popat RA, Parker SW, Krebs DE. Rehabilitation of balance in two patients with cerebellar dysfunction. *Phys Ther.* 1997;77:534–552.]

Key Words: *Balance, Balance rehabilitation, Cerebellar rehabilitation, Postural control.*

Kathleen M Gill-Body
Rita A Popat
Stephen W Parker
David E Krebs

The cerebellum controls limb, posture, and eye-head coordination and may also be involved in nonmotor functions such as cognition[1] and attention.[2] Anterior lobe (paleocerebellum or spinocerebellum) and midline disease impairs lower-limb coordination, equilibrium responses, and head and trunk synergy, whereas lateral lobe disease chiefly affects limb coordination.[3-5] Anterior and flocculonodular lobe lesions lead to oculomotor and balance impairments, with gait ataxia and functional limitations. Lesions of the flocculonodular lobe result in "central vestibular" symptoms because the peripheral vestibular system can be completely intact, but without cerebellar inhibition, integration of vestibular information is impaired.[3,6] Lesions of the vermis typically produce gait and trunk ataxia, with abnormalities of slow-phase eye movements.[6] Oculomotor impairments caused by cerebellar dysfunction may include saccadic hypermetria, impaired smooth pursuit, increased vestibulo-ocular reflex (VOR) gains, impaired fixation suppression of the VOR, and nystagmus.[3,7]

Functional limitations observed in patients with cerebellar dysfunction may include postural instability,[8,9] gait ataxia,[8] dyssynergia (the inability to perform movement involving multiple joints in one smooth pattern),[10] hypotonicity (decreased resistance to passive stretch, with difficulty fixating limbs posturally),[12] fatiguability, and weakness resulting in activity limitations.[13] The specific mechanism underlying generalized weakness and fatiguability is unclear, but these limitations have been theorized to be due to a loss of cerebellar facilitation to the motor cortex that results in a reduction of spinal motoneuron activity during voluntary movement.[14] The cerebellum also compares sensory information with motor output during voluntary movement and performs predictive compensatory modification of reflexes in preparation for movement. According to Ito,[15] learned movements are either controlled or triggered by processes occurring in the cerebellum. Horak and Diener[16] reported specific deficits in

This case report of two patients with cerebellar dysfunction describes a staged, home-based intervention approach that provides increasing challenges to body stability in standing and walking.

KM Gill-Body, PT, NCS, is Assistant Professor, Graduate Programs in Physical Therapy, MGH Institute of Health Professions, 101 Merrimac St, Boston, MA 02114 (USA) (gill-body.kathleen@mgh.harvard.edu), and Neurologic Clinical Specialist, Physical Therapy Services, Massachusetts General Hospital, Boston, Mass. Address all correspondence to Ms Gill-Body at the first address.

RA Popat, PT, NCS, was Supervisor, Physical Therapy Services, Massachusetts General Hospital, and Adjunct Assistant Professor, MGH Institute of Health Professions, at the time this report was written. She is currently a graduate student, University of Massachusetts, Amherst, Mass.

SW Parker, MD, is Chief of Otoneurology, Massachusetts General Hospital, and Assistant Professor of Neurology, Harvard Medical School, Boston, Mass.

DE Krebs, PhD, PT, is Associate Professor, MGH Institute of Health Professions; Director, Massachusetts General Hospital Biomotion Laboratory, Boston, Mass.; Instructor, Harvard Medical School; and Lecturer, Massachusetts Institute of Technology, Cambridge, Mass.

This work was supported by National Institute of Disability and Rehabilitation Research grant H133G60045 and National Institutes of Health grant RO1AG11255.

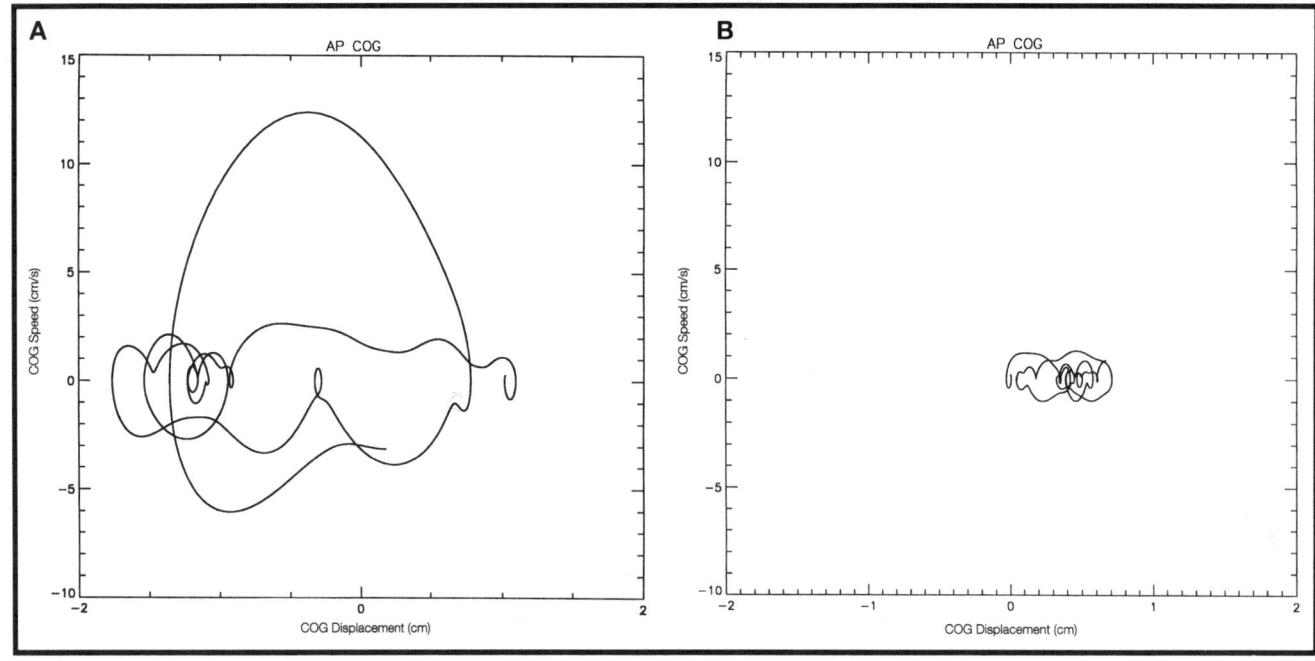

Figure 1.
Phase-plane plots during semitandem standing with eyes open for patient with resected cerebellar tumor before treatment (A) and after treatment (B). Anteroposterior (AP) center of gravity (COG) speed is plotted on the vertical axis, and AP COG displacement is plotted on the horizontal axis during a 7-second standing trial. Note the widely diverging pattern in Figure 1A, with a wide variance in both the speed and displacement of the COG, signifying an unstable movement pattern. Figure 1B, in contrast, is an example of a converging pattern with minimal variance in the speed or displacement of the COG, signifying a stable movement pattern. A similar improvement in standing stability was also observed in this patient during standing with feet together and eyes closed before and after treatment.

the use of the central set to scale the magnitude of initial postural responses based on prior experience in patients with anterior lobe disorders. Because the cerebellum is considered to be crucial to motor learning, some people believe that patients with known cerebellar dysfunction may be less responsive to physical rehabilitation.

There is limited evidence that treatment programs improve function in patients with cerebellar dysfunction. Recovery after cerebellar lesions or disease in humans is poorly documented. There is, however, strong evidence of recovery after cerebellar lesions in experimental animals, which suggests that if the cerebellum is not totally destroyed, neighboring areas of the cerebellum can adapt or compensate for the impaired region.[9,17] Possible mechanisms of recovery after central nervous system lesions may include neural sprouting, vicarious functions, functional reorganization, substitution, and plasticity.[18]

No studies have demonstrated changes in gait, balance, or locomotor function from exercise interventions for patients with cerebellar dysfunction. Rehabilitation of patients with acute cerebellar dysfunction has included Frenkel's exercises,[19] rhythmic stabilization,[20] and the use of walking aids and weights.[21] Kabat,[20] in 1955, described proprioceptive neuromuscular facilitation (PNF), including resistive exercises to help improve strength, coordination, endurance, balance, and gait, but no research studies of the efficacy of PNF for patients with cerebellar disorders have been reported. There is sparse evidence of successful treatment of chronic cerebellar dysfunction, and some clinicians regard this condition as refractive to treatment.[22] In general, rehabilitation interventions for patients with chronic cerebellar dysfunction have, in the past, been restricted to conservative management (eg, maintaining range of motion) and compensation strategies (eg, recommending that patients increase their base of support or use assistive devices to improve or replace postural stability).[23]

More recently, balance rehabilitation that increasingly challenges body stability have been advocated,[24,25] but most of the available treatment-related publications[24–27] lack adequate intervention descriptions for replication as well as scientific controls. Balliet et al[24] were among the first investigators to describe neuromuscular retraining methods for five patients with chronic cerebellar dysfunction and gait disorders. Treatment was based on the premise that the patients needed to reacquire proper motor control and associated balance through adaptation to increasingly demanding conditions. Therefore, upper-extremity use during balance and gait activities was minimized to facilitate independent balance control. Improvement in functional ambulation was often judged by the type of assistive device used, amount of upper-extremity weight bearing on the device, level of assistance required to ambulate, and maximum distance ambulated. All patients improved on all four variables. Brandt et al[25] proposed similar treatment for ataxia by progressively increasing body instability to activate "sensorimotor rearrangement." In a case report, Sliwa et al[26] reported functional improvement following rehabilitation in a patient with paraneoplastic subacute cerebellar degeneration, but they provided no details about the treatment program.

In our case report of two patients, we describe a staged, home-based intervention approach that provides increasing challenges to body stability in standing and walking. The patients had different etiologies, durations, and clinical presentations of cerebellar dysfunction. The treatment program is based on recent ideas regarding balance rehabilitation suggesting that activities that activate postural and neural control mechanisms may be most effective in achieving better overall postural control.[24-28] Such postural and neural control mechanisms may include the integration of sensory information or alternate motor control strategies to enhance postural stability. We report data regarding patient response to treatment in terms of patient self-report, clinical balance assessment, whole-body movement analysis, and posturography testing (when available).

The medical evaluation for each patient just prior to referral for physical therapy consisted of an examination by a neurologist and diagnostic testing as deemed appropriate by that neurologist. Each patient also underwent a three-dimensional movement analysis in our biomotion laboratory. A whole-body kinematic and kinetic analysis of key standing and gait activities (ie, standing, free and paced gait, and walking in place at a pace of 120 steps per minute) was completed. The motion analysis is described in detail elsewhere.[29-31] Briefly, the system consists of an 11-segment, 66-degree-of-freedom whole-body (head, arms, trunk, pelvis, thighs, shanks, and feet) kinematic model; two force plates; and software to integrate the kinematic and kinetic data.[31] Selspot II hardware* and a TRACK™ kinematic data-analysis software package† are used to acquire and analyze the three-dimensional whole-body kinematic data. Floor reaction forces are acquired from two Kistler platforms‡ and processed on the same computer as the kinematic data. Kinematic and kinetic data are sampled at 150 Hz and digitally filtered. The system accuracy is ±1 mm for linear displacement and ±1 degree for angular displacement.[32] The accuracy for the estimation of center of gravity (COG) is less than 1 cm.[30]

Stability during the standing and gait tests is quantified in several ways, including (1) using the COG and center of pressure (COP) to calculate the maximum separation that occurs between the COG and COP (or the COG-COP moment arm[30]) during gait tests, (2) standard time-distance variables, such as double-limb support time, speed, and base of support during gait, and (3) phase plane analysis[33] of standing and walking in place. Briefly, a phase-plane analysis involves plotting a variable (eg, mediolateral COG displacement) against its first time derivative (eg, speed).[33] Stable COG standing motion has a converging phase plane, whereas unstable motion has a diverging phase plane (Fig. 1). We use mathematical modeling (root mean square of the plot variance) to quantify the anteroposterior and mediolateral phase-plane plots, thereby permitting quantitative as well as qualitative analysis of the subjects' horizontal COG movement patterns during various activities.[33] Phase-plane analysis has been shown to discriminate between subjects with and without balance impairments.[33] The data collected during the whole-body movement analysis were collected as part of a larger pilot study aimed at identifying the kinetic and kinematic characteristics of postural control that change after rehabilitation. Thus, this information was not used for treatment planning purposes in the following case report of the two patients but is reported for descriptive purposes.

Patient 1—Cerebellar Dysfunction After Removal of a Cerebellar Tumor

History

A 36-year-old left-handed woman was referred for physical therapy. She complained of experiencing dizziness and unsteadiness 7 months following surgical resection of a recurrent pilocystic cerebellar astrocytoma. Six years previous to the surgery, she had severe headaches and hydrocephalus. A cerebellar tumor was identified. Following resection of the tumor, she was back at work within 8 weeks. Five years later, as a result of recurrence of the tumor, the patient had repeat surgery (debulking of residual grade I glioma located in the middle and superior cerebellar vermis and extending to the floor of the fourth ventricle) (Fig. 2). Two months after the resection, she received radiation therapy for 1 month. During radiation treatment, she developed hearing loss, which was worse on the left side. After the second surgery, she noted problems with unsteadiness and dizziness. Her sensation of dizziness worsened following the radiation therapy and was aggravated by head movements. She also reported an unsteady "drunk" sensation. She had moderate dysarthria. A 2-month trial of dexa-

---

* Selective Electronics Corp, Partille, Sweden.
† Developed at the Massachusetts Institute of Technology, Cambridge, MA 02139.
‡ Type 9281A, Kistler Instruments AG, Winterthur, Switzerland.

methasone (4 mg/d), initiated subsequent to radiation therapy to alleviate symptoms of dizziness and unsteadiness, was not effective and was gradually tapered.

The patient lived with her husband. She stopped working as a teacher following the second surgery due to hearing loss, dizziness, and unsteadiness. Due to difficulty with blurred vision during side-to-side head movements, she was not able to drive during the 7 months between surgery and the initiation of physical therapy. She was independent with basic activities of daily living but experienced increased dizziness and unsteadiness in crowded areas such as malls and supermarkets. The patient reported that she ambulated outdoors only when accompanied by her husband because of instability and difficulty crossing streets.

Prerehabilitation Findings

Four days prior to the patient's first appointment for physical therapy, she was examined by a neurologist. The patient told the neurologist that she had resolving left-sided weakness, impaired hand coordination, dizziness, and postural unsteadiness. The neurologist found the patient to be alert and cooperative. Her speech was fluent but mildly dysarthric. Extraocular movements were full, with no spontaneous or gaze nystagmus. She said that her eyes felt "unstable." Facial sensation and movement were symmetrical. Tongue and palate movements were normal. Tympanic membranes were bilaterally intact when inspected visually. Vibration and position sense were present at the toes. Finger-to-nose and heel-to-shin tests were performed accurately and smoothly. Rapid alternating movements were slightly slowed bilaterally. A Romberg's test was negative, but an increased postural sway was observed. Deep tendon reflexes were normal (2+). Gait appeared to be mildly unsteady, with a slightly widened base and a tendency to veer to the left. Step length appeared to be normal, and there was associated arm swing during ambulation. Tandem gait appeared to be unsteady, with a tendency to fall toward either side. Hallpike positional testing revealed no nystagmus and slight dizziness. The patient had impaired fixation suppression of the VOR, which was tested by having her attempt to follow a moving target with the eyes and head moving in unison with the target in the same direction. She demonstrated nystagmus during the test, suggesting that she was unable to suppress the VOR.

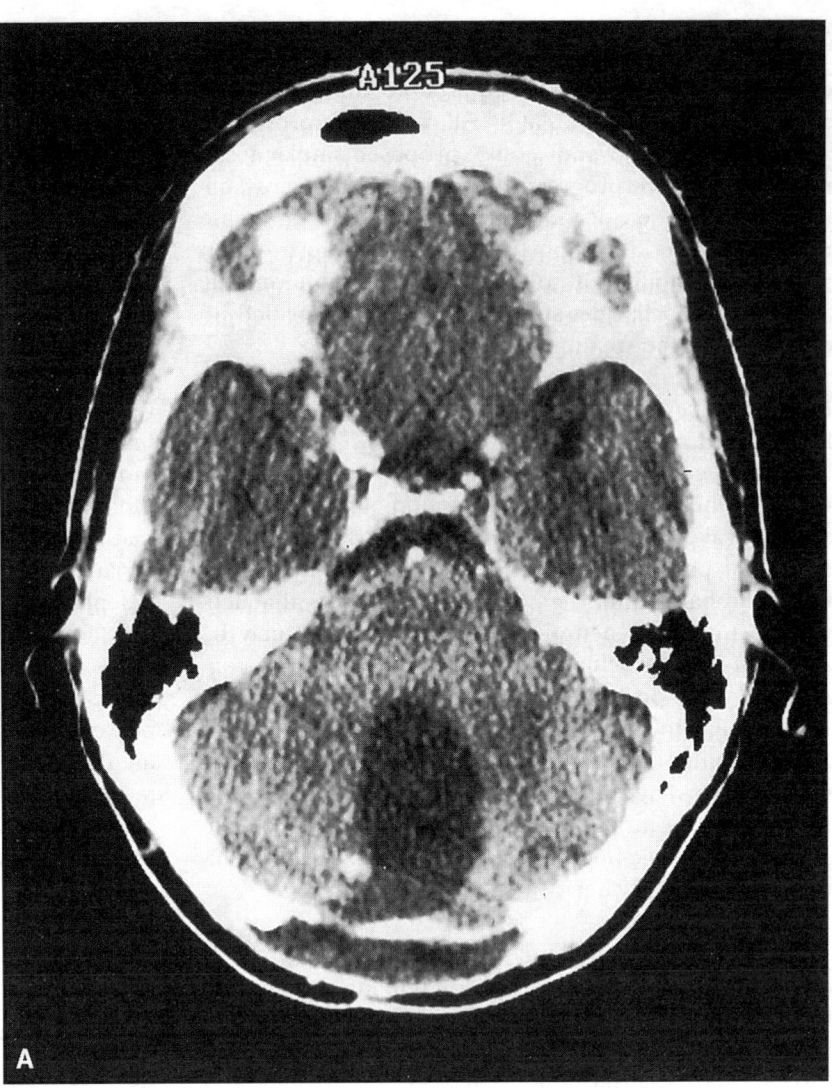

Figure 2.
Computed tomography (CT) scans for patient with cerebellar tumor resection following the second resection: (A) CT scan 6 weeks after second surgical removal of midline cerebellar astrocytoma demonstrating a cystic space replacing the inferior and midcerebellar vermis, with preservation of the cerebellar hemispheres and brain stem. (B) A more rostral section of the same CT scan demonstrating the cystic space replacing the vermis, with a rim of preserved vermis anteriorly and superiorly.

Prior to referral for physical therapy, she underwent vestibular testing, including an electronystagmogram (ENG) with caloric stimulation, sinusoidal vertical axis rotation, visual vestibular interaction rotation, and posturography testing using the Equitest™ system.[§,34] During the ENG, there were normal pursuit and saccadic eye movements, no nystagmus with eyes open and closed,

[§] NeuroCom International Inc, 9570 Lawnfield Rd, Clackamas, OR 97015.

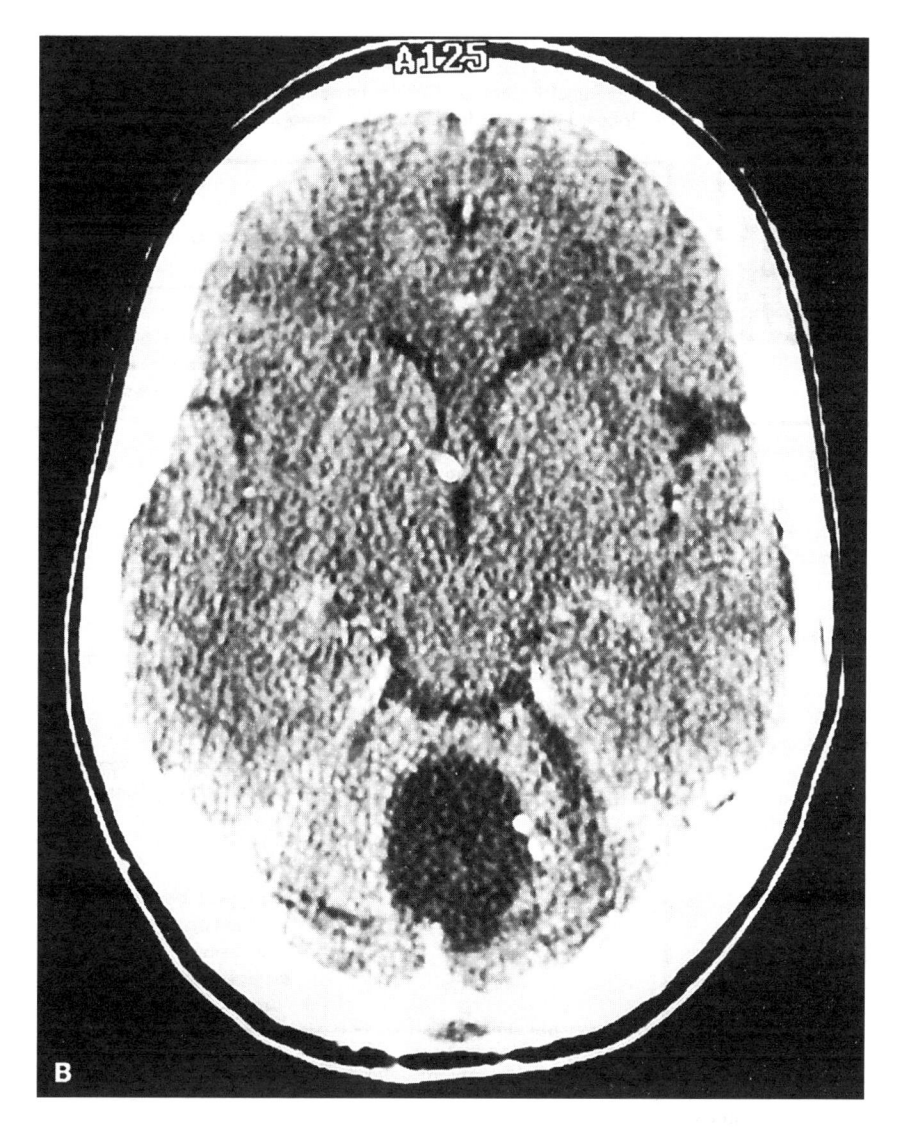

During the initial physical therapy examination, active range of motion was normal for all extremities. Cervical and lumbar spine mobility was normal and pain-free. Manual muscle test grades were normal (5/5) for all muscle groups of the upper and lower extremities. Finger-to-nose movements and heel-to-shin movements were performed quickly, smoothly, and accurately, bilaterally. Rapid alternating movements were slow on the left side. Sensation for light touch and proprioception (as tested by noting the patient's ability to accurately describe the joint position at the knees, ankles, and toes) was normal. Muscle tone was normal. She reported slight dizziness during positional testing (moving to a side-lying position to either side from the sitting position), but there was no nystagmus. Extraocular movements were normal. She was unable to visually fixate her gaze on a target when performing side-to-side head movements at frequencies greater than 1 Hz (timed with a metronome). With her head stationary, visual acuity was 20/10. With side-to-side head movements at 1 Hz, visual acuity worsened to 20/40, and was further degraded to 20/70 when head movements were performed at 2 Hz, which suggested to us that she had difficulty with VOR-mediated gaze fixation at these speeds of head movement.

and no gaze nystagmus. Sequential closed-loop caloric testing of each ear with 27°C and 44°C water stimulation produced symmetrical and appropriate nystagmus and good fixation suppression of nystagmus. Sinusoidal vertical axis rotation testing with a peak velocity of 50°/s revealed normal VOR gains, phase lead, and symmetry[34] for all seven frequencies tested (ie, 0.01, 0.02, 0.05, 0.1, 0.2, 0.5, and 1.0 Hz). Visual vestibular interaction testing demonstrated normal optokinetic tracking and a normal fixation suppression index. These findings suggested intact peripheral vestibular and brain-stem function. A discrepancy, however, existed between her ENG and rotation test results and her clinical test results with regard to suppression of the VOR. This discrepancy may be explained by the different speeds of head movement at which these various tests are performed. Posturography testing revealed falls on two out of three trials and excessive sway on the single successful trial of standing on a sway-referenced platform with eyes closed (Fig. 3).

Sensations of the frequency and intensity of dizziness were evaluated using a standardized questionnaire. The patient reported that dizziness was present for some part of every day at a 5/10 intensity (10 being the highest level of dizziness imaginable). Dizziness increased with head movements in a sitting or standing position and with attempts to focus on objects when walking. The sensation of disequilibrium was present daily at a 7/10 intensity. The patient scored 88 out of a possible 100 on the Dizziness Handicap Inventory (DHI),[35] reporting problems in eight out of nine items related to functional activities, in all seven items related to physical activities, and in eight out of the nine items related to emotional health (Tab. 1). The DHI, originally devised to measure perception of handicap in individuals with benign paroxysmal positional vertigo, is used routinely in our clinic for patients with dizziness or balance problems to document perception of handicap related to the dizziness or balance problems.

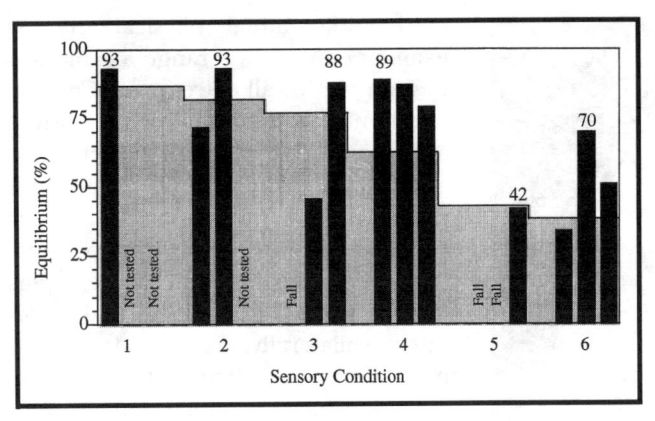

Figure 3.
Baseline (week 0) posturography (ie, sensory organization) test results for patient with cerebellar tumor resection. Equilibrium score=angular difference between the patient's calculated maximum anteroposterior center of gravity and the theoretical maximum displacement of 12.5 degrees; the result is expressed as a percentage between 0 and 100, with 0 indicating sway exceeding the limits of stability and 100 indicating perfect stability. Numerical equilibrium scores for the best performance for each trial are indicated above. Shaded areas represent norms for performance; therefore, scores above the shaded areas represent normal test scores for each test. Sensory conditions: 1=fixed platform, eyes open/fixed visual surround; 2=fixed platform, eyes closed; 3=fixed platform, eyes open/sway-referenced visual surround; 4=sway-referenced platform, eyes open/fixed visual surround; 5=sway-referenced platform, eyes closed; 6=sway-referenced platform, eyes open/sway-referenced visual surround. Not tested=repeat trials not performed; standard testing procedures are to perform only one trial for sensory conditions 1–3, unless the patient is observed to have a large amount of sway or falls, and to perform three trials for sensory conditions 4–6, unless patient appears to have successfully completed the test in fewer trials. Fall=patient fell during trial.

Table 1.
Dizziness Handicap Inventory Items[35] Reported to Be Problematic Prior to Rehabilitation and Improvements Reported After Rehabilitation for Patient With Resected Cerebellar Tumor

Physical/ Functional/ Emotional Factors	Sometimes a Problem	Always a Problem
Physical activities	Performing household chores Turning over in bed Walking down a sidewalk	Looking up[a] Walking down a supermarket aisle[b] Quick head movements Bending over
Functional activities	Getting into or out of bed	Traveling Social activities[a] Reading[a] Managing heights Strenuous housework Walking outdoors independently[b] Walking in the dark (at home)
Emotional factors		Frustration Fearful to go out alone[a] Fearful of being home alone[a] Embarrassment[a] Concentration Feelings of being handicapped Depression Increased stress on relationships

[a] Item rated as "a little improved" after rehabilitation.
[b] Item rated as "much improved" after rehabilitation.

For both patients, balance during standing and walking was evaluated using a standardized protocol that has been in place at our clinic for 5 years. Both patients were evaluated and treated by the same physical therapist. Balance assessment focused on evaluating each patient's sensory and motor organization aspects of postural control as well as automatic postural responses. These tests were selected based on the patient's neuropathology and history, and the need to identify (for treatment planning purposes) the underlying aspects of postural control that were most problematic for each patient.

In standing and walking, the patient had a tendency to be positioned posteriorly (ie, weight appeared to be shifted over the heels). She could stand with feet together and eyes closed for 60 seconds (measured with a digital stopwatch). When she was asked to maintain balance in that position and turn her head from side to side at a pace of 60 beats per minute (paced with an audible metronome), balance could be maintained for 60 seconds with a marked increase in postural sway. She was able to maintain standing balance on a 7.62-cm (3-in) compliant cushion with eyes open for 30 seconds and with eyes closed for 3.4 seconds, suggesting that she had difficulty with postural control when visual inputs were removed and somatosensory inputs were altered.

She was able to maintain balance in tandem standing with eyes open for 60 seconds. Standing on the dominant leg (determined by first asking the patient which leg would be used to kick a ball) could be performed for 30 seconds with eyes open and for 2.74 seconds with eyes closed, suggesting difficulty with postural control when visual inputs were removed and she needed to maintain her COG over a narrow base of support. Increased postural sway in the posterior direction was observed during all standing balance tests, especially when the base of support was narrowed or when visual cues were removed. This finding suggested to us that she may have had difficulty selecting appropriate sensory input for postural control. Stepping strategies (taking a step to regain balance) were delayed in response to unexpected perturbation or release in the anteroposterior direction. The timed "up and go" test[36] (performed over a 12.2-m [40-ft] walkway) was completed in 14.34 seconds without the use of an assistive device. The patient's gait appeared to be steady, and she slowed down during a 180-degree turn. Walking with eyes closed over a 6.1-m (20-ft) walkway was performed in 5.6 seconds, but with three crossed steps (one foot crossed over the other or a stagger to the side), suggesting difficulty with postural control during gait when visual inputs were removed. She was able to perform tandem gait with eyes open for only two steps but was unable to perform this task with eyes closed, suggesting difficulty with postural control during gait when the base of support was narrowed and the COG needed to be maintained within a smaller area. Walking over a 6.1-m walkway turning her head from side to side every third step was performed in 7.02 seconds, but with two crossed steps, suggesting difficulty integrating inputs related to head movements with other sensory inputs during this activity.

The patient's goals for rehabilitation included being able to drive and walk outdoors independently. She also hoped to decrease her sensation of dizziness during head movements so that she could become comfortable in crowded areas and be able to participate more in social activities.

Rehabilitation

The balance rehabilitation program designed for this patient was based on the following interpretation of the patient's condition:

1. Her impaired postural stability was related to cerebellar dysfunction resulting from pathology of the midline cerebellum. Even though she did fairly well on most of the balance tests, she exhibited increased postural sway during the tests, which could reflect difficulties with selecting appropriate sensory information for postural control. The practice of increasingly demanding balance and gait activities may help improve the patient's ability to select and use visual, somatosensory, and vestibular inputs more effectively to minimize her unsteadiness. Improved steadiness may decrease her perception of disequilibrium and improve her ability to control the COG.

2. She was most dependent on visual and somatosensory cues for her standing balance, and she demonstrated an inconsistent ability to use vestibular information for postural control in situations in which visual and somatosensory information were less available than vestibular inputs. For example, she was unable to stand on foam with eyes closed for more than a few seconds and, during posturography testing, had difficulty standing on a sway-referenced platform with eyes closed (Fig. 3), a testing situation in which vestibular inputs are primarily available for postural control. She was able, however, to stand on a sway-referenced platform with a sway-referenced visual surround (although she demonstrated excessive sway on the initial trial), a testing situation in which visual inputs are thought to be critical to resolve the imposed sensory conflict. Her vestibular function tests showed normal peripheral vestibular function. The vestibular system is modulated centrally by the cerebellum.[6] The cerebellum pathology, therefore, is the likely cause of this patient's inability to consistently use vestibular inputs effectively.

3. Her delay with stepping strategies (taking a step to regain balance) during perturbation testing (quickly pushing the patient's COG outside the base of support) in the clinic may be consistent with the scaling problems (matching the magnitude of the response to the displacement) seen in patients with cerebellar dysfunction.[16] For example, her delay in stepping backward with posterior perturbations may be due to an initial hypermetric (or exaggerated) response to the perturbation[14] (which presumably would occur in the tibialis anterior muscles), causing her COG to move anteriorly. The antagonist muscles may then contract (in a hypermetric manner as well),[16] causing a posterior displacement of her COG and perhaps leading to taking a step. The repetition of balance and gait activities may help her to better utilize somatosensory feedback to scale (or match) the magnitude of these postural responses.[16]

4. Her impaired gaze stabilization during functional activities was related to her cerebellar dysfunction. Because patients with cerebellar dysfunction can use vision to help achieve postural stability,[37] we believe that it is important to try to improve gaze stability to improve stability during gait and other activities of daily living that typically require head movement. Her impaired gaze stability may be related to either her VOR function or her inability to suppress her VOR. Therefore, activities that help the patient use alternative strategies for gaze stabilization (eg, using cervical inputs during head movements via the cervico-ocular reflex) as well as practice suppressing the VOR may be helpful.

Our balance rehabilitation treatment program for this patient consisted of the standing balance and gait exercises and activities outlined under phase 1 through phase 3 in Table 2. She performed phase 1 of the program during the first 2 weeks, phase 2 during weeks 3 and 4, and phase 3 during weeks 5 and 6. In addition, she performed eye-head coordination exercises to help improve gaze stabilization during side-to-side head movements (Appendix, page 552). A brief explanation of the rationale for each activity in the treatment program is included in Table 2. The patient attended weekly 30- to 45-minute physical therapy sessions, during which her status was reassessed, she participated in eye-head coordination exercises as well as gait and balance activities, and she was instructed in progression of her home

Table 2.
Balance Rehabilitation Treatment Program and Its Rationale for Patient With Resected Cerebellar Tumor[a]

Rationale	Treatment Activity
Phase 1	
Promote use of VOR and COR for gaze stability	Visual fixation, EO, stationary target, slow head movements
Promote use of saccadic eye movements for gaze stability	Active eye and head movements between two stationary targets
Promote VOR cancellation	EO, moving target with head movement, self-selected speed
Improve ability to use somatosensory and vestibular inputs for postural control	Static stance, EO and EC, feet together, arms close to body, head movements
Improve ability to use vestibular and visual inputs for postural control	Static stance on foam surface, EC intermittently, feet 2.54–5.08 cm (1–2 in) apart
Improve postural control using all sensory inputs	Gait with narrowed base of support, EO, wide turns to right and left
Improve postural control using visual and vestibular inputs	March in place, EO, on firm and foam surfaces, prolonged pauses in unilateral stance
Phase 2	
Promote use of VOR and COR for gaze stability	Visual fixation, EO, stationary and moving targets, slow and fast speeds, simple static background; imaginary visual fixation, EC
Promote use of saccadic eye movements for gaze stability	Active eye and head movements between two targets, slow and fast speeds
Promote VOR cancellation	EO, moving target with head movement, fast and slow speeds
Improve ability to use somatosensory and vestibular inputs for postural control	Semitandem stance, EO and EC, arms crossed
Improve ability to use vestibular inputs for postural control	Stance on foam, EC intermittently, feet 2.54–5.08 cm apart
Improve postural control using visual and vestibular inputs	Gait with EO with sharp 180° turns to the right and left, firm and padded surfaces
Improve postural control using vestibular and somatosensory inputs	March in place, EC, prolonged pauses in unilateral stance
Improve postural control using all sensory inputs	Walking sideways and backward; standing EO and EC, heel touches forward, toe touches backward
Improve postural control with head moving using all sensory inputs	Gait with EO, normal base of support, slow head movements
Phase 3	
Promote use of VOR and COR for gaze stability	Visual fixation, EO, stationary and moving targets, various speeds, complex static and dynamic backgrounds; imaginary visual fixation, EC
Promote use of saccadic eye movements for gaze stability	Active eye and head movements between two targets, various speeds
Promote VOR cancellation	EO, moving target with head movement, various speeds, complex static and dynamic backgrounds
Improve ability to use somatosensory and vestibular inputs for postural control	Semitandem stance with EC continuously, and with EO on firm and padded surfaces
Improve postural control using vestibular and somatosensory inputs	Gait with EC with base of support progressively narrowed, firm and padded surfaces; march in place slowly, EO and EC on firm and foam surfaces
Improve postural control using visual and vestibular inputs	Gait with EO, rapid sharp turns to right and left, firm and padded surfaces
Improve postural control when head is moving using all sensory inputs	Gait with normal base of support, EO, fast head movements
Improve postural control using all sensory inputs	Braiding; active practice of ankle sway movements; bending and reaching activities

[a] EO=eyes open, EC=eyes closed, VOR=vestibulo-ocular reflex, COR=cervico-ocular reflex.

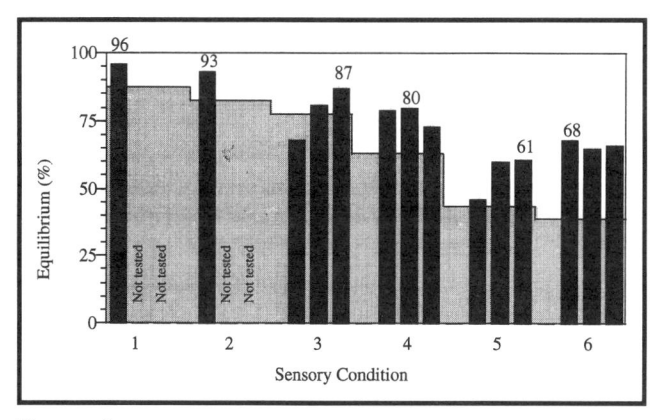

Figure 4.
Posttreatment (6-week) posturography (ie, sensory organization) test results for patient with cerebellar tumor resection. See Figure 3 legend for explanation of scores and sensory conditions.

Table 3.
Percentage of Improvement From Pretreatment Evaluation in Kinematic Indicators of Stability[a] During Standing Balance Activities and Locomotor Performance for Two Patients With Cerebellar Dysfunction

Task/Variable	Improvement (%)[b] Demonstrated by Patient With Cerebellar Tumor	Improvement (%)[b] Demonstrated by Patient With Cerebellar Xanthomatosis
Free gait		
Speed	20	10
Base of support	36	24
Whole-body COG-COP maximum moment arm[c]	4	16
Mediolateral COG-COP maximum moment arm[d]	18	18
Paced gait		
Cycle time	0	10
Double support time	28	28
Stance duration	2	18
Base of support	36	29
Whole-body COG-COP maximum moment arm	43	3
Mediolateral COG-COP maximum moment arm	24	24
Anteroposterior COG phase plane[e]		
Feet together with eyes closed	24	−54[f]
Semitandem stance with eyes open	70	No data[g]

[a] COG=center of gravity, COP=center of pressure.
[b] Improvement corresponds to a decrease in the values for all kinematic indicators of stability except speed and whole-body COG-COP maximum moment arm; for these items, improvement reflects an increase in these values.
[c] Whole-body COG-COP maximum moment arm is the difference between the body's COP and COG in the diagonal (combined anteroposterior and mediolateral) direction. A larger whole-body moment arm indicates that a state of less biomechanical stability is allowed to occur during the activity; that the patient allows the overall moment arm to get larger during an activity (and does not fall) signifies a higher level of overall balance control.[30] A 10% improvement in whole-body COG-COP maximum moment arm has been shown to represent a statistically significant and functionally meaningful difference in individuals with balance impairments.[38]
[d] Mediolateral COG-COP maximum moment arm is the difference between the body's COP and COG in the mediolateral direction. A smaller maximum moment arm in the mediolateral direction during activities in which the body's COG and COP are moving anteriorly (eg, walking forward) indicates that the individual is more stable and walking with a less variable base of support.
[e] Anteroposterior COG phase plane is a measure of the variance of the COG speed and displacement in the anteroposterior direction. A smaller value indicates less variance in the COG speed and displacement during a task, suggesting a higher overall level of stability.[33] Based on data from asymptomatic subjects, a change of more than 30% represents a meaningful change.[39]
[f] This value represents a decline in stability.
[g] No data available because the patient was unable to complete the test.

program. She had no difficulty with weekly progression of her home exercise program. She was instructed to perform the exercises at least once daily at home and to note the exercises completed, number of repetitions, and any difficulties experienced using a standard adherence tool in use at our clinic. She completed daily exercise logs, indicating that she was adherent to the home program on a once-per-day basis 5 out of 7 days per week over the 6-week course of treatment. The home program took her 30 to 40 minutes to complete.

After 6 weeks of treatment, she was reevaluated in the clinic and in the biomotion laboratory using the same measures as those used during the initial assessment. Repeat ENG and posturography tests were also performed.

Postrehabilitation Findings

At the conclusion of the 6-week treatment program, this patient reported a decrease in frequency and intensity of disequilibrium. She now felt unsteady only occasionally (ie, up to three times per week) at an intensity of 5/10 (compared with 7/10 prior to rehabilitation). There was no change in the frequency or intensity of dizziness. She scored 72/100 on the DHI (compared with 88/100 at the initial visit), reporting improvements in two physical activities, in two functional activities, and in three areas of emotional health that were reported to be problematic at the initial visit (Tab. 1). No items on the DHI were reported to be worse. The patient was now able to drive and walk outdoors independently. Balance assessment revealed no change in the ability to perform standing on foam with eyes closed or unilateral standing with eyes closed. Performance on other standing balance measures also remained the same, but there was a consistent decrease in the amount of postural sway observed. There was no change in the timed "up and go" test. Walking with eyes closed was performed in 5.39 seconds, but with three crossed steps (slightly faster). Tandem gait with eyes open could be performed for three steps (compared with two steps initially); she was still unable to perform tandem gait with eyes closed. No delay in response was observed during unexpected perturbation or release in the anteroposterior direction. There was an improvement in her ability to stabilize gaze during head rotation, as indicated by less degradation of visual acuity with head rotation at 1 Hz (20/20 compared with 20/40 initially) and at 2 Hz (visual acuity was 20/30 as compared with 20/70 initially).

Repeat ENG, sinusoidal axis rotation, and visual vestibular interaction testing showed no change when compared with testing done prior to rehabilitation. Repeat posturography testing indicated that she was able to maintain balance with normal equilibrium scores on all six test conditions (Fig. 4), thereby showing an improvement in her ability to stand on a sway-referenced platform with eyes closed.

The three-dimensional movement analysis revealed several changes indicative of improved postural stability (Tab. 3). During preferred pace (or free) gait, speed increased while base of support decreased, indicating that the patient moved more quickly and with a narrower base of support during gait. During paced gait (ie, when the speed of gait was controlled), double-limb support time and base of support decreased, implying that the patient walked in a more stable manner. The whole-body maximum COG-COP moment arm increased (whereas it decreased in the mediolateral direction) during both free and paced gait, implying a higher level of stability.[30,38] The COG phase-plane measure during semi-tandem standing improved (Fig. 1), indicating that the patient had better control of her COG displacement and speed during these tasks.[33,39]

Patient 2—Cerebellar Dysfunction Due to Cerebrotendinous Xanthomatosis

History
A 48-year-old right-handed man was referred for physical therapy with a diagnosis of cerebrotendinous xanthomatosis (CTX) resulting in balance and gait instability. Cerebrotendinous xanthomatosis is a rare autosomal recessive disorder of lipid metabolism (deficiency of liver mitochondrial enzyme required for oxidation of cholesterol to bile acids), characterized by elevations in cholestanol and cholesterol that deposit in tendons, peripheral tissues, in the spinal cord, and centrally in the cerebellum.[40] Major clinical manifestations include progressive cerebellar ataxia, subnormal intelligence, tendon xanthomas, cataracts, dementia, and limb paresis due to spinal cord pathology.[40] The onset of this progressive neurodegenerative disease typically occurs in early adulthood.[40]

This patient initially noted swelling of the Achilles tendon and gait difficulty at age 38 years. His gait instability progressed over the 10 years prior to our seeing him and resulted in a few falls during the last 2 years. His medical history included a T-12 compression fracture 4 years previously, a fracture of the left lower extremity as a result of a fall 2 years previously, and bilateral lens implants 5 years ago for cataracts. The patient had been maintained on cholesterol-lowering medication (Chenodil, 250 mg, three times daily) for the past 4 years. He had been seeing a neurologist twice a year to monitor his metabolic and neurologic status.

Transcranial Doppler testing provided evidence of occluded left vertebral artery and basilar artery disease. An electroencephalogram indicated mild generalized slowing of background activity and occasional brief episodes of more pronounced slowing over the left frontal temporal region. Sterol analysis demonstrated consistently increased concentrations of cholestanol and other sterols (however, the values were greatly reduced from values recorded 5 years previously). A computed tomography scan of the head performed approximately 3 years prior to referral for physical therapy showed cerebellar atrophy, calcification in the dentate nuclei of the cerebellum, and widening of the prepontine region consistent with brain-stem atrophy (Fig. 5). Trace to mild mitral regurgitation, with prolapse of both mitral leaflets, was shown on an echocardiogram. Carotid ultrasounds were normal. Electromyography showed no definitive electrophysiologic evidence of sensorimotor neuropathies. He lived with his mother and a younger brother, who also had CTX. He stopped driving a few years ago due to progressive visual problems related to his cataracts. He was employed as a materials handler in an industrial company but stopped working 2 years prior to his referral for physical therapy, at which time he applied for disability due to his visual problems and increasing difficulty with standing balance and walking.

Prerehabilitation Findings
A neurologist who examined him 2 months prior to his referral for physical therapy found him to be pleasant, talkative, and oriented to person, place, and time. There was mild dysarthria and decreased hearing on the right side. Extraocular movements and pursuit tracking were normal in all directions. There was a mild lateral gaze nystagmus on far excursion bilaterally. Lipid deposits measuring approximately 8 × 10 cm were present on both Achilles tendons. Deep tendon reflexes were brisk (3+) bilaterally in the upper extremities, normal (2+) at the knees, and diminished (1+) at the ankles. Babinski testing was normal bilaterally. Motor examination (performed with resisted isometric muscle testing of all muscle groups) revealed normal and symmetric upper- and lower-extremity strength. There was mild dysmetria

in the left upper extremity. There was no evidence of dystonia or choreoathetosis. Light touch, temperature, and proprioception were intact in all limbs. Vibration sense was mildly decreased in the toes and ankles bilaterally. The patient was able to walk independently without an assistive device, but his gait was wide-based (approximately 51 cm [20 in]) and appeared to be unsteady and stiff. Turns during gait were made very slowly and without rotation of the trunk. He was unable to perform tandem gait. Previous neuropsychological testing indicated that he was mildly retarded, without language or aphasic difficulties. The patient's neurologic examination findings were unchanged compared with the findings of an examination done 6 months earlier.

During the initial physical therapy examination, the patient was able to follow two-step commands but was easily distracted. Active range of motion in the upper and lower limbs was normal except for ankle dorsiflexion, which was limited to 0 degrees bilaterally (with the knee extended). Manual muscle testing of the upper and lower extremities was normal (5/5) for all muscle groups. Heel-to-shin movements were slow but accurate bilaterally. Finger-to-nose and rapid alternating movements of the upper extremity were slow and slightly dysmetric on the left side. The patient's sensation of light touch and proprioception were intact in both lower extremities.

The patient did not report any sensation of dizziness (eg, feelings of spinning or light-headedness). He reported the sensation of disequilibrium (eg, as if he might fall) approximately two or three times per week (when standing or walking) at an intensity of 6/10. A DHI was not completed due to the patient's cognitive limitations and his inability to distinguish problems related to his dizziness and balance from his visual problems. He was able to go outdoors independently, and he routinely spent 2 to 3 hours each day visiting friends. He reported feeling the need to be cautious when he was outside alone due to his gait instability and as a result decreased his walking speed and distance. He did not routinely help with household tasks but was able to help with cleaning and laundry. He found going outdoors to be particularly difficult during the winter months. As a result, he restricted walking outdoors in the winter and would go out only if he had transportation.

The patient demonstrated a forward-bent posture during standing and walking. He stood with a 20.3-cm (8-in) base of support. He said that he felt that he was steadier in this position as compared with when his feet were closer together. He was able to stand erect in response to verbal cues; however, he reported feeling unsteady and experienced the sensation of falling backward. The patient could stand with feet together and eyes closed for 19 seconds. When he was asked to maintain balance in that position and turn his head from side to side at a pace of 60 beats per minute, balance could be maintained only for 7 seconds. This finding suggested to us that the patient had difficulty when inputs related to head movement needed to be integrated simultaneously. He was able to maintain standing balance on a 7.62-cm compliant cushion with eyes open for 30 seconds and with eyes closed for 11 seconds, suggesting difficulty with postural control when vision was removed and somatosensory inputs were altered. He was unable to perform tandem standing with eyes open, suggesting difficulty maintaining the COG over a narrow base of support. He could stand on one leg for 1.5 seconds with eyes open but was unable to do so with eyes closed. This finding suggested to us that the patient had difficulty maintaining the COG over a narrow base of support even when visual inputs were available. A marked postural sway in the anteroposterior direction was observed during all standing balance tests, especially when the base of support was narrowed.

The timed "up and go" test (performed over a 12.2-m walkway) was completed in 18 seconds without the use of an assistive device. His gait appeared to be steady, although he slowed down during the 180-degree turn. Walking with eyes closed over a 6.1-m walkway was performed in 10 seconds, but with two crossed steps, suggesting difficulty with postural control during gait when vision was removed. He was unable to perform tandem gait with eyes open or closed. This finding suggested to us that the patient had difficulty maintaining the COG over a narrow base of support during gait even when visual inputs were available. Walking over a 6.1-m walkway while turning the head from side to side every third step was performed in 9 seconds, but with two crossed steps, suggesting that the patient had difficulty integrating vestibular inputs from head movements during walking. Gait on a 2.54-cm (1-in) foam walkway was steady and performed in 4 seconds with eyes open. Stepping strategies were markedly delayed in response to a sudden perturbation (a quick, high-speed push on the sternum to move the COG outside the base of support) or release (an unexpected removal of pressure from the sternum) in the posterior direction.

The patient's goals for rehabilitation included being able to walk outdoors for 4.8 km (3 miles) with a steadier gait, improved posture, and decreased risk and fear of falling.

Rehabilitation

The balance rehabilitation program designed for this patient was based on the following interpretation of his condition:

1. His primary problem of impaired postural stability was related to his cerebellar dysfunction. The pathology causing his cerebellar dysfunction was presumed to involve diffuse regions of his cerebellum rather than a specific area. Patients with cerebellar degeneration tend to have increased anteroposterior sway in standing with eyes open or closed when compared with individuals without cerebellar dysfunction, but they are able to use vision to decrease their unsteadiness.[37] This patient's postural sway did not appear to decrease even when his eyes were open during clinical balance testing (eg, standing with feet together or on foam), suggesting that he may not be using vision effectively to help decrease his unsteadiness. He may have difficulty using vision effectively for postural control due to his impaired visual acuity related to his cataracts. This patient may benefit from balance retraining that focuses on improving his use of visual cues for postural control.

2. He was not effectively using vestibular information for postural control in situations in which visual and somatosensory information were less available than vestibular inputs, as noted by his performance during balance testing (eg, standing on foam with eyes closed, walking with eyes closed). This finding was presumed to reflect abnormal integration of sensory information in the cerebellum and to be related to his cerebellar dysfunction.

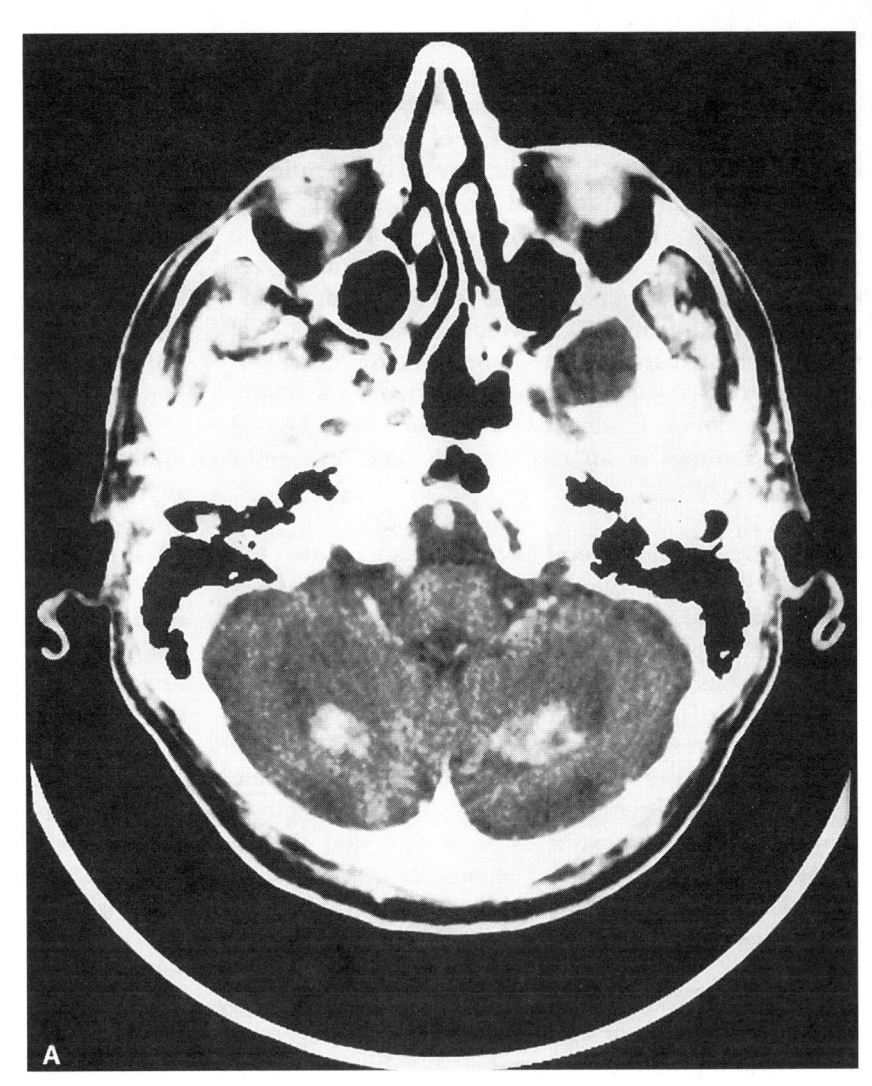

Figure 5.
Computed tomography (CT) scans for patient with cerebrotendinous xanthomatosis taken 3 years prior to referral for physical therapy: (A) CT scan demonstrating calcification of the dentate nuclei of the cerebellum. (B) CT scan demonstrating enlargement of cerebellar sulci secondary to atrophy of the cerebellar hemispheres. Enlargement of the fourth ventricle and the prepontine cistern are also shown. Findings are consistent with atrophy of the cerebellum and brain stem.

3. His difficulty with stepping strategies, supported by his performance during clinical testing with perturbation tests, may be consistent with scaling problems seen in patients with cerebellar dysfunction.[16] Alternately, it could be due to his inability to maintain balance (ie, control his COG) while standing on one leg. Repetition of specific balance and gait activities may help him to better utilize somatosensory feedback for scaling the magnitude of his postural responses.

4. His decreased ankle range of motion was related to decreased flexibility of his plantar-flexor muscles bilaterally and could contribute to his impaired postural responses (eg, inability to perform tandem standing or one-legged standing). Active stretching exercises, therefore, were included in the treatment program.

The balance rehabilitation treatment program received by the patient consisted of the standing balance and gait activities outlined under phase 1 through phase 3 in Table 4. The patient performed phase 1 of the program during the first 2 weeks, phase 2 during weeks 3 and 4, and phase 3 during weeks 5 and 6. A brief explanation of the rationale for each activity in the treatment program is included in Table 4. In addition, he was given exercises to stretch the ankle plantar flexors to help improve or preserve ankle range of motion. The patient had no difficulty tolerating progression of the exercises during weekly 30-minute physical therapy sessions. He was instructed to perform the exercises at least once daily at home and to note the exercises completed, number of repetitions, and any difficulties experienced using a standard adherence tool in use at our clinic. Due to evidence of slight cognitive impairments, his mother supervised his assigned home exercise program, which took 30 minutes to complete. The patient completed daily exercise logs, indicating that he was adherent to the home program 4 out of 7 days per week on a once-per-day basis over the 6-week course of treatment. After 6 weeks of treatment, he was reevaluated in the clinic and in the biomotion laboratory using the same measures as those used during the initial assessment.

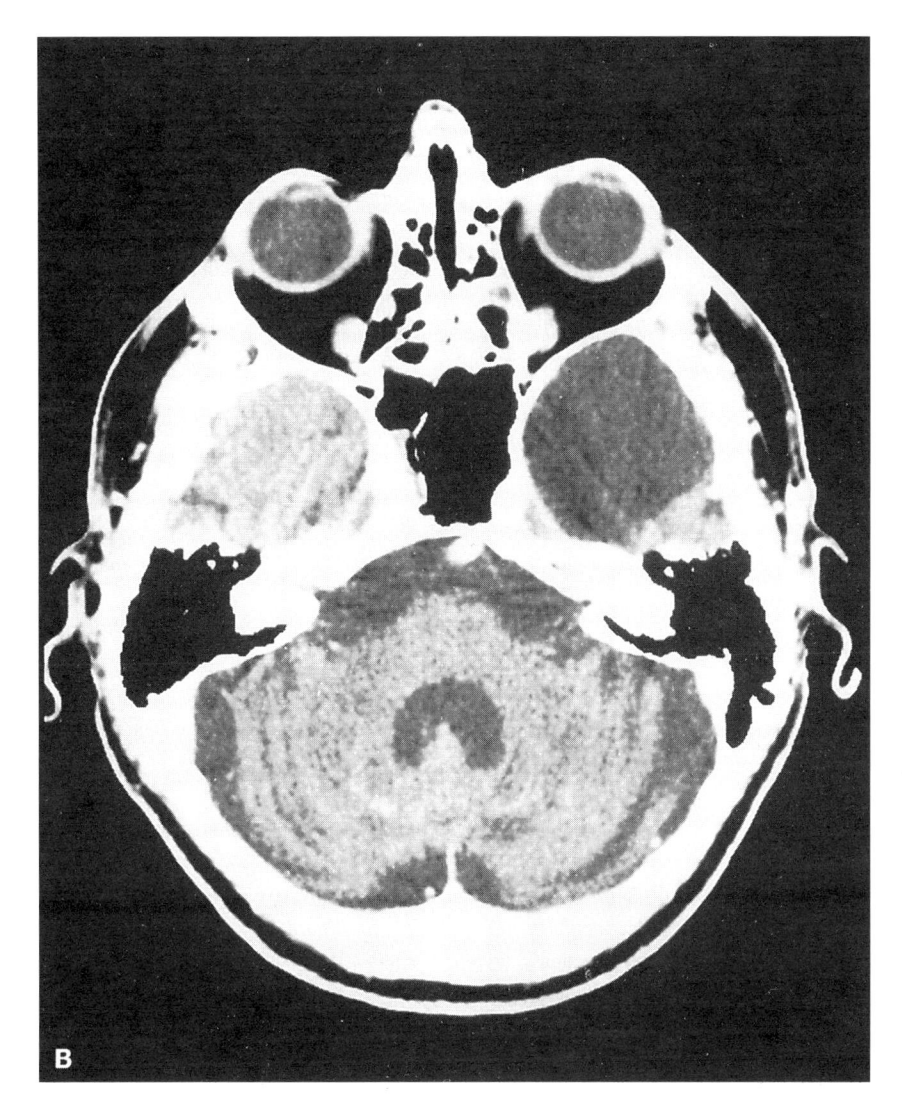

Postrehabilitation Findings

At the conclusion of the 6-week treatment program, the patient reported a decrease in both the frequency and intensity of his disequilibrium. He reported the sensation of disequilibrium only occasionally (approximately one time per week), and the intensity was reduced to 3/10 (from 6/10 initially). He was able to walk for 4.8 km several times per week, with less fear of falling. No falls had occurred. There was no change in ankle range of motion. Balance assessment revealed improvements in his ability to stand with feet together with eyes closed (60 seconds compared with 19 seconds) and with eyes closed with head rotation (17 seconds compared with 7 seconds). He improved in his ability to maintain balance with eyes closed on foam (21 seconds compared with 11 seconds). Tandem standing with eyes open could be performed for 5 seconds (as compared with 0 seconds); standing on one leg with eyes open could be performed for 3 seconds (as compared with 1.5 seconds). There was no change in his ability to stand on one leg with eyes closed. The timed "up and go" test was performed in 14 seconds (19% faster). Gait with eyes closed was performed 11% faster, with only one crossed step. The patient was able to perform tandem gait for three steps (compared to no steps before) with eyes open but was still unable to do tandem gait with eyes closed. Walking with head rotation was performed 19% faster, with no crossed steps (compared with two steps before). Walking on a foam walkway was performed 43% faster. Stepping strategies now appeared to be only minimally delayed in response to sudden perturbation or release in the posterior direction.

Several changes indicative of improved postural stability were shown with he three-dimensional movement analysis (Tab. 3). During free gait, walking speed increased while base of support decreased, indicating that the patient walked faster with a more narrow base of support. During paced gait, double-limb support time and base of support decreased, further suggesting that the patient walked in a more stable manner. The whole-body maximum COG-COP moment arm increased (whereas it decreased in the mediolateral direction) during free and paced gait, implying a higher level of stability.[30,38]

Discussion

Both patients demonstrated improvements in postural stability and function while reporting improvements in their perception of disequilibrium following 6-week individually designed programs of physical therapy. Although there were some similarities in the patients' responses to treatment, there were important differences between these two patients. This discussion will address two important questions: (1) Why did the patients have different responses to treatment, as indicated by varied performance results on test measures? and (2) If the treatment programs were related to the

Table 4.
Balance Rehabilitation Treatment Program and Its Rationale for Patient With Cerebellar Dysfunction Due to Cerebrotendinous Xanthomatosis

Rationale	Treatment Activity[a]
Phase 1	
Improve ability to use somatosensory and vestibular inputs for postural control	Static stance, EO and EC, feet together, arms close to body
Improve ability to use vestibular and visual inputs for postural control	Static stance on foam surface, EO, arms close to body, feet 7.62–10.16 cm (3–4 in) apart
Improve postural control using all sensory inputs	Gait with narrowed base of support, EO, wide turns to right and left
Improve postural control using all sensory inputs	March in place, EO, slow speed
Decrease ankle plantar-flexor tightness	Plantar-flexor stretching exercises
Phase 2	
Improve ability to use somatosensory and vestibular inputs for postural control	Static stance, EO and EC, arms crossed with head movements; semitandem stance, EO
Improve ability to use vestibular inputs for postural control	Static stance on foam, EO, feet 2.54–5.08 cm (1–2 in) apart, arms across chest
Improve postural control using visual and vestibular inputs	Gait with narrowed base of support, firm and padded surfaces
Improve postural control using all sensory inputs	Standing with alternate heel touches forward, toe touches backward; walking sideways and backward
Improve postural control with head moving using all sensory inputs	Gait with normal base of support, slow head movements, EO
Decrease ankle plantar-flexor tightness	Plantar-flexor stretching exercises
Phase 3	
Improve ability to use somatosensory and vestibular inputs for postural control	Semitandem stance, EC intermittently; static stance, EC with head movements
Improve ability to use vestibular inputs for postural control	Static stance on foam, EC with progressive narrowing of the base of support
Improve postural control using vestibular and somatosensory inputs	Gait with EC, base of support is progressively narrowed
Improve postural control using vestibular inputs	March in place, EO and EC on firm and foam surfaces
Improve postural control when head is moving using all inputs	Gait with normal base of support, EO, fast head movements
Improve postural control using all sensory inputs	Braiding; active practice of ankle sway movements; bending and reaching activities
Decrease ankle plantar-flexor tightness	Plantar-flexor stretching exercises

[a] EO=eyes open, EC=eyes closed.

improvements, why might the improvements have occurred?

The patient with the recurrent resected cerebellar tumor (initially diagnosed 6 years prior to the initiation of physical therapy) reported problems with dizziness and unsteadiness only 7 months prior to starting physical therapy. Therefore, her problems were relatively recent in onset, and she was in the subacute phase of recovery. In contrast, the patient with CTX reported progressively worsening problems with unsteadiness over 10 years. The patient with the resected cerebellar tumor may, therefore, have a greater potential for residual spontaneous recovery even though her symptoms were stable during the 7 months prior to referral for physical therapy.

Another important consideration is the difference in neuropathology between the two patients. In the patient with cerebellar tumor resection, the middle and superior vermis was predominantly affected (Fig. 2) and her functional problems were predominantly related to gait ataxia, consistent with a lesion in the vermis. In the patient with CTX, there was evidence of diffuse cerebellar atrophy, suggesting involvement of the spinocerebellum (both the vermis and intermediate zones of the hemispheres), the cerebrocerebellum, and the vestibulocerebellum (Fig. 5). In addition, there was CT scan evidence of involvement of the dentate nuclei (Fig. 5). Lesions of the deep cerebellar nuclei (such as the dentate nucleus) typically produce symptoms that are more severe than those seen with disorders restricted to the cortex.[41] This patient's clinical signs and symptoms, however, suggested greater involvement of the spinocerebellum. This patient did not have formal testing (ie, vestibular function tests) to examine central and peripheral vestibular pathways; therefore, involvement of the vestibulocerebellum cannot be ruled out.

Why might postural stability have improved in both of these patients? Bronstein et al[37] showed that although patients with cerebellar dysfunction swayed more than individuals without cerebellar dysfunction during tests with eyes open, with eyes closed, and with visual stimulation, they retain the ability to use vision to control much of their unsteadiness. Furthermore, these investigators found that on repeatedly moving the visual surround, the patients were able to suppress the destabilizing effect of visual stimuli, demonstrating the ability to adapt their responses and switch reliance to vestibulo-proprioceptive-postural loops.[37]

The patient with the resected cerebellar tumor did fairly well on balance measures at initial evaluation and therefore demonstrated minimal posttreatment changes on timed balance measures. This finding may have occurred because the patient underwent adaptation or spontaneous recovery prior to referral for physical therapy. Other considerations are that this patient was younger than the patient with CTX and that she may have already learned to use vision to control much of her unsteadiness. Her posttreatment posturography findings demonstrate her improved ability to integrate and use appropriate vestibular information in the absence of visual and somatosensory information. Why she did not improve in her ability to maintain balance while standing with feet together and eyes closed on compliant foam is unclear. This is a clinical test that is designed to simulate (to some degree) the same condition on which she improved during posturography testing. Perhaps standing on a foam surface serves more to distort than to reduce somatosensory input (such as occurs during posturography testing), making it a more difficult task for this patient. In contrast to the patient with CTX, this patient showed marked improvement in her ability to control COG speed and displacement in semitandem standing (Fig. 1). A decreased postural sway was also evident in the anteroposterior direction during assessment of the same standing posture. These findings indicate that time-based measures alone may not be adequate to accurately detect changes in postural stability in a patient such as this one, whose initial assessment revealed minimal deficits in performance.

The patient with CTX showed marked improvement in his ability to maintain balance with eyes closed on a firm surface both with and without head movements. This finding implies that the patient may have become better trained to use somatosensory inputs for postural control. He also demonstrated improved postural stability on a compliant foam surface with eyes closed, demonstrating his improved ability to use vestibular inputs. Similarly, his performance improved during tandem gait with eyes open and walking with head rotation, which suggests that he learned to use visual inputs more effectively for postural control. One possibility is that the patient, through repetition of the various activities performed, was trained to more efficiently use any available sensory input (visual, somatosensory, or vestibular). Many studies now support the idea that cerebellar circuits are modified by experience and that these changes are important for motor learning.[41] This patient, however, did not improve on COG phase-plane measures during standing with feet together and eyes open or closed, or in semitandem standing with eyes open. That the COG phase-plane measures did not improve after physical therapy quantifies the clinical observation of increased postural sway during these standing tasks. A more prolonged period of practice (eg, longer than 6 weeks) might have resulted in improvements in this patient's ability to control the speed and displacement of his COG, but further study is needed to determine whether this is true.

Although these two patients demonstrated different changes in standing postural stability after treatment, both patients demonstrated similar trends in improvements on gait stability measures (Tab. 3), despite their initial differences in performance and abilities. Briefly, free gait speed increased, whole-body COG-COP maximum moment arm increased (whereas COG-COP maximum moment arm in a mediolateral direction decreased), and the base of support decreased. When the speed of gait was controlled, the improvements demonstrated in base of support, double-limb support time, and mediolateral COG-COP maximum moment arm were of similar magnitude for the two patients.

Horak and Deiner[16] have suggested that the anterior lobe of the cerebellum in humans is not critical for normal latencies or for spatial or temporal timing of multisegmental agonists and antagonists of automatically triggered postural responses. The anterior lobe, however, appears to be critical for accurately tuning the magnitude (or scaling) of postural responses based on immediate prior experience. Use of speed feedback to scale the magnitude of postural responses is not impaired in patients such as those studied by Horak and Diener, who had various types of cerebellar dysfunction but all involving some portion of the anterior lobe.[16] Horak and Diener concluded that patients with anterior cerebellar lobe dysfunction appear to compensate for the abnormal scaling of hypermetric agonist responses by using somatosensory feedback to adjust the magnitude of later-occurring antagonist responses to the speed and amplitude of actual postural displacement. Both patients described in our case report had some involvement of their anterior cerebellar lobes, although neither patient had exclusive anterior lobe pathology.

The physical therapy program for both patients included activities in standing and during gait that would challenge their postural stability (eg, standing or walking with a narrow base of support with eyes open and closed), thereby inducing a movement strategy in response (eg, multisegmental sway, ankle sway). These experiences were probably instrumental in improving both patients' ability to effectively use somatosensory feedback for modifying the magnitude of postural responses rather than relying on prior experience or central set. This theory might also explain why both patients did better on the perturbation tests. An unexpected perturbation in the posterior direction, for example, produces an initial posterior perturbation, and the patient then has to return the COG to a more central point to stay erect or take a step if the COG has moved outside the base of support. Patients with cerebellar dysfunction have hypermetric responses to unexpected perturbations, causing them to sway more and for a longer time before returning to an equilibrium point (Bortolami SB, Wernick M, Krebs DE; unpublished research). After treatment, both patients appeared to have more timely stepping strategies when challenged with a large unexpected perturbation, suggesting that they were better able to scale the magnitude of their postural responses. Further research, including electromyographic analysis of muscle activity during perturbation tests, is necessary to determine whether this is true.

Summary

After participation in individually designed, staged programs of physical therapy, two patients with different cerebellar pathologies demonstrated improvements in symptoms, postural stability, and function, as indicated by self-report and three-dimensional movement analysis of gait activities. One patient did not demonstrate changes on time-based clinical tests but showed improvements on kinematic and kinetic variables measured during three-dimensional movement analysis of standing tasks. This finding indicates that time-based measures may not be comprehensive in detecting improvement in postural stability for all patients. We believe that it is unlikely that improvements in performance noted could be attributed to practice of the tasks, because the three-dimensional movement analysis of the gait activities included activities that were not performed as part of the treatment program (ie, paced controlled gait). Whether the trends in improvement described for these two patients using whole-body movement analysis represent trends that characterize other patients with similar pathologies cannot be determined. These conclusions can only be made after studying a large group of patients in a more controlled manner. The similarities in the two patients' responses to treatment emphasize that patients with cerebellar lesions, acute or chronic, can learn to improve their postural stability. Therefore, if the cerebellum is not totally destroyed, adaptation or compensation for the impairments produced appears to occur, perhaps in a neighboring area of the cerebellum or in another part of the brain. Further research is necessary to investigate the effectiveness of this treatment approach for patients with cerebellar dysfunction and to further understand the strategies used by persons with balance impairments to improve their postural control.

References

1 Roland PE. Partition of the human cerebellum in sensory-motor activities, learning, and cognition. *Can J Neurol Sci.* 1993;20(suppl 3):S75. Abstract.

2 Akshoomoff NA, Courchesne E. A new role for the cerebellum: cognitive operations. *Behav Neurosci.* 1992;106:731.

3 Gilman S, Bloedal J, Lechtenberg R. The symptoms and signs of cerebellar disease. In: *Disorders of the Cerebellum.* Philadelphia, Pa: FA Davis Co; 1981:189–262. Contemporary Neurology series.

4 Dichgans J, Diener HC. Different forms of postural ataxia in patients with cerebellar disease. In: Igarishi M, Black FO, eds. *Disorders of Posture and Gait.* New York, NY: Elsevier Science Inc; 1986:207–215.

5 Adams RD, Victor M. Abnormalities of movement and posture due to disease of the extrapyramidal motor systems. In: *Principles of Neurology, Part II: Cardinal Manifestations of Neurologic Disease.* New York, NY: McGraw-Hill Inc; 1989:68–75.

6 Thurston SE, Leigh RJ, Abel LA, Dell'Osso LF. Hyperactive vestibulo-ocular reflex in cerebellar degeneration: pathogeneses and treatment. *Neurology.* 1987;37:53–57.

7 Zee DS, Yee RD, Cogan DG, et al. Ocular motor abnormalities in hereditary cerebellar ataxia. *Brain.* 1976;99:207–234.

8 Cooper IS. *Involuntary Movement Disorders.* New York, NY: Harper & Row, Publishers Inc; 1969.

9 Amici R, et al. *Cerebellar Tumor Resections: Clinical Analysis and Physiopathologic Correlations.* New York, NY: S Karger and Co; 1976:35–76.

10 Holmes G. The cerebellum of man. *Brain.* 1939;62:1.

11 Oas JG, Baloh JW. Vertigo and the anterior inferior cerebellar artery syndrome. *Neurology.* 1992;42:2274–2279.

12 Iloeje SO. Measurement of muscle tone in children with cerebellar ataxia. *East Afr Med J.* 1994;71:256–260.

13 Viallet F, Bonnefoi-Kyriacou B, Massion J, et al. Quantitative assessment of postural asynergy in cerebellar pathology. In: Trouillas P, Fuxe K, eds. *Serotonin: The Cerebellum and Ataxia.* New York, NY: Raven Press Inc; 1993:343–355.

14 Bremer F. Le Cervelet. In: Roger GH, Binet L, eds. *Traite de physiologie normale et pathologique, volume 10.* Paris, France: Masson; 1935.

15 Ito M. Neurophysiologic aspects of the cerebellar motor control system. *Int J Neurol.* 1970;1:162.

16 Horak FB, Diener HC. Cerebellar control of postural scaling and central set in stance. *J Neurophysiol.* 1994;72:479–493.

17 Ito M. *The Cerebellum and Neural Control.* New York, NY: Raven Press Inc; 1984:1–7.

18 Bach-y-Rita P. Central nervous system lesions: sprouting and unmasking in rehabilitation. *Arch Phys Med Rehabil.* 1981;62:413–417.

19 Urbsheit NL, Oremland BS. Cerebellar dysfunction. In: Umphred DA, ed. *Neurological Rehabilitation.* 2nd ed. St Louis, Mo: CV Mosby Co; 1990:597–618.

20 Kabat H. Analysis and therapy of cerebellar ataxia and asynergia. *Arch Neurol Psychiatry.* 1955;74:375–382.

21 Morgan MH. Ataxia and weights. *Physiotherapy.* 1975;61:332–334.

22 Sage GH. *Motor Learning and Control: A Neuropsychological Approach.* Dubuque, Iowa: Wm C Brown Communications Inc; 1984.

23 Morgan MH. Ataxia: its causes, measurement, and management. *Int Rehabil Med.* 1980;2:126–132.

24 Balliet R, Harbst KB, Kim D, Stewart RV. Retraining of functional gait through the reduction of upper extremity weight-bearing in chronic cerebellar ataxia. *Int Rehabil Med.* 1987;8:148–153.

25 Brandt T, Krafczyks S, Mahbenden I. Postural imbalance with head extension: improvement by training as a model for ataxia therapy. *Ann NY Acad Sci.* 1981;74:636–649.

26 Sliwa JA, Thatcher S, Tet J. Paraneoplastic subacute cerebellar degeneration: functional improvement and role of rehabilitation. *Arch Phys Med Rehabil.* 1994;75:355–357.

27 Safe AF, Cooper S, Windsor ACM. Cerebellar ataxia in the elderly. *J R Soc Med.* 1992;85:449–451.

28 Shumway-Cook A, Woolacott MH. Assessment and treatment of patients with postural disorders. In: Shumway-Cook A, Woolacott MH, eds. *Motor Control: Theory and Applications.* Baltimore, Md: Williams & Wilkins; 1995:207–235.

29 Krebs DE, Lockert J. Vestibulopathy and gait. In: Spivack BS, ed. *Evaluation and Management of Gait Disorders.* New York, NY: Marcel Dekker Inc; 1995:93–116.

30 Riley PO, Hodge WA, Mann RW. Modelling the biomechanics of posture and balance. *J Biomech.* 1990;23:503–505.

31 Krebs DE, Wong DK, Jevsevar DS, et al. Trunk kinematics during locomotor activities. *Phys Ther.* 1992;72:505–514.

32 Antonsson EK, Mann RW. Automatic 6-DOF kinematic trajectory acquisition and analysis. *Journal of Dynamic Systems Measurement and Control.* 1989;111:31–39.

33 Riley PO, Benda BJ, Gill-Body KM, Krebs DE. Phase plane analysis of stability in quiet standing. *J Rehabil Res Dev.* 1995;32:227–235.

34 Parker SW. Vestibular evaluation: electronystagmography, rotational testing, and posturography. *Clin Electroencephalogr.* 1993;24:151–159.

35 Jacobson GP, Newman CW. The development of the dizziness handicap inventory. *Arch Otolaryngol Head Neck Surg.* 1990;116:424–427.

36 Podsiadlo D, Richardson S. The timed "Up and Go": a test of basic functional mobility for frail elderly persons. *J Am Geriatr Soc.* 1991;39:142.

37 Bronstein AM, Hood JD, Gresty MA, Panage C. Visual control of balance in cerebellar and parkinsonian syndromes. *Brain.* 1990;113:767–779.

38 Krebs DE, Gill-Body KM, Riley PO, Parker SW. Double-blind placebo-controlled trial of vestibular rehabilitation for bilateral vestibular hypofunction: preliminary report. *Otolaryngol Head Neck Surg.* 1993;109:735–741.

39 Danis CM. *Relationship of Standing Posture and Stability.* Boston, Mass: MGH Institute of Health Professions; 1996. Master's thesis.

40 Brown MS, Goldstein JL. Disorders of lipid metabolism. In: Petersdorf RG, Adams RD, Braunwald E, et al, eds. *Harrison's Principles of Internal Medicine.* 10th ed. New York, NY: McGraw-Hill Book Co; 1983:547–559.

41 Ghez C, Fahn S. The cerebellum. In: Kandel E, Schwartz J, eds. *Principles of Neural Science.* 2nd ed. New York, NY: Elsevier Science Inc; 1985:502–522.

Appendix.
Cerebellar Rehabilitation Eye-Head Coordination Exercises to Promote Gaze Stability for Patient With Resected Cerebellar Tumor

1. Visual Fixation on a Stationary Target
Write a word (eg, "open") on a business card. Hold the card in your hand at arm's length so that you can see the word clearly. Alternatively, you may tape the card on a wall. Keep your eyes focused on the word. Next, move just your head from side to side, keeping the word in focus at all times. Try to do this for 1–2 minutes without stopping. You should stop only if the word becomes unclear or if you get very dizzy. If the word becomes hard to read, do this exercise moving your head a little slower.
Do this exercise:
_____ while sitting
_____ while standing with your feet _____
_____ with the target (eg, card) close to you
_____ with the target across the room
_____ Practice this exercise at different speeds of head movement.
_____ Repeat the exercise moving your head up and down for 1–2 minutes.
_____ Repeat the exercises using a large pattern in the background such as a checkerboard, wallpaper, or television. First, move your head from side to side for 1–2 minutes. Rest briefly. Then, move your head vertically for 1–2 minutes.

2. Active Eye-Head Movements Between Two Stationary Targets
Hold two targets in front of you at eye level and placed approximately 20 cm (8 in) apart. First, look directly at the first target and then align your head with that target. Next, look at the second target with your eyes first and then turn your head to the second target. Be sure to keep the target in focus during the head movement. Repeat in the opposite direction; that is, start by looking at the first target and then align your head with the first target. Look at the second target with your eyes first and then turn your head to the first target. Place the two targets close enough together such that when you are looking directly at one target, you can see the other target with your peripheral vision. Practice for 5 minutes, resting if necessary.
As you do this exercise:
_____ Vary the speed of the head movement, keeping the targets in focus.
_____ Also perform this exercise with two vertically placed targets.

3. Visual Fixation on a Moving Target—Vestibulo-ocular Reflex Cancellation
Write a word (eg, "open") on a business card. Hold the card in your hand at arm's length such that you can see the word as clearly as possible. Keep your eyes focused on the word. Next, move your head and the card together from side to side, keeping the word in focus as much as possible. Try to do this for 1–2 minutes without stopping. You should stop only if the word becomes unclear or if you get very dizzy. If the word becomes hard to read, do this exercise moving the card and your head a little slower.
Do this exercise:
_____ while sitting
_____ while standing with your feet _____
_____ Practice this exercise at different speeds of head movement.
_____ Repeat the exercise moving your head up and down for 1–2 minutes.
_____ Repeat the exercises using a large pattern in the background such as a checkerboard, wallpaper, or television. First, move your head from side to side for 1–2 minutes. Rest briefly. Then, move your head vertically for 1–2 minutes.

4. Visual Fixation on a Moving Target—Gaze Stability
Write a word (eg, "open") on a business card. Hold the card in your hand at arm's length. Make sure you can see the word clearly. Next, move the card and your head horizontally (ie, from side to side) in opposite directions for 1–2 minutes, keeping the word(s) in focus all the time. (That is, when your head moves to the right, the card should move to the left; when the head moves to the left, the card should move to the right.)
Do this exercise:
_____ while sitting
_____ while standing
_____ Move your head at different speeds but keep the words in focus. Continue to do this for 1–2 minutes without stopping.
_____ Repeat the exercise moving your head and the card up and down in the opposite directions for 1–2 minutes.
_____ Repeat the exercises using a large pattern in the background such as a checkerboard, wallpaper, or television. First, move your head from side to side for 1–2 minutes. Rest briefly. Then, move your head vertically for 1–2 minutes.

5. Imaginary Visual Fixation
Look at a target (eg, word on a card) directly in front of you. Close your eyes and turn your head slightly, imagining that you are still looking directly at the target. Next, open your eyes and check to see if you have been able to keep your eyes on the target. Repeat in the opposite direction. Be as accurate as possible. Vary the speed of head movement. Practice for up to 5 minutes. This exercise can also be performed in the vertical direction.

Balance Retraining After Stroke Using Force Platform Biofeedback

Balance is a somewhat ambiguous term used to describe the ability to maintain or move within a weight-bearing posture without falling.[1,2] Balance can further be broken down into three aspects: steadiness, symmetry, and dynamic stability.[3] *Steadiness* refers to the ability to maintain a given posture with minimal extraneous movement (sway). The term *symmetry* is used to describe equal weight distribution between the weight-bearing components (eg, the feet in a standing position, the buttocks in a sitting position), and *dynamic stability* is the ability to move within a given posture without loss of balance.[3]

All of these components of balance (steadiness, symmetry, and dynamic stability) have been found to be disturbed following stroke.[2,4,5] Balance testing of patients with hemiparesis secondary to stroke has revealed a greater amount of postural sway during static stance,[1,4] asymmetry with greater weight on the nonparetic leg,[2,4] and a decreased ability to move within a weight-bearing posture without loss of balance.[2,4] Furthermore, research has demonstrated moderate relationships between balance function and gait speed ($r=-.67$ and $.42$, respectively),[6,7] independence ($r=.62$),[7] appearance (defined as "significantly abnormal," "slightly abnormal," and "nearly normal") ($r=.50$),[7] dressing ($r.55-.69$),[8] wheelchair mobility ($r=.51$),[8] and reaching ($r=.49-.78$).[9]

Thus, a principal construct within physical therapy practice is the reestablishment of balance function in patients following stroke. Recent advances in technology have resulted in the commercial availability of numerous force platform systems for the retraining of balance function in patient populations, including patients with stroke. These systems are designed to provide visual or auditory biofeedback to patients regarding the locus of their center of force (COF) or center of pressure (COP), as well as training protocols to enhance stance symmetry, steadiness, and dynamic stability. Typical force platform biofeedback systems consist of at least two force plates to allow the weight on each foot to be determined, a computer and monitor to allow visualization of the COF or COP, and software that provides training protocols and data analysis capabilities. Some units allow auditory feedback in addition to the visual feedback in response to errors in performance.

[Nichols DS. Balance retraining after stroke using force platform biofeedback. *Phys Ther.* 1997;77:553–558.]

Key Words: *Balance; Biofeedback; Posture, general; Stroke.*

Deborah S Nichols

Whether a platform system provides a COF measure or a COP measure is dependent on the strain-gauge setup within the force plates. Center of force is calculated only from the vertical forces projecting on the force plates. Center of pressure is calculated from both the vertical forces and the horizontal forces projecting on the force plates, thus accounting for horizontal shear. In the absence of postural sway, these two calculations are identical; however, when sway is present, they are similar, both allowing for the determination of symmetry, steadiness, and dynamic stability, but not identical.[10] For the purposes of this update, however, these two calculations will not be distinguished because many of the research publications do not provide sufficient detail to determine whether COF or COP was calculated.

Measures Used to Evaluate Balance Function and Progress

Three types of measures are most commonly used by force platform systems to evaluate balance function and patient progress related to balance ability: postural sway measures, symmetry measures, and limits-of-stability measures. Although each force platform system provides these measures in different units, they tend to provide a variant of each of these measures. Postural sway measures give information relative to postural steadiness; thus, a larger sway magnitude is related to greater postural unsteadiness. Sway measures include the sway area, sway path, and standard deviation or root mean square of the sway distance. The sway increase for patients following stroke has been reported to be as high as double that for age-matched peers.[7]

Symmetry measures reflect the amount of weight on each foot or the distance of the COF away from the midline. Testing of subjects following stroke has shown asymmetries in weight bearing of up to 27%, with control subjects demonstrating little asymmetry in weight bearing (ie, <7%).[5]

Finally, most units provide a measure of dynamic stability related to limits of stability. The limits of stability are the maximal distance an individual can lean in any direction without loss of balance; these limits describe a cone projecting about the feet with maximal displacement equal to 8 degrees anteriorly, 4 degrees posteriorly, and 8 degrees laterally to either side.[11] Individuals with hemiparesis secondary to stroke have been found to have reduced limits of stability. Dettman et al[12] calculated a stability index (percentage of the base of support over which the COP was moved during weight shifting without loss of balance) as a measure of limits of stability for subjects with hemiparesis and age-matched control subjects. The stability index was 2.3% for the subjects with hemiparesis and 16.6% for the control subjects. The authors also reported that the COP was shifted toward the nonparetic limb in the subjects with hemiparesis.[12]

A principal construct within physical therapy practice is the reestablishment of balance function in patients following stroke.

Balance Retraining Protocols

Balance retraining with postural biofeedback can address each of the components of function described (steadiness, symmetry, and dynamic stability). Postural steadiness can be addressed through activities that require maintenance of the COF, usually depicted by the cursor on a computer screen, within a narrow target or within a narrow range, designated by a shaded area on the screen, as weight is transferred from one target to the next (Fig. 1).

Postural symmetry can be addressed by maintaining the COF in midline, defined on the computer screen by a vertical line or cross hair (Fig. 2), or by providing visual information regarding the percentage of weight on each foot or auditory input when less than a target weight is placed on the paretic limb. The patient can be asked to perform various activities while maintaining equal weight distribution, such as coming to a standing position or reaching.

Finally, dynamic stability can be addressed by activities that require weight shifting along the anteroposterior or mediolateral plane or to selected targets displayed on a computer screen (Figs. 3 and 4). These activities often address more than one balance component; activities that encourage stance symmetry also require minimal postural sway for the patient to be successful, and activities that involve weight shifting for dynamic stability also often address postural sway and symmetry in order for the target to be reached quickly and accurately.

Effectiveness of Postural Biofeedback

Steadiness

Numerous researchers have examined the effect of postural biofeedback on stance steadiness as measured by postural sway.[1,13–16] Only a few researchers, however, have studied this effect in individuals with hemiparesis.[1,13,15] Shumway-Cook et al[1] trained subjects to main-

---

DS Nichols, PhD, PT, is Director and Associate Professor, Physical Therapy Division, School of Allied Medical Professions, The Ohio State University, 1583 Perry St, Columbus, OH 43210 (USA) (nichols.3@osu.edu).

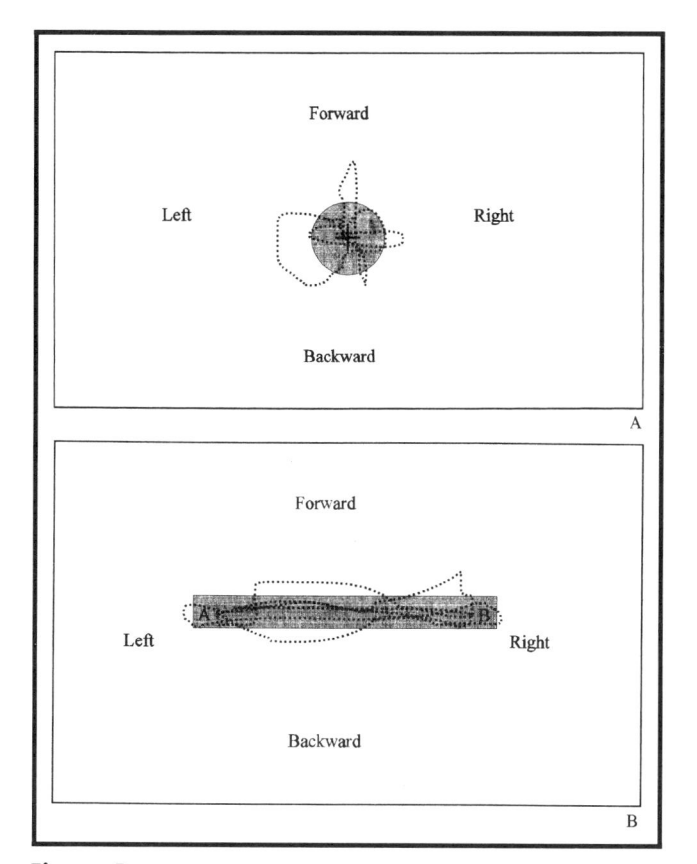

Figure 1.
Steadiness training with central target: (A) In this task, the subject is asked to maintain the computer cursor (central "+" sign) inside the shaded circle. The postural sway can be depicted on the screen as well (dotted line). Measures typically indicate the amount of time the cursor is maintained in the central target and the sway magnitude. (B) In this task, the subject is asked to shift weight repetitively from left (target A) to right (target B) while maintaining the cursor within the shaded rectangle; the sway can be depicted as well (dotted line). Time in the shaded area is calculated, as well as sway magnitude.

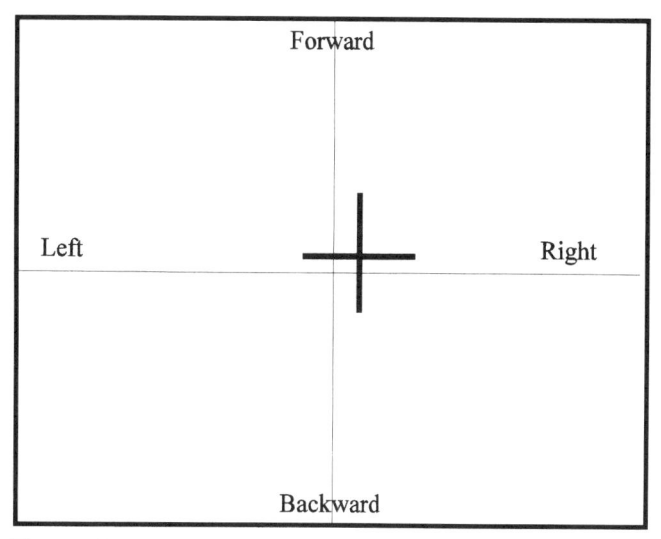

Figure 2.
Symmetry training with central target: In this task, the subject is asked to maintain the computer cursor (+) in the center of the computer screen as marked by the cross hair. The sway path may be depicted on the screen (not illustrated).

tain the cursor in the center of a small target in the middle of the computer screen with even weight distribution between the two feet. The emphasis of the training was on symmetry, but the activity required postural sway to be confined to the central target for the subject to demonstrate symmetry. There was no change in sway area following the 2 weeks of training for either biofeedback-trained or traditionally trained subjects, although symmetry was improved. Conversely, McRae et al[15] found a greater, but not statistically significant, decrease in postural sway in subjects trained with biofeedback in comparison with traditional therapy. However, the difference may not have reached statistical significance because of the small sample size; therefore, the results should be viewed with caution. Winstein et al[13] also reported a decrease in sway variability in subjects treated with postural biofeedback, but this decrease was equal to that of subjects treated by traditional physical therapy. Hocherman et al[17] examined the training effect of stance on a moving platform over time and found that subjects were able to tolerate increased amplitudes of movement over the training period. This training effect might also be interpreted as increased steadiness, but these researchers did not use sway as a measure; instead, the measure used was the maximal platform movement tolerated without falling.

Symmetry

Most studies that have evaluated the use of postural biofeedback have emphasized stance symmetry in their training protocols. Symmetry has been addressed by providing feedback on the percentage of weight on the paretic limb[13,18] and by having subjects maintain a cursor in the center of a target on the computer screen.[1,19] In several studies, functional activities were incorporated into the symmetry training: coming to a standing position with equal weight distribution,[13,19] reaching to the side and returning to a symmetrical stance,[18] and stride standing and stepping.[13,19] In all of these studies, increased stance symmetry was found following training, and in those studies that had a control group, the increase in symmetry was greater in the subjects who received the biofeedback training than in the control subjects who received traditional physical therapy.[1,13,19] In addition, increases in symmetry have been reported to be maintained at a 1-month follow-up.[17] Furthermore, dynamic stability training, involving weight shifting to successive targets, has also been found to increase stance symmetry.[19]

Wannstedt and Herman[18] identified several other issues pertinent to the use of postural biofeedback training for enhancing stance symmetry. They reported greater improvement with this training in subjects with right hemiparesis compared with subjects with left hemipare-

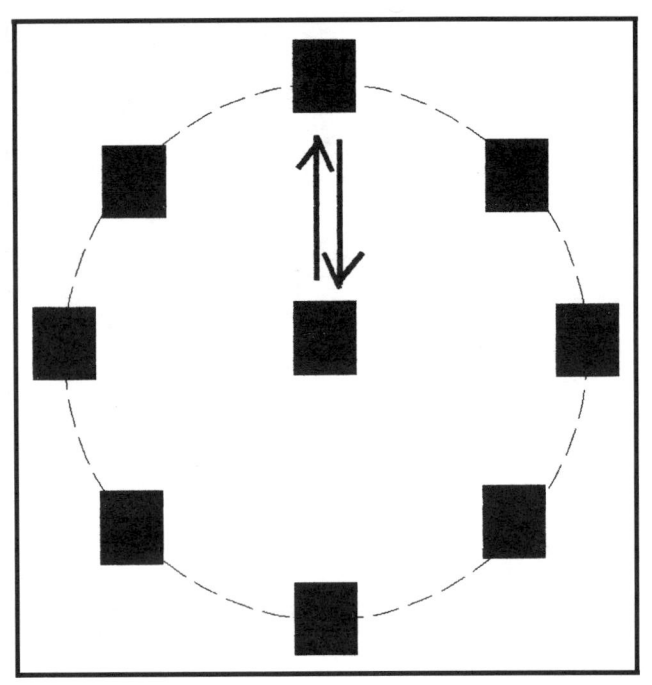

Figure 3.
Dynamic stability from center to target: A central target is surrounded by a series of targets. The subject is asked to move the center of force from the central target to a lit target and then back to the center within a given time period. Successive targets are then lit so that the subject has to shift weight successively in each direction. Transition time, path sway, and distance error can be calculated.

Figure 4.
Dynamic stability to successive targets: A series of targets in a circle are depicted on the computer screen. The subject starts at the uppermost target and has to transfer weight (depicted by the computer cursor) to each successive target as it is lit. This can be done in either a clockwise or counterclockwise manner. Transition time, path sway, and distance error can be calculated.

sis. This finding has not been addressed in any other study. They also reported that those subjects who were able to achieve symmetry in stance during the first training session with biofeedback were the only subjects to acquire the ability to maintain symmetry without feedback following their training protocol and to retain this ability 1 month later. Finally, the subjects in this study were all at least 6 months poststroke, which suggests that this type of training can be facilitatory even in persons with chronic strokes.

Dynamic Stability Training

The training of dynamic stability, referring to movement within the limits of stability, is most commonly done by having subjects shift weight so that the screen cursor, which is indicative of their COF, moves to a designated target. Two protocols have been described most consistently in the literature. One protocol involves a central target encircled by a series of targets at 45-degree angles (Fig. 3). The subject's task is to shift his or her weight forward to a lit target and back to the central target within a specified period of time, typically 7 to 10 seconds, before the next target is illuminated.[15,16,19] The transition time (time to move the COF from the starting position to the target), the sway path (cumulative distance covered), the sway error (accuracy of the weight shift from the central target to the peripheral target [calculated as a difference score: straight-line path −

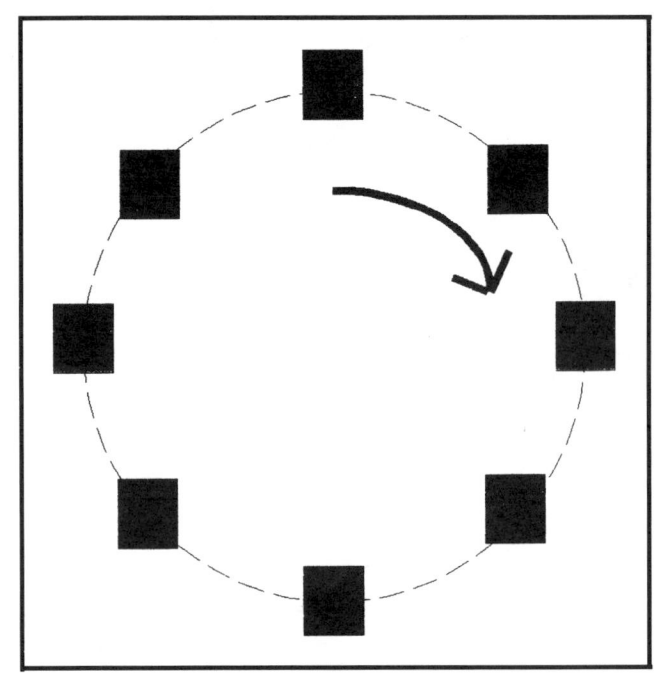

sway path]), and peripheral sway area (sway magnitude once the target is reached) are units used to evaluate patient performance.[20] The other protocol involves shifting weight around a series of successive targets oriented in a circle at 50% to 75% of the individual's limits of stability (Fig. 4); again, transition time, sway path, sway error, and peripheral sway area are the units used to evaluate subject performance.[14–16,19] This type of training has been found to decrease the magnitude of each of these variables, which indicates an increased accuracy of the weight shift in subjects without balance dysfunction,[13] older subjects with balance dysfunction,[16] and subjects with hemiparesis.[19] In addition, both subjects without balance dysfunction[14] and subjects with hemiparesis[16] have been able to extend their limits of stability with dynamic stability training. Expanding these limits should decrease the likelihood of falling, but this relationship has not been evaluated in any study. Furthermore, this type of training may affect steadiness. McRae et al[15] found a decrease in static sway following six dynamic stability training sessions in subjects with hemiparesis.

Although force platform measures of steadiness have been reported to be reliable and valid, units that use COF measures have been found to be more reliable than those that use COP measures (regression coefficients ranging from .31 to .85 for COF and from −.07 to .49 for

COP).[3] Furthermore, the dynamic measures (transition time, sway path, sway error) related to the dynamic stability activities have been found to be more reliable than static measures in subjects with hemiparesis (intraclass correlation coefficients ranging from .84 to .88 for dynamic measures and from .29 to .63 for static measures).[6]

Implications

Increased steadiness, decreased asymmetry, and enhanced dynamic stability are consistent with the therapeutic goals set for most patients with hemiparesis secondary to stroke. Thus, force platform biofeedback may be a useful tool in the treatment of these patients. The therapist designing a treatment protocol needs to keep in mind, however, that the evaluative measures, the type of training protocol used, and the therapeutic goals will have an impact on the effectiveness of this treatment modality.

I believe that the therapist needs to choose the best possible measure of patient progress. Steadiness, as measured by postural sway, has been found to be inconsistently affected by platform biofeedback. Of the studies that have examined sway following training,[1,13,15] two studies[13,15] demonstrated decreased sway and one study[1] demonstrated no change in sway. In the study by Winstein et al,[13] however, the magnitude of the decrease in sway was equal in the trained and nontrained subjects. Thus, biofeedback protocols may not be any more beneficial than traditional approaches in increasing postural steadiness but may add variability of practice to the treatment session.

Measures of symmetry and dynamic stability may, in my view, be more strongly linked to function and may be better indicators of patient progress than changes in postural sway or steadiness. Significant correlations have been found between these measures and improved transfer ability (Spearman correlations ranging from .34 to .54),[15] enhanced endurance (Spearman correlations ranging from .34 to .54),[15] and other measures of balance, including the Berg Balance Scale (Kendall coefficients ranging from −.55 to −.61)[6] and functional reach (Pearson correlation coefficients ranging from .66 to .75).[9] In two single-case studies, improved stance symmetry was associated with improvement in measures of activities of daily living and gross motor function.[19] Postural symmetry and dynamic stability also have consistently been improved by biofeedback training using force platform systems.[1,13–19] Furthermore, dynamic stability components (eg, transition time, sway error) have demonstrated better reliability than the static sway measures associated with steadiness.[6]

Although symmetry and dynamic stability have been found to correlate with many functional measures, the impact of platform biofeedback training on function is an area of considerable controversy in the existing literature. The degree to which postural biofeedback training seems to affect function appears to be related not only to the functional activity evaluated but also to the training protocol used.

Studies in which multiple activities were used, including a dynamic stability protocol, have shown the most consistent changes in patient function, including transfers,[15] home mobility (ability to move from one room to another),[15] endurance,[15] activities-of-daily-living scales,[19] gross motor function scales,[19] and gait.[16,19] Improvement in home mobility but not endurance was found in subjects following biofeedback training in comparison with a nontrained control group.[15] In an evaluation of two single-subject case studies, Sackley and Baguley[19] found substantial improvements in scores on the Rivermead Motor Assessment and a 10-point activities-of-daily-living scale with postural biofeedback that incorporated symmetry training in a standing position and in coming to a standing position, dynamic stability training to successive targets, reaching with a return to a symmetrical posture, stride standing and stepping, and bending the paretic limb while bearing weight on it. Subjects were tested over an 8-week period, using a reversal ABAB design. Improvements that were noted during the biofeedback training continued throughout the nontraining period. Thus, it appears to be important to include weight-shifting activities that challenge the limits of stability and require accuracy and speed within the retraining protocol to achieve functional improvement.

The most controversial aspect of postural biofeedback training has been its effect on gait. Although balance function and weight-bearing symmetry have been found to correlate with most gait components in subjects with hemiparesis secondary to stroke,[7] the effect of postural biofeedback on these gait components has varied considerably. In the earliest report of the effect of postural biofeedback training on gait, Winstein et al[13] identified increases in gait speed, cadence, stride length, and cycle time following biofeedback training, which were equal in magnitude to the changes identified for patients treated with traditional physical therapy, yet no change in the asymmetrical gait pattern occurred with either training protocol. More recently, McRae et al[15] reported that their nontrained subjects demonstrated greater improvement in ambulation than did subjects who trained with postural biofeedback; however, the method of evaluating ambulation was not described. In contrast, Rose et al[16] reported changes in joint angle diagrams and phase-plane portraits that reflected improved gait symmetry following balance retraining with a dynamic stability program in four subjects with hemiparesis secondary to stroke. This study, however, did not include a control group.

Thus, the type of training protocol (ie, static versus dynamic) may affect the transference of force platform biofeedback training to gait. Furthermore, improved gait symmetry has been reported with postural biofeedback during gait provided by a limb-load monitor.[21] These conflicting findings illustrate that the type of gait analyses conducted, the gait components chosen for analysis, and the training protocol used may affect the results. Moore and Woollacott[20] pointed out that studies have examined only time-distance or joint angle variables and that no studies have evaluated the magnitude of limb loading on the paretic limb. Future research, therefore, needs to address the effects of postural biofeedback training on components of gait not measured in the existing studies, such as limb loading, as well as evaluate the use of postural biofeedback during ambulation, which is possible with some commercially available units with a runway-type platform or movable footplates.

Finally, although there is considerable need for further research on the effects of force platform biofeedback on the balance components of steadiness, symmetry, and dynamic stability and its impact on functional outcome in patients with hemiparesis secondary to stroke, the research to date suggests that there is a place for this type of program in the rehabilitation of patients exhibiting postural asymmetry or decreased limits of stability following stroke. The patient's prognosis and therapeutic goals should define the role of postural biofeedback in his or her treatment program. For patients with more severe involvement, for whom postural steadiness sufficient for maintenance of stance is a primary goal, a training protocol that emphasizes postural steadiness may be sufficient; however, no research has been conducted with these types of patients. For patients with moderate involvement, for whom symmetry and dynamic stability in activities of daily living are goals, training protocols that address these postural components may be an appropriate component of the rehabilitation program and have been reported to enhance functional gains.[15,19] For patients with mild involvement, for whom symmetrical community-based ambulation is a goal, traditional force platform biofeedback may facilitate improvements in gait speed and cadence but may not address asymmetry.[13] Postural biofeedback with a limb-load monitor or force platform system that provides a runway, however, might facilitate symmetrical weight bearing during gait.[21]

References

1 Shumway-Cook A, Anson D, Haller S. Postural sway biofeedback: its effect on reestablishing stance stability in hemiplegic patients. Arch Phys Med Rehabil. 1988;69:395–400.

2 Horak F, Esselman P, Anderson M, Lynch M. The effects of movement velocity, mass displaced, and task certainty on associated postural adjustments made by normal and hemiplegic individuals. J Neurol Neurosurg Psychiatry. 1984;47:1020–1028.

3 Goldie PA, Bach TM, Evans OM. Force platform measures for evaluating postural control: reliability and validity. Arch Phys Med Rehabil. 1989;70:510–517.

4 Dickstein R, Nissan M, Pillar T, Scheer D. Foot-ground pressure pattern of standing hemiplegic patients: major characteristics and patterns of movement. Phys Ther. 1984;64:19–23.

5 Mizrahi J, Solzi P, Ring H, Nisell R. Postural stability in stroke patients: vectorial expression of asymmetry, sway activity, and relative sequence of reactive forces. Med Biol Eng Comput. 1989;27:181–190.

6 Liston R, Brouwer B. Reliability and validity of measures obtained from stroke patients using the Balance Master. Arch Phys Med Rehabil. 1996;77:425–430.

7 Bohannon RW. Gait performance of hemiparetic stroke patients: selected variables. Arch Phys Med Rehabil. 1987;68:777–781.

8 Nichols DS, Miller L, Colby LA, Pease WS. Sitting balance: its relation to function in individuals with hemiparesis. Arch Phys Med Rehabil. 1996;77:865–869.

9 Fishman MN, Nichols DS, Colby LA, Sachs L. Comparison of functional upper extremity tasks and dynamic standing balance in hemiparesis. Phys Ther. 1996;76:S79. Abstract.

10 Nichols DS, Glenn TM, Hutchinson KJ. Changes in the mean center of balance during balance testing in young adults. Phys Ther. 1995;75:699–706.

11 Nashner LM. Sensory, neuromuscular, and biomechanical contributions to human balance. In: Duncan PW, ed. Proceedings From the APTA Forum; Nashville, Tenn; June 13–15, 1989. Alexandria, Va: American Physical Therapy Association; 1990:5–12.

12 Dettmen M, Linder M, Sepic S. Relationships among walking performance, postural stability, and functional assessments of the hemiplegic patient. Am J Phys Med. 1987;66:77–90.

13 Winstein C, Garner E, McNeal D, et al. Standing balance training: effect on balance and locomotion in hemiparetic adults. Arch Phys Med Rehabil. 1989;70:755–762.

14 Hamman R, Mekjavic I, Mallinson A, Longridge N. Training effects during repeated therapy sessions of balance training using visual feedback. Arch Phys Med Rehabil. 1992;73:738–744.

15 McRae J, Panzer V, McKay M. Rehabilitation of hemiplegia: functional outcomes and treatment of postural control. Phys Ther. 1994;74(suppl):S119. Abstract.

16 Rose D, Clark S, Fujimoto K. Dynamic balance retraining: Does it transfer to gait? Journal of the American College of Sports Medicine. 1995;27(5):S5. Abstract.

17 Hocherman S, Dickstein R, Pillar T. Platform training and postural stability in hemiplegia. Arch Phys Med Rehabil. 1984;65:588–592.

18 Wannstedt GT, Herman RM. Use of augmented sensory feedback to achieve symmetrical standing. Phys Ther. 1978;58:553–559.

19 Sackley C, Baguley B. Visual feedback after stroke with the balance performance monitor: two single-case studies. Clinical Rehabilitation. 1993;7:189–195.

20 Moore S, Woollacott MH. The use of biofeedback devices to improve postural stability. Physical Therapy Practice. 1993;2:1–19.

21 Seeger B, Caudrey D. Biofeedback therapy to achieve symmetrical gait in children with hemiplegic cerebral palsy: long-term efficacy. Arch Phys Med Rehabil. 1983;64:160–162.

Advances in the Treatment of Vestibular Disorders

This article discusses the pathophysiology, evidence of treatment efficacy, and factors that contribute to improved treatment outcome in three different vestibular disorders. In patients with unilateral and bilateral vestibular loss, recent research suggests that customized, supervised exercises facilitate recovery of postural stability. These exercises are based on knowledge of normal vestibular function as well as on our understanding of the various compensatory mechanisms that can contribute to recovery. Recognizing the limitations of these compensatory mechanisms as substitutes for lost vestibular function is important in establishing treatment goals. Treatment of patients with benign paroxysmal positional vertigo (BPPV) is based on the identification of the specific canal involved and the anatomy of the labyrinth. Although patients with BPPV primarily experience brief episodes of vertigo, this disorder is also associated with postural instability, which may not resolve with remission of the positional vertigo. [Herdman SJ. Advances in the treatment of vestibular disorders. *Phys Ther.* 1997;77:602–618.]

Key Words: *Balance, Vestibular system.*

Susan J Herdman

The use of exercises in the rehabilitation of patients with vestibular disorders, a relatively old treatment approach dating to the 1940s, has for many years been based on anecdotal evidence of improved function with treatment. Recent studies[1-12] have led to a refinement of the treatments used and have documented treatment efficacy in a variety of vestibular disorders. This article will explore these advances in treatment of patients with the two most common vestibular problems who are referred for rehabilitation: (1) vestibular paresis or loss and (2) benign paroxysmal positional vertigo (BPPV).

Vestibular Paresis and Loss

The term "vestibular paresis" implies a loss of vestibular hair cells or vestibular neurons and therefore a decrease in the vestibular system's response to head movement. Unilateral and bilateral vestibular deficits both result in postural instability, disequilibrium, and oscillopsia, although these problems are usually more severe in patients with bilateral vestibular loss. Acute unilateral deficits also result in vertigo, spontaneous nystagmus, and skew deviation (vertical malalignment of the eyes due to an abnormal otolith input), which are the result of the asymmetry in the tonic firing of the vestibular neurons. This asymmetry recovers spontaneously, usually within a few days of onset, and exercises do not affect the course of recovery in patients with this condition.[13] Patients with vestibular loss usually do not have a history of vertigo or nystagmus because in most cases the vestibular loss is symmetrical. Postural instability, disequilibrium, and oscillopsia are due to the decreased gain of the vestibular response to head movement. *Gain* refers to the relationship of the input signal (in this case, head movement) to the output (the eye movement generated or postural stability). Ideally, the gain of the vestibular system would be "1." Recovery of postural stability and of vestibulo-ocular reflex (VOR) gain following vestibular loss requires both visual inputs and movement, and there is evidence that if visuomotor experience is delayed, the recovery period will be more prolonged.[13,14] This recovery may occur through an increase in the gain of the remaining vestibular response, but the substitution of other sensory and motor strategies is a major part of recovery in these patients. This recovery can be facilitated through the use of exercises.[1-3,15-23]

Treatment goals, I believe, should be specific to the patient's problems and should reflect both the direct effect of the vestibular paresis or loss and the indirect effects of the inactivity that accompanies these vestibular problems. These goals may include decreasing complaints of disequilibrium, improving postural stability in stance and during ambulation and other functional activities, improving gaze stability during head movements, and improving tolerance for activity (endurance). Effective treatment of people with vestibular deficits has recently been demonstrated in several controlled studies.[1-5]

Evidence That Exercise Facilitates Recovery Following Vestibular Loss

Although there is considerable anecdotal support that exercises are important in the rehabilitation of patients with vestibular problems,[17-23] only recently have prospective, controlled studies provided evidence that vestibular rehabilitation techniques are beneficial for patients with unilateral or bilateral vestibular losses.[1-3] These studies have primarily emphasized changes in postural stability, in disability, and in patient complaints as a result of these interventions. Horak et al[1] reported that patients with chronic, unilateral vestibular deficits had improved postural stability after a 6-week course of

---

SJ Herdman, PhD, PT, is Associate Professor, Division of Physical Therapy, Department of Orthopaedics and Rehabilitation, University of Miami School of Medicine, 5915 Ponce de Leon Blvd, Plumer Bldg, 5th Floor, Coral Gables, FL 33146-2480 (USA) (sherdman@mednet.med.miami.edu).

Table 1.
Factors Influencing Recovery Following Vestibular Paresis or Loss

Positive Influences	Negative Influences
Customized,[a] supervised exercises	Generic, unsupervised exercises
Stable unilateral vestibular deficits	Fluctuating disorders (eg, Ménière's disease)
Less severe initial disability	Head injury
Recent onset	Mixed central and peripheral lesion
	Vestibular suppressant medications

[a] Customized based on problems identified in the clinical examination.

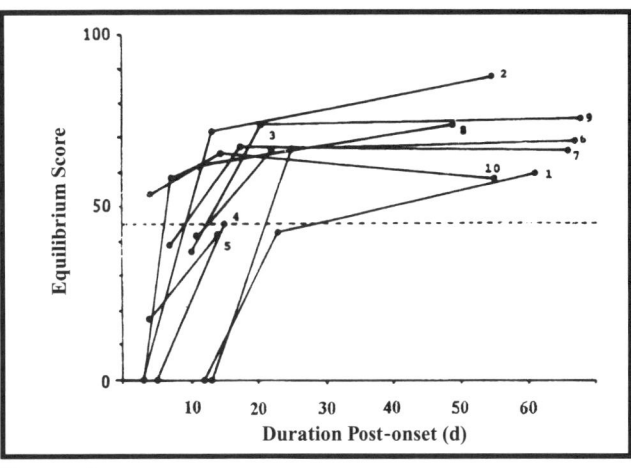

Figure 1.
Recovery of postural stability following unilateral vestibular loss in 10 patients as measured using computerized dynamic posturography. The equilibrium scores reflect anteroposterior sway, with 100 indicating perfect stability and 0 indicating loss of balance. The scores shown here are the averages from tests in which both visual and somatosensory cues were altered (tests 5 and 6; three trials each). Patients were tested as early as the third day after onset of the unilateral vestibular loss. Most patients recovered to within normal limits (above dotted line) by the third week from onset. (Adapted from Fetter et al[31] with permission.)

vestibular exercises compared with a group of patients performing general conditioning exercises. The exercises were customized for each patient and included balance and gait exercises as well as exercises incorporating combinations of head and eye movements. Krebs et al[2] studied the effectiveness of vestibular exercises on postural stability during functional activities in patients with chronic bilateral vestibular deficits. They used a placebo-controlled trial and found that patients performing customized exercises had better stability while walking and during stair climbing and were able to walk faster than patients performing isometric and conditioning exercises. Their vestibular exercise program also consisted of both balance and gait training and combinations of head and eye movements. Vestibular adaptation exercises have also been shown to produce a more rapid recovery during the acute stage following unilateral vestibular loss.[3] Adaptation exercises initiated on the third day following resection of acoustic neuroma resulted in improved postural stability in stance and during ambulation and in a decrease in the perception of disequilibrium when compared with the findings for a control group of patients.[3]

Factors influencing treatment efficacy. Several factors have been identified that affect the potential for recovery in patients with vestibular deficits (Tab. 1). The exercises used today in the treatment of patients with vestibular loss should be customized to the patient based on the results of the examination. Customized, supervised exercises for patients with vestibular disorders result in more patients achieving complete remission of symptoms (85%) compared with a generic, unsupervised exercise program that patients perform at home (64%).[4,24] Szturm et al[5] reported similar findings in a comparison of vestibular adaptation exercises with Cawthorne-Cooksey exercises,[25] which were not customized to the individual patient.

Studies suggest that patients with stable unilateral vestibular deficits (as opposed to fluctuating disorders such as Ménière's disease), symptoms provoked by movement,[4] less severe initial disability, or a more recent time of onset will have a better recovery. The effect of concurrent head injury on recovery of function is not clear. Shepard et al[26] have shown that patients with head injury tend to have a poorer prognosis, perhaps because the structures involved with central adaptation and compensation may be impaired, although many patients show a decrease in symptoms with treatment. Shepard et al[27] found that a more prolonged period of therapy was necessary if the patient had a mixed central and peripheral lesion, used vestibular suppressant medications, or had increased long-latency responses to sudden perturbations of the support surface. Shepard et al did not discuss the importance of the increased long-latency responses, but these responses may be related to the presence of central nervous system lesions in some patients. Keim et al,[28] however, reported little difference in recovery between patients with central vestibular deficits and patients with peripheral vestibular deficits. The effect of age on the rate and final level of recovery also is not clear, although studies[27,29] indicate that improvement occurs in elderly patients.

Mechanisms of Compensation Following Vestibular Loss

Understanding compensatory mechanisms and their limitations in improving postural and gaze stability should lead to more effective treatment of these patients and to a better understanding of the potential for functional recovery. The primary mechanisms of recovery of postural stability appear to be improved vestibular responses[3,30,31] and increased reliance on visual[32,33] and somatosensory cues.[30,34,35] A variety of mechanisms contribute to the recovery of gaze stability following unilateral and bilateral vestibular loss. These mechanisms include recovery of the VOR itself,[36,37] alterations in saccadic amplitude and direction,[38,39] potentiation of the cervico-ocular reflex (COR),[39–42] central preprogramming,[39,43] visual tracking mechanisms,[39] and limiting of head movement and activity.[41]

Postural Stability

Postural stability is maintained through complex interactions among sensory inputs, biomechanical constraints, and voluntary motor control. Three systems—visual, vestibular, and somatosensory—provide the main inputs to the automatic postural reflexes and contribute to voluntary postural control. Although there is considerable redundancy in the contributions of the different sensory cues to postural stability, each sensory input appears to have an optimal stimulus frequency at which it acts to stabilize balance. The vestibular system functions across both low and high frequencies of input; however, neither visual nor somatosensory cues stabilize balance at the high frequencies.[44–46]

Recovery of vestibular function. Recovery of the vestibulospinal system is difficult to measure because it is difficult to isolate that system from systems associated with postural control. Several researchers[3,30,31] have noted the recovery of the ability of patients with unilateral vestibular loss to maintain their balance when both visual and somatosensory cues are altered (Fig. 1). This finding may indicate an improved ability of patients to use remaining vestibular signals to maintain their balance, or it may be due to recovery of some vestibular neurons or to adaptation of the vestibular system.

Adaptation implies a long-term change in how the vestibular system responds to head movement. It is important to note that although adaptive capabilities decrease with aging, older individuals have considerable abilities to modify the gain of their vestibular responses.[47] Most studies of vestibular adaptation have been performed using the VOR as the outcome measure, in part because it is far easier to measure the VOR than to measure the vestibulo-spinal reflex and because the "error signal" that induces a change in the gain of the vestibular response appears to be retinal slip, that is, movement of an image across the retina.[48–50] More recent studies indicate that eye movements are important as well.[51] This error signal is processed through the cerebellum and the vestibular nuclei and changes the output of the vestibular system (Fig. 2).[52]

Several concepts about adaptation of the vestibular system are particularly important. First, adaptation is context specific. This concept was demonstrated several years ago for frequency of head movement.[53] When attempts are made to artificially increase VOR gain by

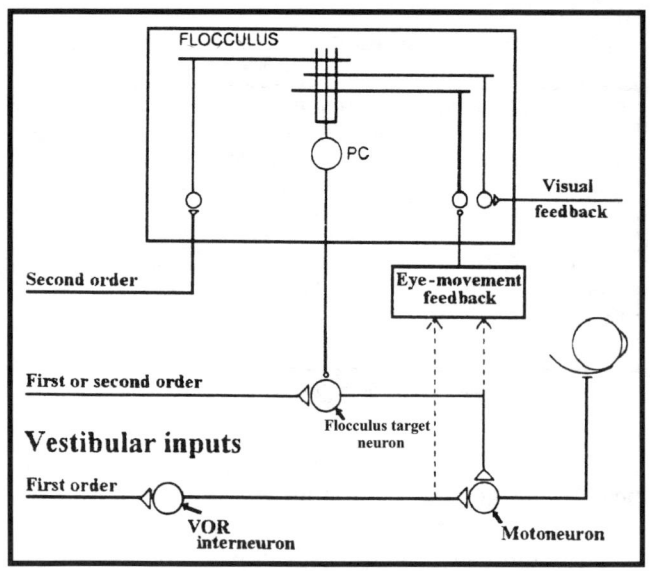

Figure 2.
Feedback loop that provides flocculus with the error signal necessary to produce a change in the gain of the vestibulo-ocular reflex (VOR). Lisberger[52] has suggested that this mechanism involves the flocculus and flocculus target neurons in the vestibular nucleus. The Purkinje cells (PC) in the flocculus receive visual, eye movement, and vestibular signals. (Adapted from Lisberger[52] with permission.)

having subjects move their head while wearing magnifying glasses, the greatest changes in gain occur at the training frequency, with smaller changes in gain occurring at other frequencies.[53] These results suggest that vestibular adaptation exercises should be performed across a wide range of frequencies to be most effective. More recently, orientation of the head during training has been shown to be a factor, presumably because the otolith input influences the effect of training.[54]

Second, although VOR gain changes occur within minutes, it takes time to induce persistent changes in VOR gain.[55] This finding has been aptly demonstrated by subjects without vestibular disorders wearing reversing prism glasses.[55] When the head turns, the reversing prisms cause the visual environment to appear to move in the same direction as the head movement instead of opposite to the direction of head movement. Within a few minutes after wearing the reversing prisms, VOR gain begins to decrease to reduce this effect. If the glasses are then removed, VOR gain rapidly returns to normal. The longer the exposure to the altered visual input, however, the longer the VOR gain changes are retained.

Third, not all head movements appear to result in adaptation. Changes in VOR gain have been demonstrated for horizontal (yaw) and vertical (pitch) head movements in humans, but there is little adaptive capability associated with head movements in the roll plane (Leigh RJ, personal communication). Although the

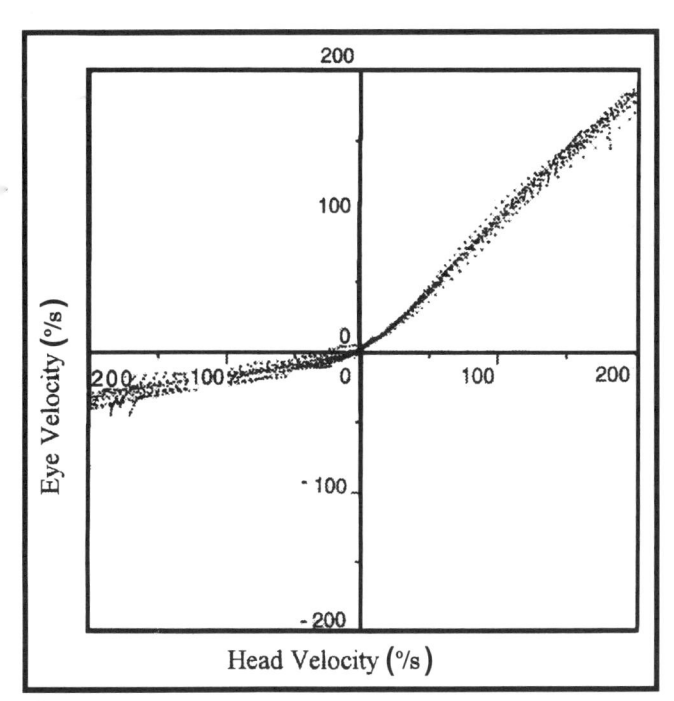

Figure 3.
Asymmetry in vestibulo-ocular reflex gain in patient with unilateral vestibular deficit becomes apparent at high speeds. Eye speed (Y-axis) is plotted against head speed (X-axis) for head rotations horizontally at speeds of up to 200°/s toward (positive numbers) and away from (negative numbers) the normal side. (Adapted from Halmagyi et al[66] with permission.)

cliché "If it makes you dizzy, it's good for you" is often used as a criterion for vestibular exercises, this may not always be appropriate; repeated head movements in the roll plane certainly make patients as well as subjects without vestibular disorders "dizzy" but will not substantially alter their long-term vestibular responses. Therapists need to take these factors into consideration when developing exercise programs for their patients.

Substitution of other mechanisms. Somatosensory cues: Black et al[30] showed that in the acute stage following resection of acoustic neuromas, subjects had decreased postural stability when somatosensory feedback from the lower extremities was distorted. This finding suggests that patients with unilateral vestibular loss may rely on somatosensory cues during that early stage of recovery. Bles and colleagues[34,35] have shown that during the course of recovery, patients with complete bilateral vestibular loss change how they rely on sensory cues for stability. Initially, they rely on visual cues as a substitute for the loss of vestibular cues, but over a 2-year period, these patients increase their reliance on somatosensory cues.

Visual cues: Visual inputs provide several different cues that affect postural stability. As a person sways, even in quiet stance, retinal slip information is used to determine body movement relative to environmental movement.[56] Changes in image size and retinal disparity, which would occur with fore-aft sway, are additional cues. Visual stabilization of balance appears to be primarily dependent on foveal vision. Some studies[32,33] indicate that patients with unilateral vestibular loss become less stable when visual cues are removed. Patients with bilateral vestibular loss also initially rely on visual cues for stability; however, this would not seem to be a particularly successful strategy during walking. Without the vestibular system, the eyes are not stable the during the head movement that occurs during ambulation and visual acuity degrades. Even at a visual acuity of 20/40, postural stability is decreased.[56,57] Patients may attempt to resolve this problem by decreasing head movements during activities such as walking.

Limitations of substitution. The stimulus frequency ranges at which somatosensory and visual cues contribute to postural stability are known only for stance and not for ambulation. Somatosensory cues appear to contribute postural stability between 1 and 3 Hz[44] and visual cues between 0.1 and 1 Hz.[45,46] The vestibular system operates over a wide range, with otolith signals contributing to postural stability at lower frequencies (<1 Hz) and the semicircular canals contributing to postural stability at higher frequencies (up to 5 Hz). Somatosensory and visual inputs, because they do not operate across the same frequencies as vestibular signals, would be only partially successful at substituting for lost vestibular cues.

When the body is relatively stable, such as while sitting or standing quietly, there is little head movement and visual and somatosensory cues are sufficient to maintain postural stability in patients with vestibular loss.[58] During locomotion, however, the frequency of head movements exceeds the compensatory ability of these systems. The dominant frequency of head movements in subjects without vestibular impairments walking in place ranges from 0.7 to 1.2 Hz for horizontal head movements and from 0.9 to 5.1 Hz for vertical head movements.[59] During running in place, the frequency of horizontal head movements increases to as high as 1.9 Hz and the frequency of vertical head movements increases to 5.8 Hz, well within the frequency range of vestibular function.[59-61] Similarly, the velocity of head movements during ambulation usually is well within the velocity range in which the normal vestibular system works (<300°/s).

There seems to a natural course as to which sensory cues are used to maintain postural stability at different stages following vestibular loss. Although visual cues become increasingly important, it is probably not optimal to foster visual dependency (eg, by teaching patients to fixate on a stationary object and to decrease their head movements while walking) because that may limit the patients' ability to learn to use remaining vestibular function and somatosensory cues. Additionally, patients may voluntarily restrict head movements. Ultimately, restricting head movements would result in decreased tolerance for functional activities and still would not provide a mechanism for postural stability during head movements. Central preprogramming of postural responses would be an effective strategy only when the required movement can be anticipated.

Gaze Stability

Gaze stability refers to the stabilization of the eye in space in order to see clearly. The purpose of the VOR is to maintain gaze stability during head movements. If the VOR and other mechanisms cannot produce an appropriate compensatory eye movement, movement of the head will cause substantial retinal slip and therefore degradation of visual acuity. In reality, compensatory eye movements do not have to match head movements perfectly because 2° to 4°/s of retinal slip can be tolerated without degradation of visual acuity.[60,62–64] The consequences of poor gaze stability are visual blurring (poor visual acuity during head movements) and also poor postural stability because the contribution of visual cues to postural stability would decrease with decrements in visual acuity.[56,57] Exercises that improve gaze stability, therefore, may help to improve postural stability by improving the patient's ability to use visual cues for balance.

Recovery of vestibular function. During the acute stage following unilateral vestibular loss, VOR gain is as low as 0.25 and 0.5 for rotation of the head toward and away from the involved side[36,37] (normal VOR gain is usually between 0.5 and 0.8). The gain of the horizontal VOR recovers quickly and is within normal limits in 1 to 3 months for slow head rotations.[36,37] The gain of the vertical VOR to slow head movements is reduced symmetrically by approximately 66%. There is some evidence that vertical VOR recovers more slowly than does horizontal VOR.[65] When patients are tested using rapid head thrusts or unpredictable head movements, however, there is no improvement in VOR gain for head movements toward the involved side, even 1 year after onset.[66] The poor compensation for rapid head thrusts toward the deficit is predicted by Ewald's Second Law, which states that the response of the horizontal canals is less efficient for ampullofugal (contralateral) head rotation than for ampullopetal (ipsilateral) head rotation.[55] This horizontal canal response is due to the discharge properties of the vestibular nerve, which can be increased above its resting rate more than it can be decreased. (The firing rate of neurons can only be decreased to zero.) In patients with unilateral vestibular deficits, a marked asymmetry in VOR gain persists to head movements exceeding 100°/s (Fig. 3). The VOR gain improves in some patients with bilateral vestibular loss but, again, only to relatively low-speed head movements.[67] As with the recovery of postural stability, the recovery of VOR gain may be due to the recovery of some of the vestibular hair cells or neurons themselves or to the adaptive capability of the remaining vestibular system.

Table 2.
Frequency of Complaints in 100 Patients With Benign Paroxysmal Positional Vertigo[a]

Complaint	Frequency (%)
Poor balance	57
Sense of rotation (vertigo)	53
Trouble walking	48
Light-headedness	42
Nausea	35
Queasiness	29
Spinning inside head	29
Sense of tilt	24
Sweating	22
Sense of floating	22
Blurred vision	15
Jumping vision	13

[a] Patients could indicate more than one complaint. (Unpublished data; RJ Tusa, MD, Dizziness and Eye Movement Center, University of Miami, Miami, Fla.)

Substitution of other mechanisms in gaze stability. Modification of saccades: Patients with bilateral vestibular deficits may decrease the amplitude of saccadic eye movements and make both slow-phase (<60°/s) and saccadic eye movements in the same direction during combined eye and head movements.[39] Both of these strategies assist in moving the eye to the target when the head moves. Similarly, patients with unilateral vestibular loss may make saccadic eye movements in the same direction as slow-phase eye movements to augment an inadequate VOR.[68] Although this strategy may enable patients to visually "capture" a target once the saccade is completed, they still would not be able to see during the saccadic eye movement.

Cervico-ocular reflex: Somatosensory receptors in ligaments and joints in the upper cervical region project to the contralateral vestibular nuclei and can produce compensatory eye movements (ie, CORs) that parallel the VOR.[69] In individuals without vestibular disorders, the gain of the COR is variable and often negligible.[43,70,71] When the COR is present in these persons, it operates only at low frequencies (<0.1). The gain of the COR in patients with bilateral vestibular loss can be as great as 0.25, and the COR produces compensatory eye movements across a wider range of frequencies (up to 0.3 Hz).[39,40] There is little evidence that the COR is altered in patients with unilateral vestibular loss.

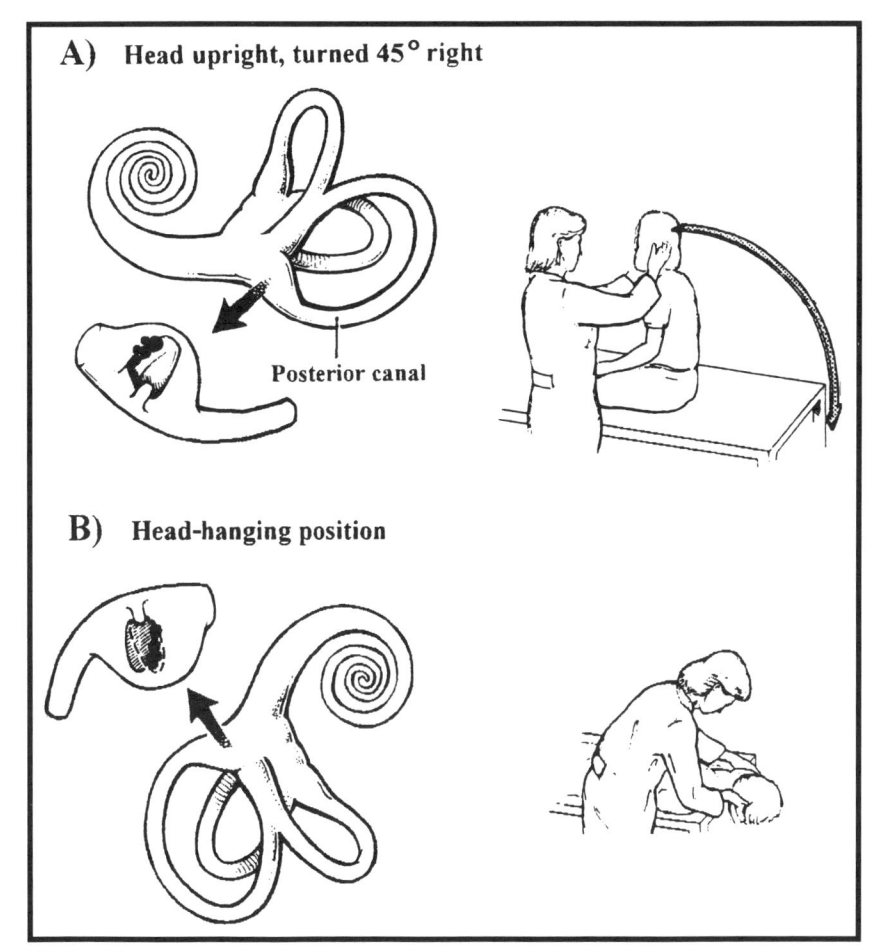

Figure 4.
Debris adhering to the cupula of the semicircular canal (shown here for posterior canal) will cause the cupula to be deflected when the person is moved from the sitting position (A) to the head-hanging position (B) in the Hallpike-Dix maneuver.

Central preprogramming: Central preprogramming of compensatory eye movements to improve gaze stability has been demonstrated primarily by comparing the gains of the compensatory eye movements during active and passive head movements.[39,43,70] Central preprogramming is effective in subjects without vestibular disorders and in people with unilateral and bilateral vestibular loss who have no central nervous system lesion.

Visual tracking: Visual tracking does not appear to be an important compensatory mechanism in the recovery of gaze stability. Kasai and Zee[39] reported that the smooth pursuit system works at the upper end of the normal range in patients with bilateral vestibular loss, that is, a gain of 1 at frequencies of less than 1 Hz and at speeds of 20° to 30°/s.

Decreased head movements: Some patients limit head movements in order to minimize oscillopsia.[41] This "learned disuse" would not be a particularly useful strategy for improving gaze stability because it would limit everyday activities and still would not provide a mechanism for seeing clearly during head movements.

Limitations of substitution. When the body is relatively stable, smooth-pursuit eye movements and the COR are sufficient to maintain gaze stability in patients with vestibular loss.[72–74] During locomotion, however, the speed and frequency of head movements exceed the compensatory ability of smooth-pursuit eye movements (<60°/s and <1 Hz) and the COR (0.3 Hz).[39,59,63] Therefore, neither tracking eye movements nor the COR will substitute completely for the lost vestibular function. Additionally, during ambulation, head movements do not occur in a predictable manner but are random. This "randomness" is an important factor because under these conditions, predictive eye movements (central preprogramming) will not help to stabilize gaze and a degradation of visual acuity would be expected in patients with vestibular loss.

Benign Paroxysmal Positional Vertigo

Benign paroxysmal positional vertigo is a biomechanical problem in which one or more of the semicircular canals is inappropriately excited, resulting in brief episodes of vertigo and in disequilibrium.[75] This disorder occurs in adults of all ages, although it is more common among older individuals, and accounts for 160,000 new cases of dizziness each year.[76,77] It is the most common cause of vertigo in patients with peripheral vestibular dysfunction and accounts for 20% to 30% of all patients seen for vertigo.[77] This disorder, therefore, represents a widespread problem, one that is, fortunately, easily treated. For patients with BPPV, the goals would be to achieve complete remission from vertigo and to improve postural stability.

Patients with BPPV experience a brief period of vertigo and nystagmus when the head is moved into particular positions. Diagnosis is based on characteristic findings, including: (1) a latency of 1 or more seconds after the head is moved into the provoking position before the onset of the vertigo and nystagmus, (2) a gradual reduction in the vertigo and nystagmus, with a duration of less than 60 seconds, (3) characteristic nystagmus, (4) reversal of the nystagmus, and a recurrence of vertigo, when the person returns to a sitting position, and (5) decreased intensity of the vertigo with repeated movement of the person into the provoking position.[75] Although in some patients there is a preceding episode of vestibular neuronitis (15%) or a history of recent head injury (18%), in most patients with BPPV, the onset is inexplicable.[75]

In addition to complaints of vertigo, many patients with BPPV identify postural instability as a major problem (Tab. 2).[78,79] Patients have reported generalized disequilibrium, unsteady gait, sensitivity to head movements and to linear accelerations, and falls.[6,80] Black and Nashner[78] reported that patients with BPPV have increased postural sway when visual feedback is altered but that they have normal postural sway when visual feedback is absent. The authors suggested that these findings indicate that patients with BPPV have developed an inability to correctly weigh which sensory cue they should rely on when maintaining balance. Voorhees,[79] however, failed to find the same postural problems and instead found that patients with BPPV had difficulty maintaining their balance when somatosensory cues were altered and visual cues were either altered or absent. Voorhees concluded that patients with BPPV have difficulty maintaining their balance using vestibular cues. One explanation for the differences in the findings of these two studies is the incidence of patients with head injury in the study by Black and Nashner[78] but not in the study by Voorhees.[79] In patients with head injuries, central nervous system damage or horizontal canal involvement secondary to the head injury could contribute to the postural instability.

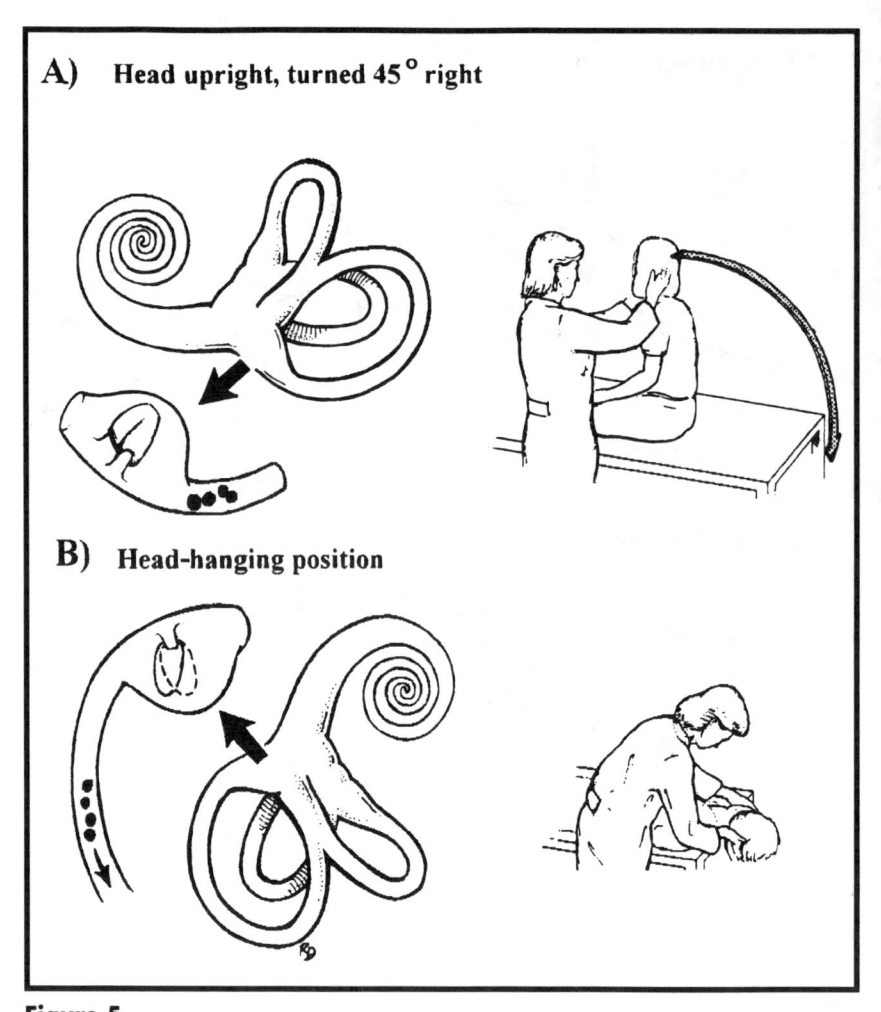

Postural instability may also occur if the BPPV is due to disruption of the anterior vestibular artery flow. The utricle's anterior and horizontal canals are supplied by the anterior vestibular artery and the saccule, and its posterior canal is supplied by the posterior vestibular artery. Disruption of the anterior vestibular artery would result in degeneration of the utricle, and therefore of the otoconia, and in horizontal canal hypofunction, but the posterior canal would still function. Cellular debris, probably otoconia, could float from the utricle into the still-functioning posterior canal, producing the symptoms of BPPV. Postural instability in patients with BPPV may be due to the abnormal signal from the semicircular canal or to an asymmetry in the signals from the utricles due to the loss of otoconia.[80,81] Identification of the underlying cause of the balance problems and appropriate treatment are critical to the successful management of these patients. In cases where the instability is due to an abnormal signal from the affected semicircular canal, new developments in our understanding of the pathophysiology of BPPV and new treatment approaches should result in more effective treatment.

Pathophysiological Basis of BPPV

Two different mechanisms have been proposed to explain the signs and symptoms of BPPV. One mechanism, "cupulolithiasis," refers to debris adhering to the cupula of the affected canal.[82] With changes in head position, gravity will cause the weighted cupula to be displaced (Fig. 4), resulting in nystagmus and vertigo. Several misgivings have been raised concerning this proposed mechanism. First, although debris has been

Figure 5.
Debris floating freely in the long arm of the semicircular canal (shown here for posterior canal) will drift to the most dependent portion of the canal when the person is moved from the sitting position (A) to the head-hanging position (B) in the Hallpike-Dix maneuver and therefore will cause the cupula to be deflected.

Table 3.
Considerations in Choice of Treatment

Treatment	Type of Benign Paroxysmal Positional Vertigo	Appropriate Canal	Consideration
Brandt-Daroff habituation	Cupulolithiasis	Posterior	Patient adherence
Liberatory maneuver	Cupulolithiasis or canalithiasis	Posterior, horizontal[a]	Neck extension, difficulty with rapid movement
Canalith repositioning maneuver	Canalithiasis	Posterior, anterior, horizontal[a]	Conversion to different canal, neck extension

[a] Modified maneuvers.

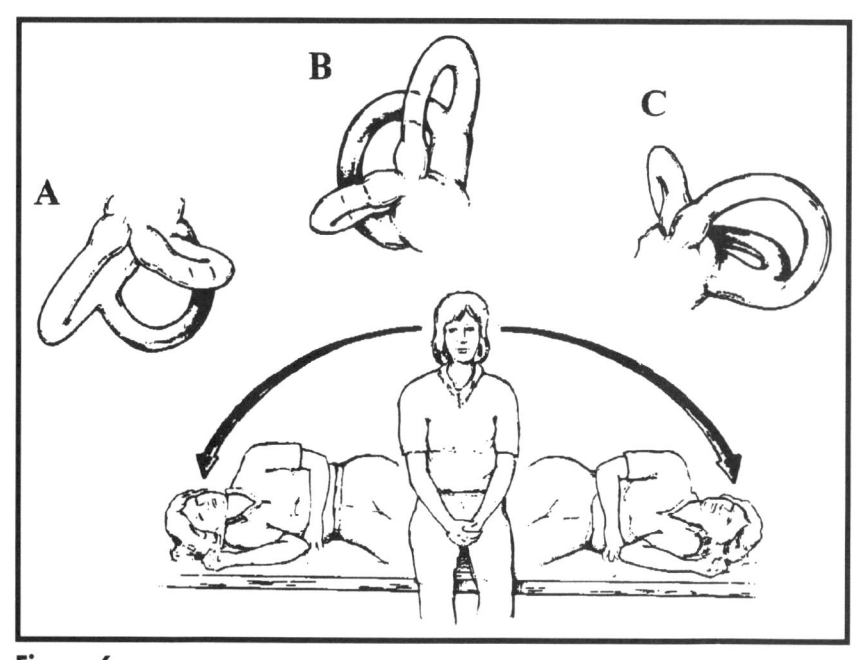

Figure 6.
Brandt-Daroff habituation exercises: The patient is first positioned sitting and then rapidly moves into the side-lying position (A). Torsional nystagmus may occur with the onset of the vertigo. The severity of the vertigo will be directly related to how rapidly the patient moves into the provoking position. The patient stays in that position until the vertigo stops, waits 30 seconds, and then sits up (B). Moving to the sitting position will usually result in vertigo, although this "rebound effect" will be less severe and of a shorter duration. Nystagmus, if it reoccurs, will be in the opposite direction. The patient remains in the upright position for 30 seconds and then moves rapidly into the mirror-image position on the other side (C), stays there for 30 seconds, and then sits up. The patient then repeats the entire maneuver 5 to 20 times, depending on the tolerance of the patient for vertigo and any accompanying nausea, or until the vertigo no longer occurs. The entire sequence is repeated three times a day until the patient has 2 consecutive days without vertigo. (Adapted from Brandt and Daroff.[86])

persists for as long as the person is kept in the provoking position, although some decrement of the nystagmus intensity may occur due to central adaptation.[84] One of the characteristics of BPPV is that the duration of the nystagmus, and of the vertigo, is typically brief, lasting less than 60 seconds.

The second mechanism, "canalithiasis," refers to debris floating within the endolymph of the semicircular canal.[7,85] When the head is moved into a position in the plane of the affected semicircular canal, the debris will move into the most dependent portion of the canal. This movement will cause the endolymph, and therefore the cupula, to move, producing vertigo and nystagmus (Fig. 5). The brief delay before the onset of the nystagmus and vertigo may be accounted for by the time it takes to overcome the inertia of the cupula. Once the debris has stopped moving, the cupula will return to its normal position within the ampulla and the nystagmus and vertigo will stop, accounting for the brief duration of the provoked signs and symptoms of BPPV. Support for this theory comes from the direct observation of debris in the affected canal of persons with BPPV.[8]

Several factors should be taken into consideration in choosing the appropriate treatment for patients with BPPV. These factors include whether the person is likely to have cupulolithiasis or canalithiasis, which canal is involved, comorbid problems, and the ability of the patient to adhere to the requirements of the treatment (Tab. 3).

Evidence That Treatment Facilitates Recovery in BPPV

Treatments based on cupulolithiasis.
The Brandt-Daroff exercises were developed based on the theory that the signs and symptoms of BPPV are due to cupulolithiasis and that the posterior canal is affected (Fig. 6).[86] These exercises originally were believed to produce habituation of the vertigo. Brandt and Daroff,[86] however, noted that the response to treatment occurred immediately in some patients, and they suggested that the debris was physi-

found adhering to the cupula in persons with a history of BPPV, similar deposits have been noted in persons without a history of positional vertigo.[83] Second, if the debris were adhering to the cupula, the nystagmus should occur as soon as the person is in the provoking position, but often there is a delay of onset of several seconds or more. Of even greater concern is that the deflection of the cupula should result in nystagmus that

cally dislodged from the cupula. Given the limitations of the Brandt-Daroff exercises, it is surprising that this treatment was shown to be effective for 95% of patients with BPPV within 2 weeks.[86] One possibility is that all patients in the study had cupulolithiasis of the posterior canal. This explanation, however, would seem to be unlikely. A second possibility is that some remissions were spontaneous and were not related to the treatment. Spontaneous recovery is common in patients with BPPV,[9,87] and this factor was not controlled for in the study by Brandt and Daroff.[86]

A second treatment, also based on cupulolithiasis, is the Liberatory maneuver (Fig. 7).[9,10] This treatment is presumed to dislodge debris from the cupula of the posterior canal in patients with cupulolithiasis. The treatment may also cause debris to move through the long arm of the posterior canal, into the common crus, and into the vestibule, thus also relieving symptoms. Semont et al[9] and other authors[10,11] have reported a remission rate following this treatment of between 70% and 95%. Unfortunately, most studies have not used a control group. One innovative study[10] examined the effectiveness of the Liberatory maneuver on a series of 10 patients using the patients as their own control. The patients were first treated with the Liberatory maneuver, but on the *unaffected* side. None of the patients had any relief from their vertigo. The patients were then treated using only the post-Liberatory maneuver instructions that they were to keep the head upright for 48 hours, including sleeping in a sitting position. Again, at the end of a week, all patients were symptomatic. The patients were then treated using the Liberatory maneuver on the affected side. At the end of 1 week, all patients were symptom-free. Although the number of subjects in this study was small, the results suggest that this maneuver may be an effective treatment.

Treatment based on canalithiasis. In patients in whom the BPPV is due to canalithiasis, the most appropriate treatment appears to be the canalith repositioning maneuver (Fig. 8).[7] Some controversy exists as to the efficacy of this treatment. In the original studies,[7,11] in which 85% to 95% remissions of symptoms were reported, there were no control groups. At least some of

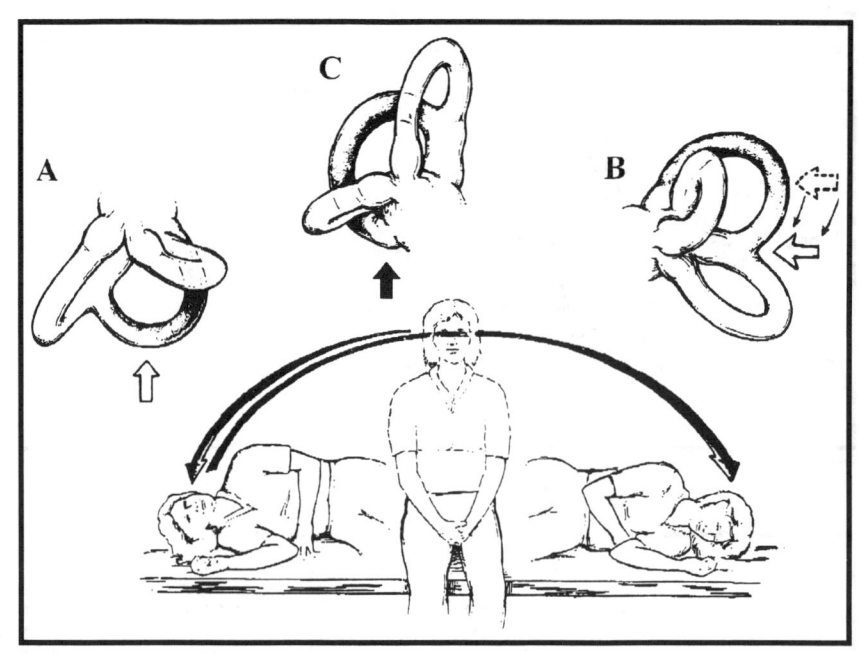

Figure 7.
Liberatory maneuver: The patient is quickly moved into the provoking side-lying position with the head turned into the plane of the posterior canal and is kept in that position for 2 to 3 minutes (A). The patient is then rapidly moved up through the sitting position and down into the opposite side-lying position, with the therapist maintaining the alignment of the neck and head on the body (B). (The face is then angled down toward the bed.) Typically, nystagmus and vertigo reappear in this second position. If the patient does not experience vertigo in this second position, the head is abruptly jostled once or twice using a small amplitude of movement, which often will provoke vertigo and nystagmus, presumably by freeing the debris. The patient stays in this position for several minutes. The patient is then slowly taken into a seated position (C). The maneuver can be repeated if the patient is symptomatic and has nystagmus when returned to the sitting position. The patient must keep the head upright for 48 hours (including while sleeping) and must avoid the provoking position for 1 week following the treatment. Although this treatment was developed based on the theory of cupulolithiasis, it may be effective in patients with canalithiasis as well. The arrows (B) indicate that the debris in the long arm of the posterior canal may move toward the common crus when the patient is moved into the opposite side-lying position. (Adapted from Herdman et al.[11])

the effects attributed to the maneuver, therefore, could have been due to spontaneous recovery. More recently, in two studies,[88,89] treatment effects were compared using untreated control groups. One research group[88] concluded that there was no difference between the remission rates of patients treated for 1 month using the canalith repositioning maneuver (n=16) and the control group (n=22). This study has been criticized because the researchers did not use the maneuver as it is commonly performed and because treatment effects were assessed 1 month after treatment, by which time recurrence of symptoms (which can occur in 10%–20% of all subjects) may have been a factor. Furthermore, advocates of the canalith repositioning maneuver suggest that one of the benefits of this treatment is the *rapid* relief of symptoms. In a different study using the canalith repositioning maneuver as originally proposed, Li[89] found that 70% of the treated group (n=27) had no nystagmus when evaluated 1 week after treatment compared with none of the untreated control group (n=23).

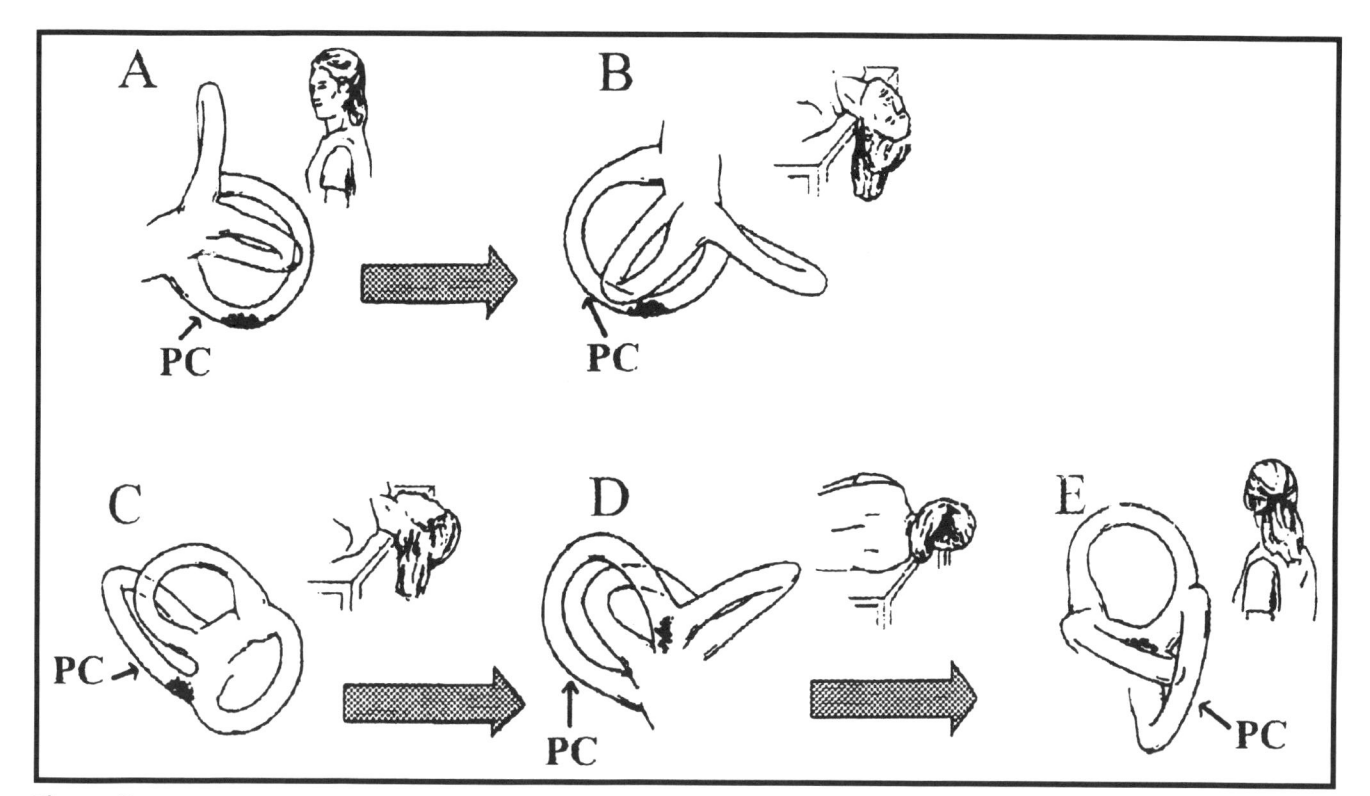

Figure 8.
Canalith repositioning maneuver for benign paroxysmal positional vertigo affecting the posterior semicircular canal on the left side. The location of debris within the posterior canal is indicated by the arrows. Note that the debris should always move away from the ampulla of the posterior canal, therefore resulting in nystagmus that always beats in the same direction. The patient is positioned sitting, and the head is turned 45 degrees toward the affected side (A) and then is quickly moved into the Hallpike-Dix position with the affected ear down (B). The patient is kept in that position for 2 to 3 minutes. The patient's head is then slowly rotated through extension until the opposite ear is down (C). Next, the patient is turned onto the side with the head rotated down 45 degrees (D). The patient remains in that position for 2 to 3 minutes and then slowly returns to the sitting position (E). Epley[7] suggests that the maneuver should be repeated until no nystagmus is observed when returning to a sitting position. The maneuver should be repeated if the direction of the nystagmus reverses. Immediately after the treatment, the patient is fitted with a soft collar and advised not to lie down, bend over, or move the head vertically for the next 48 hours. The patient is to avoid lying on the affected side for the subsequent 5 days. PC=Purkinje cells. (Adapted from Herdman and Tusa.[12])

Table 4.
Identification of Canal Involvement Based on Direction of Nystagmus During Hallpike-Dix Test[a]

Canal	Eye Muscle (Excited)	Right Hallpike-Dix Position	Reversal Phase	Return to Sitting Position
Right posterior	Ipsilateral superior oblique, contralateral inferior rectus	Upbeat, counterclockwise	Down and clockwise	Down and clockwise
Right anterior	Ipsilateral superior rectus, contralateral inferior oblique	Downbeat, counterclockwise	Up (and clockwise)	Up (and clockwise)
Left anterior	Ipsilateral superior rectus, contralateral inferior oblique	Downbeat, clockwise	Up (and counter-clockwise)	Up (and counter-clockwise)
Right horizontal	Ipsilateral medial rectus, contralateral lateral rectus	Horizontal[b]	Horizontal	Horizontal
Left horizontal	Ipsilateral medial rectus, contralateral lateral rectus	Horizontal[b]	Horizontal	Horizontal

[a] Direction of fast-phase eye movement of nystagmus generated by excitation of different canals (1) when patient is moved into the right Hallpike-Dix position, (2) during the reversal phase, and (3) after the patient returns to the sitting position. "Clockwise" and "counterclockwise" refer to direction of movement of the superior pole of the eye.
[b] Ageotropic if cupulolithiasis, geotropic if canalithiasis; Hallpike-Dix is not best provoking position; affected side is determined by intensity of symptoms.

The difference in the findings of these two studies may be due to the precise maneuver used.

Herdman et al[11] found that if patients with posterior-canal BPPV (n=30) were moved from the original provoking position (Fig. 8B) to the contralateral Hallpike-Dix position (Fig. 8C) and then returned to a sitting position, the remission rate was 50%. In comparison, the remission rate was 83% in a similar group of patients (n=30) who were rolled onto the contralateral side with the head turned 45 degrees toward the floor (Fig. 8B–D) before sitting up. This position facilitates the movement of the debris into the common crus. Li also advocated the use of a vibratory stimulus applied to the mastoid of the affected ear to presumably facilitate the movement of the debris through the canal during the treatment. The remission rate after one treatment, however, is no different from that reported by other researchers who did not use mastoid vibration during the maneuver.[87,89–91] Another variable in these studies may be which canal was involved, as the studies do not identify the direction of the nystagmus as part of the inclusion criteria.

One of the complications of the canalith repositioning maneuver is the possibility of conversion of BPPV of the posterior canal to BPPV involving the anterior or horizontal canal.[12] In a study of 85 consecutive patients with posterior-canal BPPV who were treated with the canalith repositioning maneuver, 5 patients had anterior-canal positional vertigo (n=2) or horizontal-canal positional vertigo (n=3) after undergoing the treatment.[12] The authors suggest that although movement of the debris into a different canal may occur during the treatment, it may also occur when the patient first lies down following the treatment. Observation of the direction of the nystagmus during treatment will ensure that the debris moves in the appropriate direction during the actual maneuver. For example, in posterior-canal BPPV, if the debris moves away from the cupula and toward the common crus, the nystagmus should always be in the same direction; a reversal of the nystagmus would indicate that the debris has moved toward the cupula or into the anterior canal. In patients who do not respond to treatment, careful observation of the direction of the nystagmus during reexamination is necessary to correctly identify which canal is involved.

Canal Involvement

Benign paroxysmal positional vertigo was originally thought to be a disorder of the posterior semicircular canal.[92,93] This belief was based on the direction of the nystagmus observed when the patient was moved into the provoking position (Tab. 4).[92,93] Signals from the posterior semicircular canal go to the ipsilateral superior oblique and contralateral inferior rectus muscles. Excitation of the receptors of the posterior canal results in a slow downward movement of the eyes, with a slow movement of the superior pole of the eye away from the affected side. These movements are followed by a quick resetting eye movement in the opposite direction. Thus, the direction of the nystagmus (which is always named by the direction of the fast phase) is "upbeating" and torsional, fast-phase beating toward the affected ("down-side") ear.

More recently, BPPV involving the anterior and horizontal canals has been reported.[6,94,95] As with BPPV involving the posterior semicircular canal, the direction of the nystagmus occurring when the person is moved into a provoking position is the basis for identifying the particular canal involved (Tab. 4). The anterior canal projects to the ipsilateral superior rectus muscle and to the contralateral inferior oblique muscle; the nystagmus, therefore, is "downbeating" and torsional. If the down-side ear is affected, the direction of the torsional component will be the same as in posterior-canal BPPV. That is, the superior pole will beat toward the down-side ear. The differentiation between anterior- and posterior-canal BPPV, therefore, must be made based on the direction of the vertical component of the nystagmus. If the nystagmus is downbeating and torsional, with the fast phase of the torsional component beating toward the "up-side" ear, it suggests that the affected anterior canal is in the up-side ear. The horizontal canal excites the ipsilateral medial and contralateral lateral rectus muscles, and in horizontal-canal BPPV, the nystagmus is horizontal when the patient is moved into the provoking position.[95] The best position is side-lying, not the Hallpike-Dix position, because of the alignment of the horizontal canal with respect to the pull of gravity. The direction of the nystagmus will depend on whether the debris is adhering to the cupula or is floating freely in the endolymph of the long arm of the canal (Fig. 9).

The identification of which of the semicircular canals is involved is most easily made by observing the direction of the nystagmus when the patient is first moved into the provoking position. In some patients, the nystagmus observed when the patient is first moved into the provoking position will reverse ("secondary nystagmus"). In addition, some patients will develop nystagmus when they return from the provoking position to a sitting position. The direction of the secondary nystagmus occurring in the provoking position and of the nystagmus that occurs when the patient returns to the sitting position can also be used to identify canal involvement (Tab. 4).[6] The secondary phase of nystagmus probably reflects the discharge of the velocity storage system. Velocity storage (storage of the velocity signal of the eye movement in the brain stem) for torsional nystagmus is poor. For this reason, in posterior- and anterior-canal

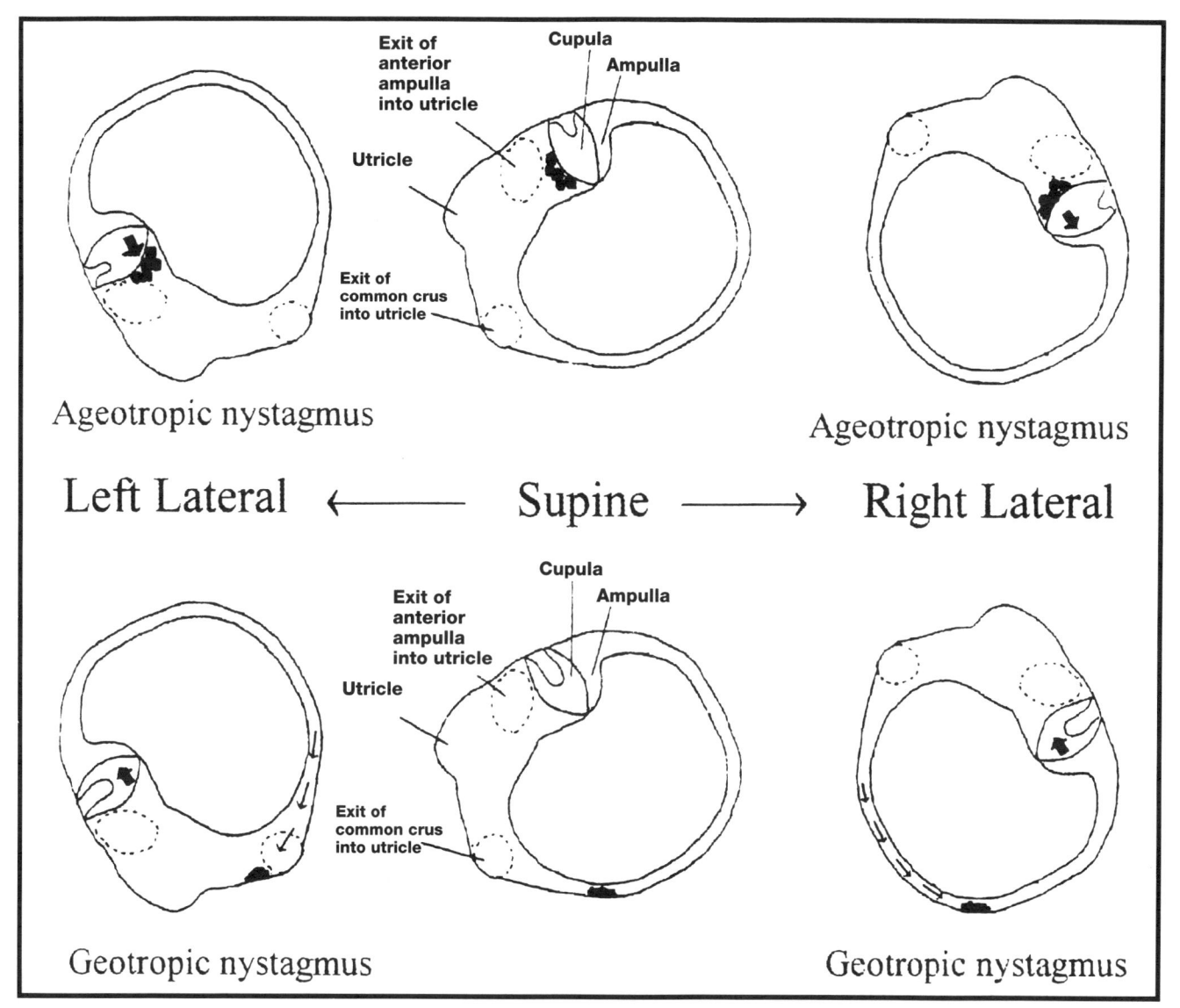

Figure 9.
The best position to provoke vertigo and nystagmus in horizontal-canal benign paroxysmal positional vertigo is to move person from the sitting to the side-lying position. The direction of the nystagmus will depend on whether the debris is adhering to the cupula (ageotropic nystagmus) or is floating freely in the endolymph of the long arm of the canal (geotropic nystagmus). (Adapted from Baloh et al.[95])

BPPV, the secondary phase is typically vertical. Nystagmus occurring when the person returns to a sitting position is due to movement of the cupula in the opposite direction; for the vertical canals, this nystagmus can have both vertical and torsional components. Posterior-canal involvement appears to be most common in patients with BPPV, occurring in more than 63% of all patients, with horizontal-canal BPPV being relatively uncommon (Tab. 5).[6] In that series of 77 consecutive patients with BPPV, however, the particular canal involved could not always be determined (24%). In most of the patients, the nystagmus was torsional, suggesting vertical-canal involvement, but because there was no vertical component, the differentiation between posterior canal and anterior canal could not be made. Additionally, some patients closed their eyes, and although nystagmus could be detected through the eyelids, the direction was not clear.

Because of the orientation of the canals, and because of the potential for movement of debris within each canal in canalithiasis, Brandt-Daroff exercises are unlikely to be appropriate for anterior-canal BPPV, although a modification of the exercises has been suggested for horizontal-canal cupulolithiasis. In this modification, the position changes are performed with the head at neutral on the body rather than turned 45 degrees away from the affected side.

The canalith repositioning maneuver has also been adapted for the treatment of patients with anterior- and horizontal-canal BPPV. In anterior-canal BPPV, the maneuver would be the same as for posterior-canal BPPV (Fig. 8), but for horizontal-canal BPPV, a modification of the maneuver must be used, designed to move the person's head in the plane of the horizontal canal (Fig. 10).[81] The efficacy of this maneuver is not known because horizontal-canal BPPV is relatively unusual and no studies have been reported. More recently, a modification of the Liberatory maneuver has been proposed for the treatment of patients with horizontal-canal BPPV due to canalithiasis.[96] De la Meilleure et al[96] described six patients in whom successful remission of symptoms was achieved with one treatment. For this treatment, with the patients positioned supine with the head flexed 30 degrees, the head was first turned toward the affected side (again, based on intensity of vertigo and nystagmus). The head was kept in this position for 5 minutes and then rapidly turned 180 degrees to the opposite side (keeping the neck flexed 30° at all times). After 5 minutes, the patients sat up. The researchers asked the patients to avoid lying down for the subsequent 48 hours and to avoid shaking the head.

Summary

Significant changes in the use of vestibular exercises have been made in the last 5 years based on the direct outcome of controlled studies on the use of exercises in the treatment of vestibular loss and of BPPV. Furthermore, the exercises used in these treatments have become more sophisticated, reflecting an increased knowledge of the physiology and anatomy of the vestibular system and the mechanisms of recovery and compensation following vestibular dysfunction. The limitations of the mechanisms that substitute for the vestibular system in maintaining postural and gaze stability indicate that exercises to improve remaining vestibular function should be emphasized in the rehabilitation process.

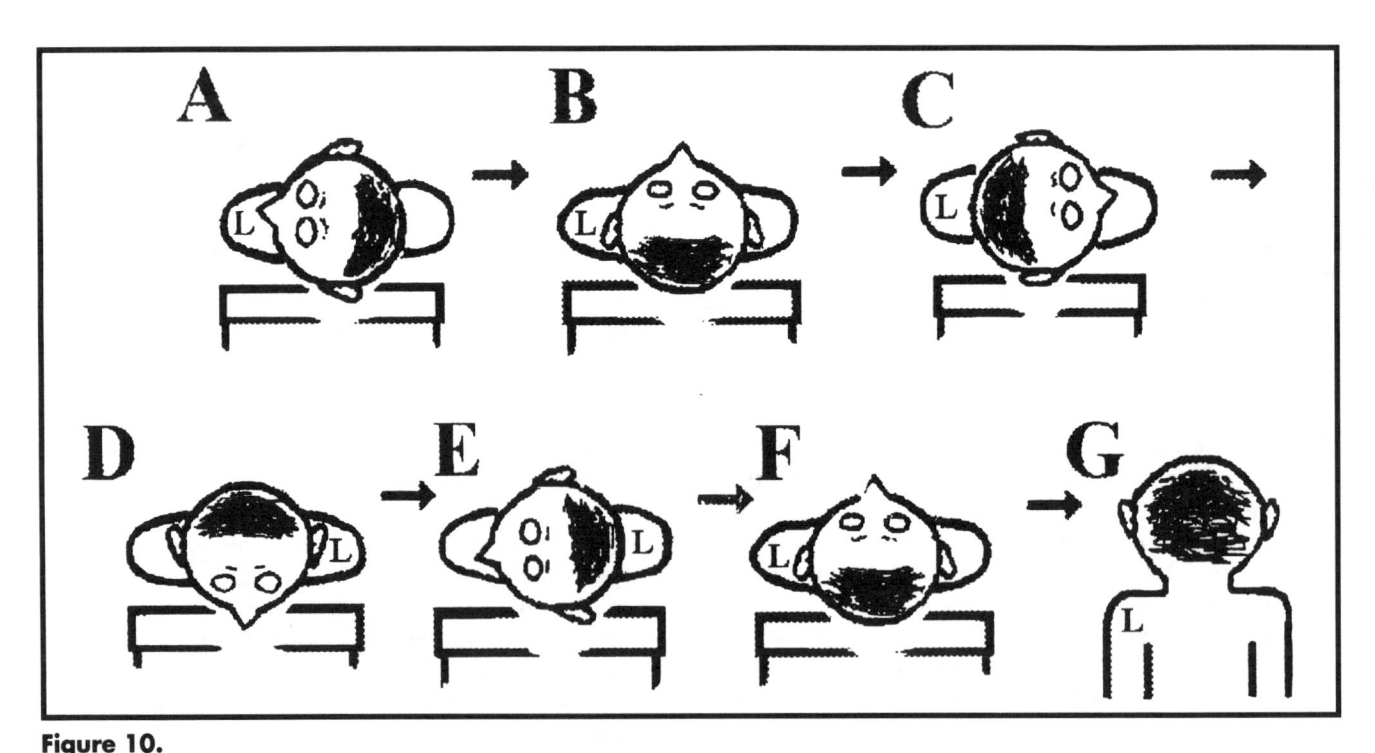

Table 5.
Percentage of Canal Involvement in Benign Paroxysmal Positional Vertigo[85]

Canal Involved	Percentage
Posterior	63
Anterior	12
Horizontal	2
Unknown (vertical?)	23

Figure 10.
Canalith repositioning maneuver for benign paroxysmal positional vertigo (BPPV) affecting the horizontal semicircular canal on the left side. The patient turns the head toward the affected side and moves quickly into the supine position (note that the head should be flexed slightly in order to position the horizontal canal in parallel with the pull of gravity) (A). After the nystagmus and vertigo stop, the head is turned to the right (B, C) and the patient is rolled toward the right and into a prone position (D) (if the patient experiences vertigo, the movement should be stopped until the vertigo stops). The head is then turned to the patient's right (E), and the patient is rolled again to a supine position (F). The patient then sits up (G). As with the canalith repositioning maneuver for posterior-canal BPPV, the patient then should keep the head upright for 48 hours. (Reprinted with permission from Herdman SJ. Physical therapy in the treatment of patients with benign paroxysmal positional vertigo. *Neurology Report.* 1996;20(3):46–53.)

References

1 Horak FB, Jones-Rycewicz C, Black FO, Shumway-Cook A. Effects of vestibular rehabilitation on dizziness and imbalance. *Otolaryngol Head Neck Surg.* 1992;106:175–180.

2 Krebs DE, Gill-Body KM, Riley PO, Parker SW. Double-blind, placebo-controlled trial of rehabilitation for bilateral vestibular hypofunction: preliminary report. *Otolaryngol Head Neck Surg.* 1993;109:735–741.

3 Herdman SJ, Clendaniel RA, Mattox DE, et al. Vestibular adaptation exercises and recovery: acute stage after acoustic neuroma resection. *Otolaryngol Head Neck Surg.* 1995;113:77–87.

4 Shepard NT, Telian SA. Programmatic vestibular rehabilitation. *Otolaryngol Head Neck Surg.* 1995;112:173–182.

5 Szturm T, Ireland DJ, Lessing-Turner M. Comparison of different exercise programs in the rehabilitation of patients with chronic peripheral vestibular dysfunction. *J Vestib Res.* 1994;4:461–479.

6 Herdman SJ, Tusa RJ, Clendaniel RA. Eye movement signs in vertical canal benign paroxysmal positional vertigo. In: Fuchs AF, Brandt T, Buttner U, Zee D, eds. *Contemporary Ocular Motor and Vestibular Research: A Tribute to David A Robinson.* Stuttgart, Federal Republic of Germany: Georg Thieme Verlag; 1994:385–387.

7 Epley JM. The canalith repositioning procedure: for treatment of benign paroxysmal positional vertigo. *Otolaryngol Head Neck Surg.* 1992;107:399–404.

8 Parnes LS, Price-Jones RG. Particle repositioning maneuver for benign paroxysmal positional vertigo. *Ann Otol Rhinol Laryngol.* 1993;102:325–331.

9 Semont A, Freyss G, Vitte E. Curing the BPPV with a Liberatory maneuver. *Adv Otorhinolaryngol.* 1988;42:290–293.

10 Ireland D. The Semont maneuver. In: *Proceedings of the XVIIth Bárány Society Meeting.* Prague, Czechoslovakia: Bárány Society; 1994:367–370.

11 Herdman SJ, Tusa RJ, Zee DS, et al. Single treatment approaches to benign paroxysmal positional vertigo. *Arch Otolaryngol Head Neck Surg.* 1993;119:450–454.

12 Herdman SJ, Tusa RJ. Complications of the canalith repositioning procedure. *Arch Otolaryngol Head Neck Surg.* 1996;122:281–286.

13 Fetter M, Zee DS. Recovery from unilateral labyrinthectomy in rhesus monkeys. *J Neurophysiol.* 1988;59:370–393.

14 LaCour M, Roll JP, Appaix M. Modifications and development of spinal reflexes in the alert baboon (*Papio papio*) following an unilateral vestibular neurectomy. *Brain Res.* 1976;113:255–269.

15 Igarashi M, Levy JK, O-Uchi T, et al. Further study of physical exercise and locomotor balance compensation after unilateral labyrinthectomy in squirrel monkeys. *Acta Otolaryngol.* 1981;92:101–105.

16 Igarashi M, Ishikawa K, Ishii M, et al. Physical exercise and balance compensation after total ablation of vestibular organs. In: Pompeiano O, Allum JHJ, eds. *Progress in Brain Research.* Amsterdam, the Netherlands: Elsevier Science Publishers BV; 1988:395–401.

17 McCabe BF. Labyrinthine exercises in the treatment if disease characterized by vertigo: their physiologic basis and methodology. *Laryngoscope.* 1970;80:1429–1433.

18 Hecker HC, Haug CO, Herndon JW. Treatment of the vertiginous patient using Cawthorne's vestibular exercises. *Laryngoscope.* 1974;84:2065–2072.

19 Dix MR. The rationale and technique of head exercises in the treatment of vertigo. *Acta Otorhinolaryngol Belg.* 1979;33:370–384.

20 Zee DS. Vertigo. In Johnson R, ed. *Current Therapy in Neurological Disease.* St Louis, Mo: CV Mosby Co; 1985:8–13.

21 Herdman SJ. Exercise strategies for vestibular disorders. *Ear Nose Throat J.* 1989;68:961–964.

22 Shumway-Cook A, Horak FB. Vestibular rehabilitation: an exercise approach to managing symptoms of vestibular dysfunction. *Seminars in Hearing.* 1989;10:196–209.

23 Telian SA, Shepard NT, Smith-Wheelock M, Kemink JL. Habituation therapy for chronic vestibular dysfunction: preliminary results. *Otolaryngol Head Neck Surg.* 1990;103:89–95.

24 Cass SP, Borello-France D, Furman JM. Functional outcome of vestibular rehabilitation in patients with abnormal sensory-organization testing. *Am J Otol.* 1996;17:581–594.

25 Cawthorne T. Vestibular injuries. *Proc R Soc Med.* 1946;39:270–272.

26 Shepard NT, Telian SA, Smith-Wheelock M. Habituation and balance retraining therapy. *Neurol Clin.* 1990;5:459–476.

27 Shepard NT, Telian SA, Smith-Wheelock M, Raj A. Vestibular and balance rehabilitation therapy. *Ann Otol Rhinol Laryngol.* 1993;102:198–205.

28 Keim RJ, Cook M, Martini D. Balance rehabilitation therapy. *Laryngoscope.* 1992;102:1302–1307.

29 Norre ME, Beckers A. Vestibular habituation training for positional vertigo in elderly patients. *J Am Geriatr Soc.* 1988;36:425–429.

30 Black FO, Shupert CL, Peterka RJ, Nashner LM. Effects of unilateral loss of vestibular function on the vestibulo-ocular reflex and postural control. *Ann Otol Rhino Laryngol.* 1989;98:884–889.

31 Fetter M, Diener HC, Dichgans J. Recovery of postural control after an acute unilateral vestibular lesion in humans. *J Vestib Res.* 1991;1:373–383.

32 Takemori S, Ida M, Umegu H. Vestibular training after sudden loss of vestibular function. *ORL J Otorhinolaryngol Relat Spec.* 1985;47:76–83.

33 Norre ME, Beckers A. Vestibular habituation training: exercise treatment for vertigo based on habituation effect. *Otolaryngol Head Neck Surg.* 1989;101:14–19.

34 Bles W, Vianney de Jong JMB, de Wit G. Compensation for labyrinthine defects examined by use of a tilting room. *Acta Otolaryngol (Stockh).* 1983;l95:576–579.

35 Bles W, Vianney de Jong JMB, Rasmussens JJ. Postural and oculomotor signs in labyrinthine-defective subjects. *Acta Otolaryngol (Stockh).* 1984;406:101–104.

36 Allum JHJ, Yamane M, Pfaltz CR. Long-term modification of vertical and horizontal vestibulo-ocular reflex dynamics in man. *Acta Otolaryngol (Stockh).* 1988;105:328–337.

37 Paige GP. Nonlinearity and asymmetry in the human vestibulo-ocular reflex. *Acta Otolaryngol (Stockh).* 1989;108:1–8.

38 Dichgans J, Bizzi E, Morasso P, Tagliasco V. Mechanisms underlying recovery of eye-head coordination following bilateral labyrinthectomy in monkeys. *Exp Brain Res.* 1973;18:548–562.

39 Kasai T, Zee DS. Eye-head coordination in labyrinthine-defective human beings. *Brain Res.* 1978;144:123–141.

40 Barnes GR. Head-eye coordination in normals and patients with vestibular disorders. *Adv Otorhinolaryngol.* 1979;25:197–201.

41 Chambers BR, Mai M, Barber HO. Bilateral vestibular loss, oscillopsia, and the cervico-ocular reflex. *Otolaryngol Head Neck Surg.* 1985;93:403–407.

42 Gresty MA, Hess K, Leech J. Disorders of the vestibulo-ocular reflex producing oscillopsia and mechanisms compensating for loss of labyrinthine function. *Brain.* 1977;100:693–716.

43 Bronstein AM, Hood JD. The cervico-ocular reflex in normal subjects and patients with absent vestibular function. *Brain Res.* 1986;373:399–408.

44 Diener HC, Dichgans J, Guschlbauer B, Mau H. The significance of proprioception on postural stabilization as assessed by ischemia. *Brain Res.* 1984;296:103–109.

45 Diener HC, Dichgans J, Bruzek W, Selinka H. Stabilization of human posture during induced oscillations of the body. *Exp Brain Res.* 1982;45:126–132.

46 Dichgans J, Brandt T. Visuo-vestibular interactions: effects on self-motion perception and postural control. In: Held R, Leibowitz HW, Teuber HL, eds. *Handbook of Sensory Physiology*. Berlin, Federal Republic of Germany: Springer; 1978:755–804.

47 Paige GD. Senescence of human visual-vestibular interactions: smooth pursuit, optokinetic, and vestibular control of eye movements with aging. *Exp Brain Res.* 1994;98:355–372.

48 Gauthier GM, Robinson DA. Adaptation of the human vestibulo-ocular reflex to magnifying lenses. *Brain Res.* 1975;92:331–335.

49 Miles FA, Eighmy BB. Long-term adaptive changes in primate vestibulo-ocular reflex, I: behavioral observation. *J Neurophysiol.* 1980;43:1406–1425.

50 Shelhamer M, Tiliket C, Roberts D, et al. Short-term vestibulo-ocular reflex adaptation in humans, II: error signals. *Exp Brain Res.* 1994;100:328–336.

51 Tiliket C, Shelhamer M, Roberts D, Zee DS. Short-term vestibulo-ocular reflex adaptation in humans, I: effect on the ocular motor velocity-to-position neural integrator. *Exp Brain Res.* 1994;100:316–327.

52 Lisberger SG. The neural basis for learning of simple motor skills. *Science.* 1988;242:728–735.

53 Lisberger SG, Miles FA, Optican LM. Frequency-selective adaptation: evidence for channels in the vestibulo-ocular reflex. *J Neurosci.* 1983;3:1234–1244.

54 Tiliket C, Shelhamer M, Tan S, Zee DS. Adaptation of the vestibulo-ocular reflex with the head indifferent orientations and positions relative to the axis of the body. *J Vestib Res.* 1993;3:181.

55 Leigh RJ, Zee DS. *The Neurology of Eye Movements*. Philadelphia, Pa: FA Davis Co; 1991.

56 Brandt T, Paulus WM, Straube A. Visual acuity, visual field, and visual scene characteristics affect postural balance. In: Igarashi M, Black FO, eds. *Vestibular and Visual Control of Posture and Locomotion Equilibrium*. Basel, Switzerland: S Karger AG, Medical and Scientific Publishers; 1985:93–98.

57 Paulus WM, Straube A, Brandt T. Visual stabilization of posture: physiological stimulus characteristics and clinical aspects. *Brain.* 1984;107:1143–1163.

58 Herdman SJ, Sandusky AL, Hain TC, et al. Characteristics of postural stability in patients with aminogycoside toxicity. *J Vestib Res.* 1994;4:71–80.

59 Grossman GE, Leigh RJ, Bruce EN, et al. Performance of the human vestibulo-ocular reflex during locomotion. *J Neurophysiol.* 1989;62:264–272.

60 Demer JL, Goldberg J, Porter FI. Effect of telescopic spectacles on head stability in normal and low vision. *J Vestib Res.* 1991;1:109–122.

61 Saito A, Okada Y, Yoshida A. Recovery of gaze disturbance in bilateral vestibular loss. *ORL J Otorhinolaryngol Relat Spec.* 1989;51:305–310.

62 Westheimer G, McKee SP. Visual acuity in the presence of retinal-image motion. *J Opt Soc Am.* 1975;65:847–850.

63 Demer JL, Amjadi F. Dynamic visual acuity of normal subjects during vertical optotype and head motion. *Invest Ophthalmol Vis Sci.* 1993;34:1894–1906.

64 Demer JL, Honrubia V, Baloh RW. Dynamic visual acuity: a test for oscillopsia and vestibulo-ocular reflex function. *Am J Otol.* 1994;15:340–347.

65 Yamane M, Allum JHJ, Pfaltz CR. Vertical and horizontal vestibuloocular reflex dynamics following unilateral vestibular deficit. In: Graham MD, Kemink JL, eds. *The Vestibular System: Neurophysiologic and Clinical Research*. New York, NY: Raven Press; 1987:557–564.

66 Halmagyi GM, Curthoys IS, Cremer PD, et al. Head impulses after unilateral vestibular deafferentiation validate Ewald's Second Law. *J Vestib Res.* 1990/1991;1:187–197.

67 Black FO, Shuppert CL, Peterka RJ, Nashner LM. Effects of unilateral loss of vestibular function on the vestibulo-ocular reflex and postural control. *Ann Otol Rhinol Laryngol.* 1989;98:884–889.

68 Segal B, Katsarkas A. Long-term deficits of goal-directed vestibulo-ocular function following total unilateral loss of peripheral vestibular function. *Acta Otolaryngol (Stockh).* 1988;106:102–110.

69 Hikosaka O, Maeda M. Cervical effects on abducens motoneurons and their interaction with vestibulo-ocular reflex. *Exp Brain Res.* 1973;18:512–530.

70 Barnes GR. Visual-vestibular interaction in the control of head and eye movement: the role of visual feedback and predictive mechanisms. *Prog Neurobiol.* 1993;41:435–472.

71 Sawyer RN, Thurston SE, Becker KR, et al. The cervico-ocular reflex of normal human subjects in response to transient and sinusoidal trunk rotations. *J Vestib Res.* 1994;4:245–249.

72 Leigh RJ, Brandt T. A reevaluation of the vestibulo-ocular reflex: new ideas of its purpose, properties, neural substrate, and disorders. *Neurology.* 1993;43:1288–1295.

73 Leigh RJ, Sharpe JA, Ranalli PJ, et al. Comparison of smooth pursuit and combined eye-head tracking in human subjects with deficient labyrinthine function. *Exp Brain Res.* 1987;66:458–464.

74 Demer JL. Evaluation of vestibular and visual oculomotor function. *Otolaryngol Head Neck Surg.* 1995;112:16–35.

75 Baloh RW, Honrubia V, Jacobson K. Benign positional vertigo: clinical and oculographic features in 240 cases. *Neurology.* 1987;37:371–378.

76 Froehling DA, Silverton MD, Mohr DN, et al. Benign positional vertigo: incidence and prognosis in a population-based study on Olmsted County, Minnesota. *Mayo Clin Proc.* 1991;66:596–601.

77 Bloom J, Katsarkas A. Paroxysmal positional vertigo in the elderly. *J Otolaryngol.* 1989;18:96–98.

78 Black FO, Nashner LM. Postural disturbances in patients with benign paroxysmal positional nystagmus. *Ann Otol Rhinol Laryngol.* 1984;93:595–599.

79 Voorhees RL. The role of dynamic posturography in neurotologic diagnosis. *Laryngoscope.* 1989;99:995–1001.

80 Buchele W, Brandt T. Benign paroxysmal positional vertigo and posture. In: Bless W, Brandt T, eds. *Disorders of Posture and Gait*. Amsterdam, the Netherlands: Elsevier Science Publishers BV; 1986:101–111.

81 Epley JM. New dimensions of benign paroxysmal positional vertigo. *Otolaryngol Head Neck Surg.* 1980;88:599–605.

82 Schuknecht HF. Cupulolithiasis. *Arch Otolaryngol.* 1969;90:765–778.

83 Moriarty B, Rutka J, Hawke M. The incidence and distribution of cupular deposits in the labyrinth. *Laryngoscope.* 1992;102:56–59.

84 Boumans LJJM, Rodenburg M, Maas AJJ. Gain of the adaptation mechanism in the human vestibulo-ocular reflex system. *ORL J Otorhinolaryngol Relat Spec.* 1988;50:319–329.

85 Hall SF, Ruby RR, McClure J. The mechanisms of benign paroxysmal vertigo. *J Otolaryngol.* 1979;8:151–158.

86 Brandt T, Daroff RB. Physical therapy for benign paroxysmal positional vertigo. *Arch Otolaryngol.* 1980;106:484–485.

87 Gyko K. Benign paroxysmal positional vertigo as a complication of bedrest. *Laryngoscope.* 1988;98:332–333.

88 Blakley BW. A randomized, controlled assessment of the canalith repositioning maneuver. *Otolaryngol Head Neck Surg.* 1994;110:391–396.

89 Li JC. Mastoid oscillation: a critical factor for success in the canalith repositioning procedure. *Otolaryngol Head Neck Surg.* 1995;112:670–675.

90 Harvey SA, Hain TC, Adamiec LC. Modified Liberatory maneuver: effective treatment for benign paroxysmal positional vertigo. *Laryngoscope.* 1994;104:1206–1212.

91 Welling DB, Barnes DE. Particle repositioning maneuver for benign paroxysmal positional vertigo. *Laryngoscope.* 1994;104:946–949.

92 Bárány R. Diagnose von krankheitserscheinungen im bereiche des otollithebapparates. *Acta Otolaryngol (Stockholm).* 1921;2:434–437.

93 Dix MR, Hallpike CS. Pathology, symptomatology, and diagnosis of certain disorders of the vestibular system. *Proc R Soc Med.* 1952;45:341–354.

94 McClure J. Horizontal canal BPV. *J Otolaryngol. 1985;14:30–35.*

95 Baloh RW, Jacobson K, Honrubia V. Horizontal semicircular canal variant of benign positional vertigo. *Neurology.* 1993;43:2542–2549.

96 De la Meilleure G, Dehaene I, Depondt M, et al. Benign paroxysmal positional vertigo of the horizontal canal. *J Neurol Neurosurg Psychiatry.* 1996;60:68–71.

Balance Special Series

The Role of Vision and Spatial Orientation in the Maintenance of Posture

This article reviews and analyzes the role of vision and spatial orientation in maintaining posture and balance. The key issues that relate to the development of postural control across the life span are discussed. Use of vision as a critical source of information that specifies spatial orientation in the environment is considered. We argue that the visual system functions as part of the perception-action cycle as promoted in ecological psychology by James Gibson. We compare and contrast theory and evidence of both standard and ecological accounts of how the visual system perceives the information and the findings relative to the role of the retinal vision in processing and acting on information related to motion. Changes in the ambient optical array (optical flow) as a non-force field are compared with gravity-based perturbations relative to the possible influence of the non-force field to changes in the motor system. Finally, a summary of some of our own work is presented, with comments about implications for further research and possible applications to clinical practice. [Wade MG, Jones G. The role of vision and spatial orientation in the maintenance of posture. *Phys Ther.* 1997;77:619–628.]

Key Words: *Posture, Spatial orientation, Vision.*

Michael G Wade

Graeme Jones

Endurance, power, and high levels of coordination and control are all necessary to execute skilled behavior and are used in a complementary fashion to provide postural stability. The reflexes that an organism possesses at birth provide a short-term safety net that permits the acquisition of nutrients and a limited and constrained connection to the organism's new environment. Without some control of posture, the organism cannot acquire the capacity to optimally explore and interact with its environment. Diminished or absent postural control can greatly disadvantage or threaten the very existence of the organism, or limit its potential to a less-than-optimal level of development. Postural stability is both the anchor and the launching pad for much of the activity of the organism. In humans, postural control provides stability, exhibited in the form of balance in a variety of body configurations (eg, seated, bipedal stance), whether stationary, preparing to move, in motion, or preparing to stop.

Earlier reviews of posture and balance by Williams[1(pp261–281)] separated what is sometimes called "static balance" from "dynamic balance." In a rather simplistic fashion, balance has traditionally been measured either by an individual's stationary position in quiet upright stance (static balance) or by tasks such as locomoting across a balance beam or walking a tightrope (dynamic balance). We view this dichotomy as artificial because it affords few interesting theoretical or practical insights. Instead, we argue that just as the development of postural stability can be defined as a continuum between early infant reflex activity and the maturing human's infinite number of voluntary motor activities, so should assessment of balance and posture be viewed across a continuum from static to dynamic balance, based on context.

Our present task is to describe the role of vision in the control of balance and postural stability. First, we consider critical factors in the role of posture and balance from a life-span developmental perspective, both as an important attribute of the developing organism and as the changes that emerge as a function of age. Second, we discuss the role of posture and balance in a changing environment and then review the way in which vision contributes to posture and balance in the context of what we term the "triad" of posture and locomotion—namely, the somatosensory, vestibular, and visual systems. We argue that of this triad, the visual system is the least well understood and has been the recipient of the least inquiry, compared with the extensive literature on the somatosensory and vestibular systems. Third, we discuss how perceptual systems derive spatial orientation, and we determine how crucial this derivation is with respect to the acquisition of information for postural control and balance. We extend this discussion further by reviewing competing theories of vision and posture.

We contrast the traditional model of a neurologically based system that is essentially computational, viewing the nervous system as a controller of the musculoskeletal system, with another view[2] that posits that information for the coordination of control and movement is directly perceived. This latter perspective views posture and balance as managed by an integrated musculoskeletal system that is heterarchical (shared) rather than hierarchical and advances the theoretical ideas of perception proposed by the late James Gibson.[3,4] Finally, we present, in summary form, data from our own laboratory on the development and maintenance of posture in younger and older adults and individuals with disabilities.

We will use the data from our laboratory to illustrate an overarching framework that seeks a more ecologically valid understanding of the role of the visual system in the control of posture and to argue aggressively for viewing the perceptual systems as the link between the environment and the active organism. With this perspective in mind, we will conclude with some comments regarding implications and possibilities for clinical practice.

Critical Factors in the Development of Posture

Postural stability is essential in the everyday activities involved in leading an independent lifestyle. Early and late in life, postural stability is of great concern because postural problems often result in injuries, especially among elderly persons, and in the expense of care and rehabilitation. Postural stability is modulated by postural control, which is exhibited in the form of postural adjustments.[5–7] These adjustments can occur prior to (anticipatory adjustments) or during (associated adjustments) voluntary movement and are thought to minimize the displacement of the center of gravity caused by voluntary movement[5] and also to affect voluntary movement directly.[6,7] Thus, postural control is dependent, to a large degree, on the goal of the voluntary movement

---

MG Wade, PhD, is Professor and Director, School of Kinesiology and Leisure Studies, College of Education and Human Development, University of Minnesota, 111 Cooke Hall, 1900 University Ave SE, Minneapolis, MN 55455 (USA) (mwade@tc.umn.edu). Address all correspondence to Dr Wade.

G Jones, is a doctoral candidate in kinesiology, School of Kinesiology and Leisure Studies, College of Education and Human Development, University of Minnesota.

and on the contextual setting[8] or environment in which it takes place. Bipedal upright stance and movement are inherently unstable, with about two thirds of the body's mass positioned over the lower extremities.[9] Although this body configuration facilitates actions such as reaching, grasping, and seeing, there are potential drawbacks, such as falling, especially for older individuals who are slower to react to rapid unexpected body perturbations.[10] This may be a factor in the changes in voluntary movement strategies that occur with aging, which can be characterized as slower, stiffer movements, with a wider base of support. For example, elderly persons often reach for objects with one hand while firmly grasping an external support such as a countertop with the other hand. Another example occurs when an elderly person climbs stairs, using a handrail for postural support.

At the other end of the life span, infants who are afforded postural stability and support from "walkers" or parents can produce voluntary movements that would not be possible on their own. Despite the differences in behaviors between infants and elderly persons, one common link is that behavior tends to emerge from intrinsic and extrinsic resources available to an individual. Thus, more often than not, decrements in one component of behavior do not linearly map onto a corresponding decrement in overall behavior. There is a certain degree of exploration that occurs, resulting in a compensation for the decrement. For instance, in infant development, independent upright stance requires adequate musculoskeletal development, which emerges at approximately 12 to 14 months of age.[11] Although infants attempt to explore their environments (crawling and sitting), independent behavior is constrained by the rate of musculoskeletal development.

Numerous studies of postural stability have focused on static, discrete postural tasks such as upright stance[12–14]; however, postural control is also a continuous process that demands responses to a constantly changing environment. Whether postural studies of discrete actions relate to real-world events is sometimes questionable. This is not to say that discrete postural tasks are not useful in developing an understanding of typical and atypical response characteristics, but rather that behavior, expressed via more natural movements, represents adaptive coordinative responses, most based in the context of continuous environmental, biological, and task constraints. Postural control, in our view, should therefore be considered on a continuum between stationary posture and movements. Furthermore, we suggest that this is a more valid approach to studying postural stability, and it can provide greater insight into the processes by which people manipulate and respond to their environments during goal-directed behaviors.

The Relationship Between Posture and Voluntary Movement

The relationship between posture and movement is an inclusive subset of a larger set of relationships between perception and action. Not only do actions within an environment lead to increases in perception, perception in turn leads to knowledge of potential behaviors within the environment (ie, affordances).[3] For example, exploratory behavior within an environment, such as a child playing with a new toy, produces sensory stimulation that is textured by the dynamics of the action-environment cycle and that results in movement modifications based on this feedback.[15,16] Given that the action-perception cycle is critical to the organism-environment interaction, Stoffregen and Riccio[17] have argued that an important goal of postural control is to provide stability to both sensory and motor systems, which optimizes the influx of sensory information while moving. For example, studies have shown that the stabilization of head motion is a fundamental feature of locomotion[18] and upright stance.[19] The ability to maintain an invariant head position relies on the constraining influence of the degrees of freedom available in the skeletal system.

In maintaining upright stance, an organism interacts physically with a surface and is subject to a gravitational force. This interaction (usually occurring on the soles of the feet) can be seen as a pivotal point around which the sum of three-dimensional inertial force vectors acting as torques of segments around joints is minimized[20] such that the gravitational force vector is within a functional base of support. This interpretation can be extended to movements such as locomotion, where although the sum of the gravitational forces is often outside the base of support, it is a deliberate functional behavior and the creation of these forces is used to aid movement progression.[21]

The ability to modulate posture and voluntary movement serves to enhance the acquisition of environmental information, not only from visual mechanisms but also from somatosensory and vestibular mechanisms. Investigation of each of these systems separately is possible; however, in our view, it is the nature of the integration of these systems that holds the key to a better understanding of how the postural system works.

How these three systems integrate across the life span is not well understood. Certain traits, however, are evident. Howard,[22] for example, proposed that the somatosensory and visual systems are primarily sensitive to low-frequency stimulation. Warren[23] has suggested that these systems are associated with postural sway (under 0.5 Hz) and gait (under 1.0 Hz). The visual system affords far more sensitive information than the vestibu-

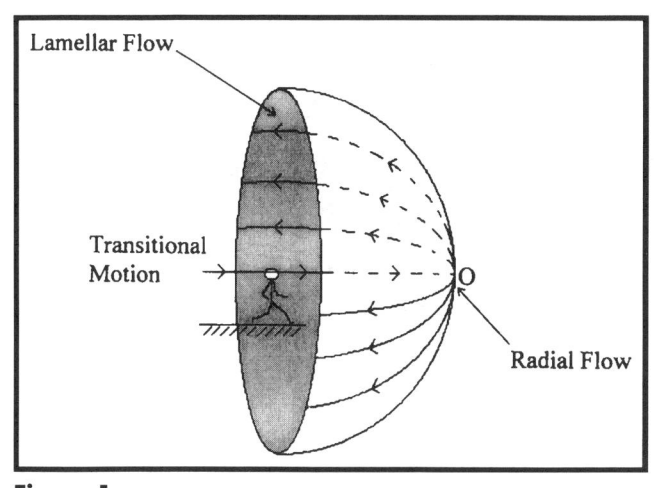

Figure 1.
A three-dimensional representation of the lines of flow of the optical flow field generated by pure transitional movement through the environment. As the flow lines approach the locomoting subject, the optical array close to point "O" flows outward in a radial fashion, transforming into lamellar flow as it passes the subject.

lar system,[24] which itself appears to be more sensitive to high-frequency movement.[22] All three systems specify information that is used for spatial orientation, and there often seems to be a redundancy in the specification of postural state.[4] Nevertheless, the importance of any one perceptual system cannot be underestimated. We believe, for example, that elderly drivers who wear hearing aids appear to be more susceptible to automobile accidents; this may also hold true for the army of cell phone users.

The importance of joint kinesthesia in postural control has also been demonstrated in quiet upright stance, where subjects experienced a loss of upright stability while they stood on compliant[25] and sway-referenced surfaces.[26] The degradation of perceptual and sensory systems has been linked to potential postural problems; accordingly, a large body of research has focused on identifying predictive variables for postural problems.[27,28] This attempt to identify predictive variables has been only moderately successful, with mostly low correlations present between predictor scores and outcome. This finding may be due to factors such as the functional heterogeneity (idiosyncracies) of the subjects studied. The finding stems from compensatory motor strategies, which rely very little on feedback from immature or degraded perceptual and sensory systems, and thus maximize feedback from intact perceptual systems. Such factors make research on atypical populations a daunting task, however, one that carries a potentially high reward.

Theoretical Issues

Vision is the third component of the triad of posture and locomotion (somatosensory, vestibular, and visual systems) and is an important source of information. The visual system acts not only via the clarity with which it "sees" (visual acuity) but also via the information that is generated by the individual's motion through the environment. The acquisition of such dynamic information generates field-of-view information for self-motion, the critical issue being active motion.[29] The traditional model of the visual system (referred to as the "two-mode theory of vision"[30]) asserts that spatially distributed information comes to the individual via the ambient mode, which is responsible for orientation and locomotion, and the focal mode, which is responsible for object recognition and identification.[30] Thus, *focal vision* refers to a system that seeks to answer the question "What is it?" and presumably generates a conscious awareness and registers events predominantly in the central retina.[31]

Ambient vision answers the question "Where is it?" and has been termed by Schmidt[31] as "motor vision." Although stimulation of the peripheral retina generally results in the use of the ambient motor vision, and the focal mode is by and large a consequence of stimulation of the central visual field (foveal), ambient vision is available and can stimulate both the central and peripheral retinal locations.[31] A large body of literature exists on age-related changes within the visual system.[32] Decreased visual acuity, restrictions of the visual field, increased susceptibility to glare, and poorer depth perception as a function of age have all been studied.[32]

The visual system of elderly persons has a decreased sensitivity to low spatial frequencies, and elderly individuals therefore require more contrast to detect spatial differences.[33] This diminished sensitivity to low spatial frequencies may be partly responsible for some problems of decreased postural stability, because locomotion and postural stability are thought to depend in part on low-frequency visual information, mediated by inputs from the peripheral visual system.

The peripheral field of view is known to decrease as a function of age, and the importance of peripheral vision in postural control has been demonstrated in numerous studies.[28,34] The traditional two-mode theory[30] asserts that postural sway, as a specific case of self-motion, is controlled primarily by the ambient visual system. The assumption is that the retinal periphery fails to detect radially structured information from the optical flow that relates to postural control and is sensitive only to lamellar flow. The types of flow are illustrated in Figure 1. This assumption implies that it is not only the retinal region that determines postural stability, but also the nature and structure of the light itself that is perceived by the periphery of the retina.[29]

The late psychologist James Gibson[3] proposed a different perspective from the traditional two-mode theory of vision. Gibson's[3] ecological theory anchors visual perception to the optic array and emphasizes the importance of optical information retrieved from various sectors of the optic array. The ambient optic array is essentially a pattern of differential reflectances that converge at every point in the visual field. For Gibson, perceiving is a "value rich ecological object"[3(p140)] that involves the whole person in the acquisition of information, not just simply the head. Thus, Gibson's theory of ecological optics involves the use of optical variables to specify different types of self-motion. Advocates of the traditional two-mode theory appear to have neglected the value of different types and magnitudes of information available from the optic array, and instead have emphasized that the differential stimulation of different regions of the retinal area can be used to explain the perception of self-motion.

As we locomote in the world, an optical flow field is generated that contains a variable geometric structure (Fig. 1).[3] Figure 1 illustrates how an optical flow field radiates outward from a point in the optic array that is spatially coincident with the direction of motion[35(p55)] and is projected to the center of the retina. At the peripheral edges of the field of view, the optical flow field is nearly parallel to the line of motion. This flow structure at the periphery has been termed "lamellar flow,"[35] as opposed to radial flow. Thus, optical information for the control of posture is a function not only of retinal location but also of the geometric structure of the light rays that form the optical flow field.[35] This ecological interpretation of visual perception challenges the traditional two-mode theory of vision.

Proponents of the ecological perspective[24,35,36] have demonstrated that the visual system is sensitive to various kinds of optical information. The important point worth noting here is that postural control and the perception of self-motion are concerned not only with the sensitivity of the retina, both at the center and at the periphery, but also with the structure of the light in the optical flow field, which may be either radial or lamellar. A subject's sensitivity to optical information specifying postural state can be evaluated in a experiment using a moving room (Fig. 2).

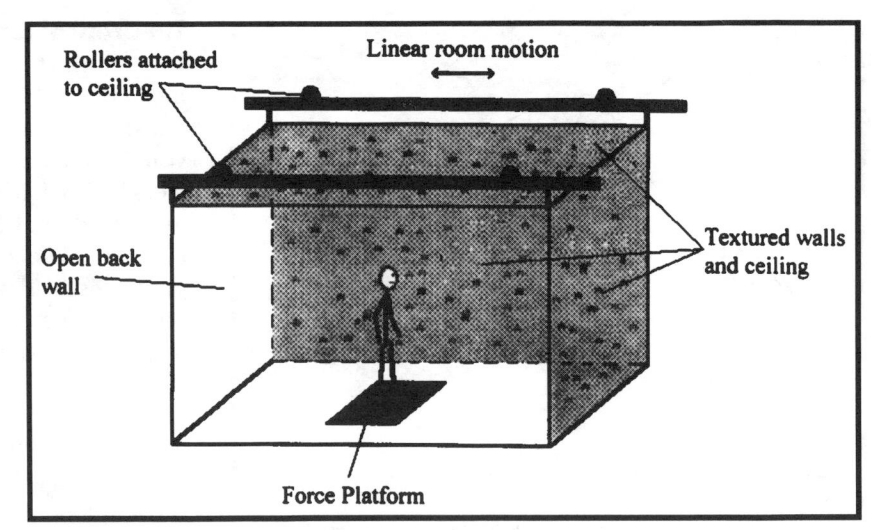

Figure 2.
The moving room with the near side wall removed. The room is attached to rollers mounted on the ceiling, enabling the room to oscillate around a stationary subject.

Subjects assume a quiet upright stance within the room as it is translated or oscillated toward or away from them. This room movement artificially generates an optical flow field pattern that is similar to the pattern experienced when translating through the environment (Fig. 1). Smaller translations of the moving room can also produce optical flow field patterns that are often experienced in upright bipedal stance. Lee and Lishman,[24] in their early work, demonstrated that these translations induce compensatory sway.

A newer feature of some moving rooms is their ability to translate the front and side walls independently, generating special optical flow fields. For example, movement of only the front wall of the moving room will generate only a radial optical flow field, whereas movement of the side wall will generate only a lamellar field. Using this feature of the moving room, we can examine the influence of certain optical flow field patterns on postural state. Lee and Lishman,[24] for example, suggested that compensatory sway corresponding to whole-room movement was controlled primarily via the ambient mode (ie, the periphery).

In examining the nature of the information that is useful for the control of stance or upright posture, Stoffregen[35] has demonstrated that the retinal periphery itself shows no particular facility for detecting posturally relevant information if the information is radially structured. Lamellar flow striking the periphery of the retina, however, provides posturally relevant information—the sensitivity of the periphery to lamellar flow.[36] Thus, the two-mode theory of visual perception, which relies primarily on the location on the retina where the visual information is detected, is an insufficient explanation for visual control of motion.

Two experiments described by Wolpert[37] tested the hypothesis that the type of information available in the two sectors of the optic ray is differentially informative as to the type of task the observer is required to perform. Wolpert's experiments on detection of descent demonstrated that the central region of the retina (the fovea) is more sensitive to self-motion than is the periphery of the retina. This finding contrasts with the traditional two-mode theory, which claims that the central region of the retina should be less sensitive to self-motion than the periphery.

A second experiment required subjects to detect acceleration.[37] Again, a central visual field detecting lamellar flow structure was more informative than the regularly expanding structure for detecting increasing speed of self-motion. The findings in these two experiments question the assumptions of the two-mode theory, because they suggest that peripheral vision is less sensitive than central vision, based on the structure of the optical flow. Of the three systems that influence the control of posture—somatosensory, vestibular, and visual—it is the visual system that seems to be least well understood.

The role of the visual system in maintaining posture and balance has been constrained by the traditional two-mode theory of vision, and this is certainly an area in need of further research. Kugler and Turvey[38] have suggested that postural equilibrium is maintained and influenced by both force flow fields and non-force flow fields (optical flow) acting on an organism.[38] Research using a gravity-based system, such as a hydraulic platform,[39] is more widely published than investigations utilizing a non-force flow field, such as that generated by the visual system in a locomoting animal or human or such as when the environment moves around a stationary organism.

Spatial Orientation

The importance of spatial orientation for the pickup of information is exemplified in an article by Marendaz et al.[40] They showed that subjects in upright, supine, and sitting immobilized postures take different amounts of time to search a visual array and locate targets. This finding suggests that nonvisual information (somatosensory and vestibular) contributes to spatial orientation, which directly affects the acquisition of information.

A knowledge of one's spatial orientation has often been directly associated with a vertical gravitational force vector.[41] Howard[42] has suggested that the gravitational vector is used as a reference for movement. Recently, this view has been challenged by Riccio and Stoffregen,[43,44] who contend that the gravitational force vector is relevant only for the maintenance of balance. For example, gravity acts to accelerate the body downward, which in upright bipedal stance causes loading on joints and stimulation of receptors on the soles of the feet. This loading carries information for balance because deviations of body segments away from being parallel to the gravitational vector result in an increase in torques around some joints.[16] Lee and Aronson[45] suggested that information carried in the form of an optical flow field contains not only information about the environment but also information concerning the body's orientation within that environment. These authors have termed this information "visual exproprioception" and have suggested that it can be used for the maintenance of postural control.

Any comprehensive theory of vision must address how coordination of the eyes with the head and the trunk occurs. Research[3,46] shows that far more information is gained when subjects move than when subjects do not move. Larish and Anderson[46] compared subjects who actively locomoted within an environment with subjects who passively viewed a three-dimensional video display. After a period of time, both displays were blacked out and, after a variable period of time, subjects were asked to describe the orientation. Subjects who actively moved around their environment were more accurate in predicting orientation. These data suggest that active movement not only allows for increases in perception but also permits subjects to extrapolate future events. There also seems to be a link between perception when a subject is active and incidence of motion sickness. Reason and Brand[47] reported that passive observers (airline passengers) are more likely to experience motion sickness and disorientation than pilots flying the plane.

Classical theories of motion sickness are built on the premise that it is caused by conflicts in the information picked up by the different sensory systems.[48] In particular, sensory conflict theory proposes that information from the retinal periphery in provocative situations disagrees with information from other perceptual systems, and thus does not allow individuals to make inferences about their world. Recently, Riccio and Stoffregen[48] challenged this notion, proposing that the perceptual systems display adaptations to the environment and that changes in environmental dynamics result in necessary changes in posture. In their view, motion sickness is the result of prolonged postural instability. It would seem that the degree of disruption is a function of the degree of similarity between the ranges of imposed and natural motion. Riccio and Stoffregen[48] argue that an intact vestibular system may be a prerequisite for motion sickness. This implies that the greatest disturbances in postural control occur when optical information is in the range of postural control frequencies. Thus, while investigating motion sickness, Riccio and Stoffregen[48] make a potentially important connection to postural control. In the case of active perception, controllers (eg, pilots) are able to anticipate environmental changes that minimize postural instability and reduce considerably any nauseating effects.

The environment is richly endowed with information that can be used not only to derive spatial orientation but also to form a reference for coordination of movements.[49,50] For example, successful batters must time the initiation of their swings with the oncoming ball within a small temporal window. Lee et al[51] demonstrated that some patients with left hemiplegia (with no comprehensional or perceptual difficulties), who displayed slow and jerky arm coordination movements, were able to coordinate their movements when provided with an external stimulus, such as hitting or catching a ball that was rolled toward them. This information is derived mainly in the form of visual information, which more often than not is used to anticipate contact with an object.[49,50]

Recent Research and Its Implications for Practice

Traditional theories of cognition view perception in the context of a computer-like information processing system that is much in step with the formal accounts of the "seeing" eye. The computer analogy fits well when describing visual perception in terms of the physics of the eye and its neurological connections. This theoretical approach has merit and a rich history of research, but it has provided no insights into what we refer to as "dynamic visual perception."[32] Dynamic visual perception considers not just the seeing eye and the associated physics and neurology, but rather a visual system that coordinates the anatomical location of the eyes in the head, the head on the shoulders, and an articulated muscle-joint system that has evolved as a special-purpose design for bipedal locomotion. Such an anatomical system requires control of posture across a range of continuous activities that include stopping, starting, locomoting, and changing direction. The ambient optic array is one in which the sight lines move up and down in a sinusoidal or quasi-sinusoidal fashion as the joint system both flexes and dampens to the motion induced by movement, proximal from the point of the seeing eye, to a distal point at the articulators of the ankle-foot joint system. None of these "sight lines" in real-world activities are fixed horizontal points connecting one point of spatial orientation to another. This view has been described by Owen and Lee,[52] and research on problems of posture in the context of natural biological motion requires a different kind of investigative approach (more descriptive than experimental) that seeks a better understanding of the links between the organism and the environment through which it moves. To describe this linkage, Gibson[2] coined the term "perception-action cycle."

When considering perception and action, and the linkages between them, the focus is on a visual system that both perceives and calibrates the movement articulators (the limbs) in response to the totality of the environment in which the organism finds itself. Thus, locomoting through a terrain that continuously changes in both texture and gradient requires continuous calibration of the movement system, based on information received as the individual locomotes. Most people perform these activities with remarkable ease, suggesting that our perceptual systems (ie, the totality of the perceptual landscape) both detect and adjust to the environment directly as they are perceived. Thus, information about changes in surface texture and sound of the air are continuously and directly monitored to maintain stability, safety, and the realization of the specific goal.

In the more immediate context of vision and postural stability, it is the sensitivity of the individual's visual-perceptual system that detects the real-time changes in the dynamical properties of the ongoing event. Thus, when we pose questions about posture and balance that we plan to investigate in the laboratory, we ask how and in what ways is the organism sensitive to visual-perceptual information that mediates and influences postural stability. Using the moving room (Fig. 2) pioneered by Lee and co-workers[24,45] and a force platform acting as a stabliograph, we have tested different groups of subjects in different experimental conditions of optical flow and recorded their responses to these flow fields.

The methods we used required subjects to adopt a standardized upright posture standing on a force platform. From this position, either a rotating disk at eye level[53] or a moving room[54] in which the front (radial flow) and side walls (lamellar flow) could move independently or together (global flow) generated an optical flow field that specified motion to the subject. These methods have been described in more detail by Wade[53] and Wade et al.[54]

Our research suggests that using a moving room protocol and recording changes in center of pressure (COP) as a function of optical flow detects differences between persons without impairments and individuals who have been diagnosed as functionally mentally handicapped[53] and that persons aged 65 years and older are more sensitive to optical flow presented globally compared with persons in their third, fourth, and fifth decades of life.[54] More recently, we have turned our attention to individuals diagnosed with multiple sclerosis at different stages of functioning, as classified by the Tinetti index.[55] Although this work is preliminary,[54] our long-range goal is to determine how changes in sensitivity of the perceptual apparatus might play a role in calibrating the motor system to changes in environmental (perceptual) information. We also hope to map more clearly the specifics of the optical flow field and the sensitivity of the retina to the flow field itself.

For some groups of subjects, sensitivity to the overall perception-action cycle may be present outside the normal range of frequencies. Maintaining upright posture in an essentially stationary mode is normally recorded between 0 and 2 Hz,[56] whereas individuals with cognitive or genetic abnormalities may exhibit different frequency oscillations. Yoneda and Torumasu,[56] using spectral analysis techniques, found differences in the power spectrum of the COP of individuals without impairments and patients with Mèniére's disease, benign paroxysmal positional vertigo, and vestibular neuritis in upright quiet stance with eyes open or closed. Current work in our laboratory is focusing on a study of optical flow fields that not only specify motion in the anteroposterior plane but that also can be used to determine sensitivity to the coupling effects on subjects as a moving room oscillates at a particular frequency. Again, the subject stands on a force platform, and we record how tightly the individual can couple his or her postural motion to the oscillatory motion of the room, as recorded by motion of the COP.

Our long-range goal is to determine whether there exists a signature represented by the mechanical state of the postural system measured stabliographically. A signature would be represented or characterized by a somewhat unique set of postural measures, which would differentiate an individual's postural profile as a function of a particular pathology or disease. Such measures (dependent variables) might be direction and range of the movement of the COP or the frequency range of an individual's postural sway while standing upright or responding to an optical flow field perturbation. Frequency, direction, and magnitude of such responses may assist in defining a profile of an individual's postural status as it relates to functional preference. These postural data may provide new insights into the treatment that might be devised for individuals in need of rehabilitation for a cognitive disability or recovering from physical or neurological trauma.

Our work assesses the role of optical flow as a mediator of postural stability in these different groups of subjects with different functional problems. If we can devise a specific clinical profile (postural signature), measured via a response to an optical flow field, there is potential for such a protocol to be used clinically to detect problems of posture and locomotion. This protocol may apply not only to individuals with motor deficits, as a function of birth or genetic pathology, but also those seeking recovery from a stroke or similar neuromuscular deficit that requires rehabilitation. When we suggest the clinical implications of research investigating posture from an ecological perspective, the underlying assumptions are fundamentally different from the responses of subjects perturbed using a gravity-based system.[39] What we have discussed focuses on the subjects' response to a non-force flow field. Although the responses for both force and non-force flow fields can be recorded as either biomechanical or electrophysiological deviations, the origin of the perturbations are very different. Movement of the COP is sensitive to non-force manipulations such as optical flow and requires a different kind of analysis than do the more usual recordings of ground reaction forces and muscle activity when a hydraulic platform perturbs the subject. We are suggesting here that the way subjects respond to the perturbation due to a nongravitational force field should be "food for thought" for clinical practice.

The role of vision in both calibrating and maintaining posture and balance provides support for the dynamical systems theory. This approach views the coordination and control of human locomotion and voluntary motor activity more in terms of an organism's ability to self-organize as a function of task and environment, rather than being controlled by internal mechanisms such as motor programs. This idea, although relatively new to the field of physical therapy,[57,58] is finding increasing theoretical and research support by investigators who are seeking a more complete description of how the system utilizes the many degrees of freedom available in the musculoskeletal system and constrains and organizes these degrees of freedom in such a way as to produce functional and skillful motor activity. This is true for movement across a wide spectrum of activities, from natural locomotion to the fine motor skills and manipulations of expert surgeons and skilled performers.

References

[1] Williams HG. *Perceptual and Motor Development*. Englewood Cliffs, NJ: Prentice-Hall Inc; 1983.

[2] Epstein W, Sheena R. *Perception of Space and Motion*. New York, NY: Academic Press Inc; 1995.

[3] Gibson JJ. *The Ecological Approach to Visual Perception*. Boston, Mass: Houghton Mifflin Co; 1979.

[4] Gibson JJ. *The Senses Considered as Perceptual Systems*. Boston, Mass: Houghton Mifflin Co; 1966.

[5] Riach CL, Lucy SD, Hayes KC. Adjustments to posture prior to arm movement. In: Johnson B, ed. *International Series on Biomechanics, Biomechanics X-A*. Champaign, Ill: Human Kinetics Inc; 1987:459–463.

[6] Cordo PJ, Nashner LM. Properties of postural adjustments associated with rapid arm movements. *J Neurophysiol*. 1982;42:287–302.

[7] Nouillot P, Bouisset S, Do MC. Do fast voluntary movements necessitate anticipatory postural adjustments even if equilibrium is unstable? *Neurosci Lett*. 1992;147:1–4.

8 Paillard J. Posture and locomotion: old problems and new concepts. In: Amblard B, Berthoz A, Clarac F, eds. *Posture and Gait: Development, Adaptation, and Modulation: Proceedings of the 9th International Symposium on Postural and Gait Research.* Amsterdam, the Netherlands: Elsevier Science Publishers BV; 1988:v–xii.

9 Winter DA, Patla AE, Frank JS. Assessment of balance control in humans. *Med Prog Technol.* 1990;16:31–51.

10 Kirshen AJ, Cape RDT, Hayes KC, et al. Postural sway and cardiovascular parameters associated with falls in the elderly. *Journal of Clinical Experimental Gerontology.* 1984;6:219–222.

11 Wild D, Nayak USL, Issacs B. Description, classification, and prevention of falls in old people at home. *Rheumatol Rehabil.* 1981;20:153–159.

12 Woollacott MH, von Hosten C, Rosblad B. Relation between muscle response onset and body segmental movements during postural perturbations in humans. *Exp Brain Res.* 1988;72:593–604.

13 Horak FB, Nashner LM, Diener HC. Postural strategies associated with somatosensory and vestibular loss. *Exp Brain Res.* 1990;82:167–177.

14 Maki BE. Biomechanical approach to quantifying anticipatory postural adjustments in the elderly. *Med Biol Eng Comput.* 1993;31:355–362.

15 McDonald PV, Oliver SK, Newell KM. Perceptual-motor exploration as a function of biomechanical and task constraints. *Acta Psychol (Amst).* 1996;88:127–165.

16 Riccio GE. Information in movement variability about the qualitative dynamics of posture and orientation. In: Newell KM, Corcos DM, eds. *Variability and Motor Control.* Champaign, Ill: Human Kinetics Inc; 1994:317–357.

17 Stoffregen TA, Riccio GE. Responses to optical looming in the retinal center and periphery. *Ecological Psychology.* 1990;2:251–274.

18 Grossman GE, Leigh RJ, Bruce EN, et al. Performance of the human vestibuloocular reflex during locomotion. *J Neurophysiol.* 1989;62:264–272.

19 Riach CL, Starkes JL. Visual fixation and postural sway in children. *Journal of Motor Behavior.* 1989;21:265–276.

20 Riccio GE, Stoffregen TA. Affordances as constraints on the control of stance. *Human Movement Science.* 1988;7:265–300.

21 McMahon TA. *Muscles, Reflexes, and Locomotion.* Princeton, NJ: Princeton University Press; 1984.

22 Howard IP. The perception of posture, self-motion, and the visual vertical. In: Boff KR, Kaufman L, Thomas JP, eds. *Handbook of Perception and Human Performance.* New York, NY: John Wiley & Sons Inc; 1986:18.1–18.62.

23 Warren WH. Self-motion: visual perception and visual control. In: Epstein W, Sheena R, eds. *Perception of Space and Motion.* New York, NY: Academic Press Inc; 1995:263–325.

24 Lee DN, Lishman JR. Visual proprioceptive control of stance. *Journal of Human Movement Studies.* 1975;18:87–95.

25 Ackner SL, Di Fabio RP. Influence of sensory inputs in standing balance in community-dwelling elders with a recent history of falling. *Phys Ther.* 1992;72:575–584.

26 Manchester D, Woollacott MH, Zederbauer-Hylton N, et al. Visual, vestibular, and somatosensory contributions to balance control in the older adult. *J Gerontol.* 1989;44:118–127.

27 Maki BE, Holliday PJ, Fernie GR. A posture control model and balance test for the prediction of relative postural stability. *IEEE Trans Biomed Eng.* 1987;34:797–810.

28 Berg WP, Alessio HM, Mills EM, et al. Correlates of recurrent falling in independent community-dwelling older adults. *Journal of Motor Behavior.* In press.

29 Wolpert L. Field of view information for self-motion perception. In: Warren R, Wertheim AH, eds. *Perception and Control of Self-Motion.* Hillsdale, NJ: Lawrence Erlbaum Associates Inc; 1990:101–122.

30 Held R. Two modes of processing spatially distributed visual stimulation. In: Schmitt FO, ed. *The Neurosciences: Second Study Program.* New York, NY: Rockefeller University Press; 1970:317–323.

31 Schmidt RA. *Motor Control and Learning: A Behavioral Emphasis.* 2nd ed. Champaign, Ill: Human Kinetics Inc; 1988.

32 Brownlee MG, Banks MA, Crosbie WJ, et al. Consideration of spatial orientation mechanisms as related to elderly fallers. *Gerontology.* 1989;35:323–331.

33 Lord SR, Clark RD, Webster IW. Visual acuity and contrast to sensitivity in relation to falls in an elderly population. *Age Ageing.* 1991;20:175–181.

34 Stoffregen TA. The role of optical velocity in the control of stance. *Perception and Psychophysics.* 1986;39:355–360.

35 Stoffregen TA. Flow structure versus retinal location in the optical control of stance. *J Exp Psychol.* 1985;11:554–565.

36 Koenderink J, Van Doorn A. Exterospecific component of the motion parallax field. *J Opt Soc Am A.* 1981;71:953–957.

37 Wolpert L. *Field of View Versus Retinal Region in the Perception of Self-motion.* Columbus, OH: Ohio State University; 1987. Doctoral dissertation.

38 Kugler PN, Turvey MT. *Information, Natural Law, and the Self-assembly of Rhythmical Movement: Theoretical and Experimental Investigations.* Hillsdale, NJ: Lawrence Erlbaum Associates Inc; 1987.

39 Nashner LM. Strategies for organization of human posture. In: Igarashi M, Black FO, eds. *Vestibular and Visual Control on Posture and Locomotor Equilibrium.* Houston, Tex: Karger & Basel; 1985:1–8.

40 Marendaz C, Stivalet P, Barraclough L, et al. Effect of gravitational cues on visual search for orientation. *J Exp Psychol Hum Percept Perform.* 1993;19:1266–1277.

41 Schone H; Strausfeld C, trans. *Spatial Orientation: The Spatial Control of Behavior in Animals and Man.* Princeton, NJ: Princeton University Press; 1984.

42 Howard IP. *Human Visual Orientation.* New York, NY: John Wiley & Sons Inc; 1982.

43 Riccio GE, Stoffregen TA. Gravitoinertial force versus the direction of balance in the perception and control of orientation. *Psychol Rev.* 1990;97:135–137.

44 Stoffregen TA, Riccio GE. An ecological theory of orientation and the vestibular system. *Psychol Rev.* 1988;95:3–14.

45 Lee DN, Aronson E. Visual proprioceptive control of standing in human infants. *Perception and Psychophysics.* 1974;15:529–532.

46 Larish JF, Anderson GJ. Active control in interrupted dynamic spatial orientation: the detection of orientation change. *Perception and Psychophysics.* 1995;57:533–545.

47 Reason J, Brand JJ. *Motion Sickness.* London, England: Academic Press Inc (London) Ltd; 1975.

48 Riccio GE, Stoffregen TA. An ecological theory of motion sickness and postural instability. *Ecological Psychology.* 1991;3:195–240.

49 Tresilian JR. Visual modulation of interceptive action: a reply to Savelsbergh. *Human Movement Science.* 1994;14:129–132.

50 Lee DN, Young PE, Reddish S, et al. Visual timing in hitting an accelerating ball. *Q J Exp Psychol [A]*. 1983;35:333–346.

51 Lee DN, Lough S, Lough F. Activating the perceptuo-motor system in hemiparesis. *J Physiol (Paris)*. 1984;349:28.

52 Owen BM, Lee DN. Establishing a frame of reference for action. In: Wade MG, Whiting HTA, eds. *Motor Development in Children: Aspects of Coordination and Control*. Boston, Mass: Martinus Nijhoff; 1986:341–360.

53 Wade MG. Impact of optical flow on postural control in normal and mentally handicapped persons. In: Vermeer A, ed. *Motor Development: Adapted Physical Activity and Mental Retardation*. Basel, Switzerland: S Karger AG, Medical and Scientific Publishers; 1990:21–29.

54 Wade MG, Linquist R, Taylor JR, et al. Optical flow, spatial orientation, and the control of posture in the elderly. *J Gerontol*. 1995;50B:P51–P58.

55 Roehrs T. *The Influence of Optical Flow on the Postural Control of Persons With Multiple Sclerosis*. Twin Cities, Minn: University of Minnesota; 1996. Master's thesis.

56 Yoneda S, Tokumasu K. Frequency analysis of body sway in the upright posture. *Acta Otolaryngologica. (Stockh)*. 1986;102:87–92.

57 Scholz JP. Dynamic pattern theory: some implications for therapeutics. *Phys Ther*. 1990;70:827–843.

58 Woollacott MH, Shumway-Cook A. Changes in posture control across the life span: a systems approach. *Phys Ther*. 1990;70:799–807.

Evaluation of Postural Stability in Children: Current Theories and Assessment Tools

Children with many types of motor dysfunction have problems maintaining postural stability. Because maintenance of postural stability is an integral part of all movements, therapists evaluate and treat to improve postural stability in these children. This article reviews current pediatric assessment tools for postural stability and issues affecting testing this construct in children. The tests and measurements are classified according to their testing purpose and the National Center for Medical Rehabilitation Research disablement framework, focusing on the impairment and functional limitation dimensions. Postural stability is defined from a systems perspective with tests related to the sensory, motor, and biomechanical systems described. Reliability and validity information on the measurements is discussed. Relatively few measurements of postural stability in children are available that have acceptable reliability and validity documentation. Suggestions for research on test development in this area are discussed. [Westcott SL, Lowes LP, Richardson PK. Evaluation of postural stability in children: current theories and assessment tools. *Phys Ther.* 1997;77:629–645.]

Key Words: *Balance, Evaluation, Motor dysfunction, Pediatrics, Postural stability, Tests and measurements.*

Sarah L Westcott

Linda Pax Lowes

Pamela K Richardson

To begin a discussion on evaluation of postural stability in children, it is necessary to define the construct. For the purpose of this article, *postural stability* is defined as the ability to maintain or control the center of mass (COM) in relation to the base of support (BOS) to prevent falls and complete desired movements.[1–3] Balancing is the process by which postural stability is maintained. The ability to maintain a posture, such as balancing in a standing or sitting position, is operationally defined as static balance. The ability to maintain postural control during other movements, such as when reaching for an object or walking across a lawn, is operationally defined as dynamic balance. Both static and dynamic postural control are thought to be important and necessary motor abilities.[2,3] Children with many types of disabilities, ranging from learning disabilities with mild motor problems to cerebral palsy with more severe motor problems, have been shown to have dysfunction of postural control.[4–14] These children may exhibit clumsiness and frequent falls during regular daily motor activities or may not be able to maintain a sitting or standing position independently. Physical therapists and occupational therapists have historically placed a high priority on the treatment of patients with postural control problems because this control appears to be an integral part of all motor abilities; therefore, improvements in postural control should lead to improvements in all movements.[1,3]

We will classify the tests and measurements of postural stability that we discuss using three theoretical frameworks, which describe (1) the purpose of an evaluation, (2) the dimension evaluated according to a disablement scheme, and (3) the body systems cooperating to control balance. A brief description of each framework follows.

We believe that there are three primary reasons that therapists assess clients: (1) for discriminative purposes, (2) for predictive purposes, and (3) for evaluative purposes.[15,16] Discriminative tests are designed to determine whether the problem makes the individual different from the typical individual and are used to quickly and easily screen the individual for further diagnostic testing or to test in greater depth to qualify an individual for services. Predictive tests are used to classify people into categories that indicate what their future status will be on the variables tested. Evaluative testing is done to determine change over time or effectiveness of therapy.

The disablement scheme we will use to classify the tests was adopted by the National Center for Medical Rehabilitation Research of the National Institutes of Health.[17] Within this framework, there are defined dimensions for treatment for individuals with disabilities. These dimensions include pathophysiology, impairments, functional limitations, disability, and societal limitations. We will describe tests and measurements from the impairment and functional limitation dimensions only. The purpose of impairment dimension testing is for determination of impairments that are influencing a person's motor ability so that specific relevant therapeutic techniques can be chosen to remediate these problems. Evaluation of the effects of these treatments then needs to follow. We believe that therapists should first examine changes at the impairment dimension because that is one dimension at which treatment should have an effect. Judgments, however, about whether therapy has been effective, in our view, should also be based at the functional limitations dimension. We therefore will present functional tests that have components related to postural stability.

Specific to the construct of postural stability, we will assume a general systems theory of motor control.[1–3,18] According to this theory, there are many systems within the body that work in concert to keep the COM within the BOS when maintaining static postures and to move the COM in relation to the BOS in a controlled manner when engaged in dynamic tasks. The primary systems involved for the process of balancing are (1) the sensory system (visual, cutaneous and proprioceptive [called "somatosensory"], and vestibular senses), which either cues the child that a response needs to be made to maintain control or gives feedback to alter the balance action during a voluntary motor task, (2) the motor system, which creates the movement to maintain posture, and (3) the biomechanical system, which includes the bony and joint frame on which movements are made and the muscles that create the movement torques. Other systems may also play a role in the maintenance of posture[2,3,18]; however, these three systems are primary systems that are within the scope of physical therapists and occupational therapists. The tests and measurements are organized under these system headings.

To be useful, any measurement needs to have adequate reliability and validity.[19,20] For each assessment dis-

---

SL Westcott, PhD, PT, is Assistant Professor, Allegheny University of the Health Sciences, Broad and Vine Streets, Philadelphia, PA 19102 (USA) (westcotts@allegheny.edu). Address all correspondence to Dr Westcott.

LP Lowes, PhD, PT, PCS, is Assistant Professor, Texas Woman's University, Houston, Tex.

PK Richardson, PhD, OT, is Occupational Therapist, California Children's Services, Santa Barbara, Calif.

cussed, reliability information will be provided. As a general scheme, reliability coefficients can be interpreted as follows: coefficients less than .50 reflect poor reliability, coefficients between .50 and .75 reflect moderate reliability, and coefficients above .75 reflect good reliability.[19] The type of reliability coefficient that was calculated, the type of measurement, and the variability of the data, however, should also be considered in the final determination.[19] Validity of the assessments described will be reported when studies exist. Many times, however, validity has not been examined formally and must then be judged on a face and content level by the therapist. Determination of responsivity of a test or measurement is one form of validity.[20,21] *Responsivity* describes the ability of the test or measurement to reflect clinically important change when that change has occurred in the individual tested.[20] This ability is very important for evaluative tests and measures. Very little research on the responsivity of tests has been done.

Before we move to a specific discussion of the available tools for evaluation of postural stability in children, there are several overall recommendations for improving the reliability and validity of measurements. Past experiences of people, their current attention to a task, the actual task being undertaken, and the environment in which the task is being done may influence postural stability.[22–29] Efforts should be taken, especially when using measurements for evaluative purposes, to be aware of, and when possible control, the variables that could affect the measurements.

Awareness of the environmental conditions during specific tests of postural stability could also provide insights for therapy. For example, the type of perturbation is an environmental condition that can affect the balancing response. Balancing can be triggered by sensory input from an unpredicted perturbation, such as the surface moving or by a bump to the body. These are examples of sensory input initiating motor output, and therefore they have been termed "feedback" postural activity.[30,31] In contrast, maintenance of postural stability can be disrupted in a predictable manner when we perturb ourselves, such as when we initiate a movement. Postural adjustments related to voluntary movement in some instances in both children and adults been shown to be initiated prior to the start of the movement.[24,29,32–34] This anticipatory postural muscle activity helps to achieve smooth execution of the desired movement. Because there is no initial sensory input triggering this anticipatory postural muscle activity, it has been termed "feedforward" postural control.[30,31] Haas et al[31] found, in children who were developing in a typical manner and who ranged in age from 7 months to 14 years 8 months, that feedback postural control develops earlier than feedforward postural control. They reported, however, that the development of feedback control is not complete when feedforward control appears.[31] This finding suggests that the control system for feedforward versus feedback postural stability may be different. Therefore, if an individual only shows problems with feedforward postural stability, the therapist may not want to spend time in therapy applying unpredictable perturbations to provoke balancing responses.

We believe that for children, therapists need to be aware of the developmental sequence of postural control, especially for discriminative testing. In typically developing children, the growth of postural stability proceeds in a cephalocaudal fashion, with the infant achieving control of the head, then the trunk, and finally postural stability in standing.[2,22–24] Extensive studies on the development of standing balance from a sensory and motor developmental perspective have been done.[29,35–41] This research has shown that, from a motor systems perspective, the sequence of activation of muscles reacting to a specific type of perturbation—pulling the floor backward or forward under the feet—appears to be generally in place as early as 18 months of age.[28,35,37] The timing and amplitude, however, of these coordination patterns or motor response strategies are not mature. The coordination of the postural response goes through a transitional stage at 4 to 6 years of age, reaching adultlike maturity by 7 to 10 years of age.[28,35,37] This transition of postural responses at 4 to 6 years of age results in less-coordinated motor patterns in terms of timing and selection of strategy. This finding has been hypothesized to be related to the growth spurt that occurs in most children during these years, resulting in alteration of the child's biomechanical characteristics.[37]

The ability of the sensory systems to detect imbalance during standing also follows a developmental sequence.[28,35,37] Infants and young children (aged 4 months to 2 years) are dependent on the visual system to maintain balance.[34,42–44] When children of this age are placed in a room with movable walls, they consistently fall in the direction that the walls are moved.[44] At 3 to 6 years of age, children begin to use somatosensory information appropriately.[35–38] Finally, at 7 to 10 years of age, children are able to resolve a sensory conflict (mismatched information coming from somatosensory and visual receptors) and appropriately utilize the vestibular system as a reference.[35–38] Interestingly, at 7 to 10 years of age, the gait pattern also reaches full maturity.[45] Because children who are developing in a typical fashion change from a dominant reliance on visual input to an ability to rely on somatosensory input and utilize the vestibular system as a reference in conditions of sensory conflict, the therapist must take into consideration the developmental level of the child when making judgments about sensory system deficits of postural stability.

For all tests and measurements, information on developmental sequence, if available, will be noted.

Individual discussions of the currently available tests for evaluating postural stability at the impairment and functional limitation dimensions in children follows. For quick reference, Tables 1 and 2 summarize a few details about all tests described.

Impairment Dimension Measurements of Postural Stability

Methods of Measuring the Sensory Systems

The tests described in this section are designed to assess the three sensory systems (visual, somatosensory, vestibular) that contribute to postural stability. The rationale underlying the use of these tests is that accurate assessment of sensory systems can identify deficits in sensory processing that affect the ability to execute an appropriate postural response.

Assessment of sensory components of balance is rooted in diagnostic tests for evaluating the vestibular system. The vestibular system has two components related to maintenance of posture—one to maintain visual clarity (the vestibulo-ocular component) and the other to facilitate postural reactions in the neck, trunk, and limbs (the vestibulospinal component).[46–48] Interaction of the vestibular system with other sensory systems is measured in differing degrees in the various tests. Tests such as past pointing, the Romberg test, and tandem walking have been used by physicians and by physical therapists and occupational therapists to obtain gross estimates of the function of the vestibular system.[49] Although these tests may provide information on postural stability, uncontrolled effects of cerebellar, visual, or musculoskeletal dysfunction can affect an individual's performance on these tests.[49,50] These tests, therefore, are not specific or sensitive enough to assess vestibular function in isolation.[49,50]

Similar problems are found with other commonly used clinical assessments of postural stability, such as tiltboard tip tests. One standardized version of a tiltboard test requires the therapist to tip the tiltboard while the child stands with feet together and hands on hips.[51] The therapist observes how far the tiltboard can be tipped before the child loses balance or steps off. The therapist measures the tilt against a backdrop marked with angles. This test has been done with both eyes open and eyes closed. Performance on this test reflects the child's ability to balance in varying sensory conditions. The eyes-open test should reflect balancing with use of all three senses, whereas the eyes-closed test requires interaction from the somatosensory and vestibular senses.[4] This test was originally developed because children with postural instability have difficulty balancing in this situation and sometimes demonstrate an uncontrolled fall.[4–6,52] Although this tiltboard test is of some clinical use in determining a child's responses to external perturbations of postural stability ("feedback" tests), in our opinion, it is not a test that systematically discriminates problems with individual sensory inputs. The tiltboard tip tests have good interrater reliability (Spearman $r=.98$), but poor test-retest reliability in both children with and without balance dysfunction (intraclass correlation coefficients [ICC]=.52–.82 and .49–.54, respectively)[52] (Spearman $r=.45$).[51] Children's performance on this balance task appears to fluctuate from one session to another, and in the eyes-closed test, a learning effect appears to be present in repeated trials of the task.[51,52] These findings suggest that this test should not be used for evaluative purposes. Because results appear to differentiate between children with and without disabilities,[4,5,51,52] however, this test may be an appropriate screening tool for determination of the need for further evaluation of postural stability.

A clinical test of vestibular function, particularly the vestibulo-ocular component, that has been widely used by pediatric therapists is the Postrotary Nystagmus Test (PRN).[53] In this test, the child sits on a rotating platform with the neck flexed forward to 30 degrees to stimulate the horizontal semicircular canals. The child is spun by the therapist for 20 seconds, after which duration of nystagmus is observed. According to Ayres,[53] either hypoactive or hyperactive nystagmus is indicative of vestibular dysfunction. The interrater reliability of measurements obtained with the PRN is good (Pearson $r=.83$); however, the test-retest reliability is poor (Pearson $r=.49$).[53–55] The validity of the PRN has been questioned due to procedural problems (testing is done in a lighted room with eyes open, which provides visual as well as vestibular stimulation), as well as concerns regarding the reliability of the normative data obtained for postrotary nystagmus.[56,57]

Vestibulo-ocular reflex (VOR) testing permits measurement of reflexive eye movements driven by the vestibular system. The individual being tested is rotated while seated in a chair in a dark room. Surface electromyographic (EMG) activity is recorded from eye muscles during and after the rotation. Although this method of testing provides measurements of the function of the horizontal semicircular canals, it does not measure the status of the vertical canals or the otoliths, or on a larger scale the vestibulospinal component.[50] Vestibulo-ocular reflex testing is most effective at measuring peripheral vestibular function.[49] Because vestibular processing deficits in children appear to be most commonly due to central nervous system dysfunction,[4,50] however, this test is less effective in identifying vestibular deficits in a

Table 1.
Impairment Tests of Postural Stability in Children[a]

Test Type	Test Name	Age Range (y)	Outcome Variable	Reliability Interrater	Reliability Intrarater	Test-Retest	Construct Validity	Normal Data	Recommended Use
Sensory system	Tiltboard tip[51,52]	4–9	Tilt (°)	r_s=.98		r_s=.45 ICC=.49–.82	Sig diff DD		Discriminative
	PRN[53–55]	3–10	Time nystagmus	r_p=.83		r_p=.49		5–9 y (N=226)	Discriminative (peripheral vestibular)
	Posturography[6–11,28,35,52,66]	1.5–10	Sway by sensory condition	Computer scored			Sig diff LD, CP DS, EP PM, HI		Discriminative
	P-CTSIB[14,38,39,59–62]	4–9	Time/sway and sensory system scores	r_s=.69–.90		r_s=.45–.78 ICC=.55–.88	Sig diff LD, CP r_s=.63–.68	4–9 y (N=120)	Discriminative
Motor system	Observe during P-CTSIB[51,59,62,67]	4–12	Strategy use (ankle, hip, step, crouch)	Kappa= .39–.68	Kappa= .54–.69	Kappa= –.10–.36			None
	COMPS[68,70]	5–9	Movement quality during six tasks	ICC=.76–.88		ICC=.79–.92	Sig diff DCD	5–9 y (N=56)	Discriminative Perhaps evaluative
	Side reach[71,72]	5–12	Balance strategy quality (head, trunk, arm, and leg position)	r_p=.98			Sig diff LD		Discriminative
	Posturography[7,8,28,32–35]	1.5–10	EMG timing, amplitude, sequence	Computer scored			Sig diff CP, DS		Discriminative
Biomechanical system	MMT[82–85]	3–adult	Ordinal strength score	ICC=.90	ICC=.80–.96 Kappa= .65–.93		Sig diff DMD		Discriminative
	HHD[62,79,86–92]	3–adult	Muscle force	ICC=.84–.99	r_p=.74–.99	ICC=.75–.99	Sig diff CP, DS	5–11 y (N=98)	Discriminative
	Standard goniometry[94–99]	Any age	ROM (°)	ICC=.25–1.00	ICC=.33–.97 SEM=2.3–6.7				Discriminative
	Video goniometry[79,100]	Any age	ROM (°)	ICC=.84–.99					Discriminative

[a] Abbreviations used: r_p=Pearson Product-Moment correlation coefficient, r_s=Spearman rho correlation coefficient, ICC=intraclass correlation coefficient, SEM=standard error of measurement, sig diff=statistically significant difference, DD=developmental delay, LD=learning disability, CP=cerebral palsy, DS=Down syndrome, EP=epilepsy, PM=premature, HI=hearing impairment, DCD=developmental coordination disorder, DMD=developmental motor disorder, PRN=Postrotary Nystagmus Test, P-CTSIB=Pediatric Clinical Test of Sensory Interaction for Balance, COMPS=Clinical Observation of Motor and Postural Skills Test, MMT=manual muscle test, HHD=hand-held dynamometry, ROM=range of motion.

Table 2.
Functional Limitation Tests of Postural Stability in Children[a]

Test Type	Test Name	Age Range	Outcome Variable	Reliability Interrater	Reliability Intrarater	Reliability Test-Retest	Validity Construct[b]	Validity Concurrent[c]	Normal Data	Recommended Use
Developmental	AIMS[102]	0–18 mo	Movement quality	r_p=.96–.98	r_p=.99	r_p=.95–.99		r_p=.84–.99 (BSID, PD, MS)	1–18 mo (N=2,400)	Discriminative Predictive Evaluative
	MAI[103,105,106]	0–12 mo	Risk score; movement quality	r_p=.51–.78		r_p=.16–.87 Kappa=.75–.97	67%–74% correct for predicting CP; 35%–63% correct for TD			Discriminative Predictive Evaluative
	BSID II[104]	0–42 mo	No. of motor skills	r_p=.75–.96	Fisher z=.84–.88	r_p=.78–.87	No sig diff BSID	r_p=.57–.77 (BSID, MSCA)	1–42 mo (N=1,700)	Discriminative Evaluative
	PDMS[81]	0–83 mo	Motor skill performance	r_p=.94–.99		r_p=.80–.99	Sig diff DP	r_p=.26–.78 (WHGM, BSID)	1–83 mo (N=617)	Discriminative Evaluative
	BOTMP[80]	4.5–14.5 y	Motor skill performance	r_p=.90–.98		r_p=.56–.81	r_p=.57–.86 (age) Sig diff MR, LD	r_p=.52–.69 (SCSIT)	4.5–14.5 y (N=765)	Discriminative Evaluative
	GMFM[76]	2–5 y	Quality of motor skills	ICC=.87–.99	ICC=.92–.99	ICC=.85–.98	Responsive to change			Discriminative Evaluative
Activities of daily living (ADL)	PEDI[107] (not including Social Function section)	0.5–7.5 y	No. of ADL skills, caregiver assistance, modifications	ICC=.79–1.00			ICC=.74–.96 (rehabilitation team to family)	r_p=.61–.97 BDIST WP	0.5–7 y (N=412)	Discriminative Evaluative
	CHAQ[108,109]	1–19 y	Independence of ADL			r_s=.80 ICC=.87–.96		Kendall tau=.77 (SFC)		Evaluative
	JASI[110]	8–18 y	Independence of ADL							None yet, needs more research
Single-item tests	FRT[61,111–113]	5–15 y	Distance reached	ICC=.98 Kendall tau=.85	ICC=.83–.97	ICC=.64G–.75 (TD) ICC=–.31–.34 (DD)			5–15 y (N=116)	Discriminative
	TUG[62,75]	3 y–adult	Time to get up, walk 3 m, and sit down	ICC=.99						Discriminative
	FST[114–116]	12–30 y	Time doing functional mobility tasks in standing position	ICC=.60–1.00						Discriminative

[a] Abbreviations used: r_p=Pearson Product-Moment correlation coefficient, r_s=Spearman rho correlation coefficient, ICC=intraclass correlation coefficient, TD=typically developing, DD=developmental delay, MR=mental retardation, LD=learning disability, AIMS=Alberta Infant Motor Scale, MAI=Movement Assessment of Infants, BSID II=Bayley Scales of Infant Development–2nd edition, PDMS=Peabody Developmental Motor Scales, BOTMP=Bruininks-Oseretsky Test of Motor Impairment, GMFM=Gross Motor Function Measure, PEDI=Pediatric Evaluation of Disability Index, CHAQ=Childhood Health Assessment Questionnaire, JASI=Juvenile Arthritis Status Index, FRT=Functional Reach Test, TUG=timed "up and go" test, FST=Functional Standing Test, BSID=Bayley Scales of Infant Development–1st edition, MSCA=McCarthy Scales of Children's Abilities, WHGM=West Haverstraw Gross Motor Test, SCSIT=Southern California Integration Test, WF=Wee Fim, BDIST=Battelle Developmental Inventory Screening Test, SFC=Steinbrocker Functional Classification.

[b] Sig diff=statistically significant difference between typically developing subjects and indicated population with disability.

[c] Correlation coefficients reported compare the test with other tests named.

pediatric population. Additionally, the equipment required for VOR testing makes it relatively impractical for clinical use.

The measurement of postural sway in the presence of sensory conflicts provides a means for evaluating deficits in central sensory organization.[35,38] *Sensory organization* is the ability of an individual to select from among the redundant sensory inputs to identify the sensory system that is providing the most accurate input for maintaining postural stability. Forssberg and Nashner[35] described the technique of sensory organization posturography testing, in which postural sway is measured in response to varying visual and somatosensory conditions. This technique permits systematic study of visual, somatosensory, and vestibular inputs for postural orientation. The individual stands on a computer-controlled movable force platform facing the center of a three-sided movable visual enclosure. The support surface and visual surroundings can be rotated in proportion to body sway, thus providing inaccurate visual and somatosensory inputs regarding the orientation of the body's COM. Body sway is measured while the individual stands for 30 seconds under six sensory conditions: (1) eyes open, normal surface (all three sensory systems providing accurate information about body position), (2) eyes closed, normal surface (only somatosensory and vestibular information available), (3) visual conflict, normal surface (sensory conflict due to inaccurate visual information but accurate somatosensory and vestibular information), (4) eyes open, somatosensory conflict (sensory conflict due to inaccurate somatosensation), (5) eyes closed, somatosensory conflict (no vision; inaccurate somatosensation, so vestibular information must be used), and (6) visual conflict, somatosensory conflict (only vestibular system providing accurate information).[28,35]

This method has been used to document developmental changes in sensory organization strategies in children[28,35] as well as deficits in sensory organization strategies in children who have motor deficits as a result of learning disabilities,[6,50] cerebral palsy,[7] Down syndrome,[8] epilepsy,[9] prematurity,[10] and hearing impairments.[4,11] Different diagnoses appear to present either no sensory deficit or different patterns of sensory deficits.[4-10,50] Platform posturography measurement of sensory organization is being used with increasing frequency in clinics, despite the high cost of the apparatus.

Several less expensive platform force-plate measurement systems have been used to document sensory deficits in children with exposure to high lead levels early in life[12] and in children with autism.[13] Interrater reliability has not been reported. Studies of test-retest reliability, if completed, have not been published in peer-reviewed journals. Evidence for construct validity has been obtained by comparing the performance of typically developing children and with that of children who have deficits in postural stability.[12,13]

Another test of sensory function related to balance, the Pediatric Clinical Test of Sensory Interaction for Balance (P-CTSIB), was developed to provide an inexpensive, clinical alternative to platform posturography.[59,60] The P-CTSIB, which is based on a suggestion from the field of physical therapy,[58] uses the same six sensory conditions that are used in platform posturography. Visual conflict is provided by use of a hatlike apparatus made of a lightweight dome. The dome allows some diffuse light to come through, but impedes the peripheral vision. As the child sways, the dome moves in synchrony with the head to simulate the moving visual surround of the platform posturography tests.[59] Somatosensory conflict is provided by having the child stand on a layer of medium-density closed-cell foam, which dampens somatosensory input during somatosensory conflict conditions. Both the amount of time the child can stand in a feet-together position and an observational measurement of anteroposterior sway are recorded.

These raw measurements are then combined for each of the six conditions and transformed into an ordinal scale spanning inability to balance in the condition to balance for the maximum of 30 seconds with less than 5 degrees of sway. These ordinal scores are then summed across sensory conditions to yield sensory system scores that are thought to provide the tester with information about whether the child can process and use each of the three sensory systems (visual, somatosensory, and vestibular). Interrater reliability[59] and test-retest reliability[60,61] have been established for this tool for both children with and without disability. Although interrater reliability for sway measurements is moderate to good (Spearman r=.69–.90),[59] test-retest reliability is lower (Spearman r=.51–.88).[60,61] Pilot norms have been established for typically developing children.[38,39] Overall, it appears that this is an easy test for typically developing children aged 4 to 9 years to perform. The children are able to stand for 30 seconds with less than 5 degrees of sway in all conditions except the last two conditions, where the time may drop by a few seconds and the sway increases by several degrees, especially in the younger children. The P-CTSIB has been used to identify sensory organization differences between children who are typically developing[38,39] and subsets of children with learning disabilities[14] and cerebral palsy,[56] which demonstrates some construct validity for the test. Scores on the P-CTSIB also correlate with functional activities related to postural stability (Spearman r=.63–.68); therefore, performance on the test reflects functional ability to some extent.[62] Due to the level of interrater reliability and the beginning normative and validity information, this test could be useful for discriminative purposes. Due to what we consider to be the moderate test-retest reliability, however, we do not believe that this test is appropriate for evaluative purposes.

Methods of Measuring the Motor System

Evaluation of motor coordination is the core of the pediatric physical therapists' and occupational therapists' expertise and practice.[63] Observational analysis of motor coordination during balancing is one method of evaluating this system. Due to the complexity of the musculoskeletal system and the variable environmental conditions in which we move, the motor coordination component of balancing has an infinite number of options for muscle activation for maintenance of postural stability. This multitude of options could make observational analyses of motor coordination very difficult due to the variability of potential responses. The general systems theory of motor control[12,18,23] postulates that there are predetermined motor strategies that help to reduce the complexity of choice of a coordinated motor response.[64–66]

Experiments that moved the floor surface forward or backward showed three basic coordination patterns during standing in adults and children: (1) an ankle strategy (primary sway centered on the ankle joint), (2) a hip strategy (primary sway centered on the hip joint), and (3) a stepping strategy (increasing the BOS).[66] Choice of these strategies is related, in part, to the strength of the perturbation, with a strong perturbation causing the stepping response, a weaker perturbation causing the hip response, and a very weak perturbation eliciting an ankle response. Other influences on choice of strategy include the surface on which the individual is balancing and availability of sensory cues.[66]

Therapists have observationally evaluated motor coordination during maintenance of postural stability by placing the child on a movable surface, tilting or moving the surface under the child, and subjectively grading the motor response observed due to the perturbation. This information is often reported as "clinical observations" and is intended to document whether the child has the appropriate balancing motor strategies (ie, head and trunk righting, arm and leg counterbalancing, and protective extension). These three motor strategies are similar to the ankle, hip, and stepping strategies, respectively, documented through the research on balancing in standing noted earlier. This type of assessment has not been examined for reliability. In an effort to improve this type of assessment, a few tests have been developed to assess in a standardized manner the motor coordination related to postural stability.

Generalizing the use of the three defined standing strategies (ankle, hip, stepping)[66] to balance on one leg[51] and to the systematically altered sensory input conditions of the P-CTSIB,[59] researchers coded in real time the use of these strategies. Interrater reliability during one-leg standing was poor to moderate (Kappa=−.10–.36).[51] During the P-CTSIB, the interrater reliability was questionable in children who were typically developing (percentage of agreement=92%–100%, but noncomputable Kappas), in part due to limited variability of motor coordination patterns observed.[59] The children appeared to use primarily an ankle strategy. Further research on children with cerebral palsy observationally scored balancing motor strategies as an ankle, hip, or crouch strategy (defined as flexion of the hips and knees in an attempt to lower the COM) during the P-CTSIB, except both P-CTSIB examiners scored independently.[62] (With the P-CTSIB, one examiner spots the child and the other examiner sits back several feet to judge sway of the child against the grid backdrop.) These scores were compared, and the reliability was moderate (weighted Kappa=.68).[62] Videotapes were made of the children during this study. These videotapes were later coded by viewing the tape once, and comparisons were made among three raters who independently scored the videotapes and with each rater scoring the videotapes on two different occasions.[67] The interrater and intrarater reliability was moderate among the three raters using the videotapes (weighted Kappa=.51–.58 and .54–.69, respectively). These researchers noted that repeated viewing of the videotapes may improve the reliability, but a more detailed analysis of the strategy through use of EMG may be necessary.[67] Further modification and testing of this system of coding motor coordination responses are needed, in our view, before this can be a viable measurement system.

The Clinical Observations of Motor and Postural Skills (COMPS)[68] was based on Ayres' original nonstandardized clinical observations used in conjunction with the Southern California Sensory Integration Tests.[69] Item administration and scoring have been standardized, yielding good interrater and test-retest reliability (ICC[3,1]=.76–.88 and .79–.92, respectively).[70] Construct validity has been demonstrated by showing statistically significant differences between scores of children with developmental coordination disorders and children who were typically developing.[70] The test is composed of six items: (1) slow motion, (2) finger-nose touching, (3) rapid forearm rotation, (4) prone extension, (5) quadruped testing of the asymmetrical tonic neck reflex, and (6) supine flexion posture. Children are rated on their motor coordination during the activities. This test provides a summary of feedforward motor coordination during these activities, including maintenance of postural stability during dynamic movements (items 1, 2, and 3) as well as static movements (items 4, 5, and 6). The COMPS would be recommended for discriminative testing, and perhaps as an evaluative measure at the impairment dimension. The test could also be used diagnostically if the tester accepts the theoretical constructs behind each of the items and designs treatment accordingly.

Fisher and Bundy[71,72] developed a flat-board and tiltboard reach test for measuring motor coordination during balancing. This test is different from the tiltboard tip test discussed earlier because the type of motor coordination used to maintain balance is the measured variable. The child is videotaped standing on either a flat board or a tiltboard with feet slightly apart and reaching as far laterally as he or she can for a toy held by the examiner. A standardized method for scoring head and trunk position and arm and leg counterbalancing was developed and found to have good interrater reliability (Pearson $r=.98$) when videotaped images were scored.[71] Test-retest reliability has not been examined. Construct validity has been established because the test discriminates between children with learning disabilities and children who are developing in a typical fashion.[72] This test is unique because it provides a measurement of a feedforward postural response during the relatively functional task of reaching laterally. With the results, identification of motor coordination problems may be localized to head, trunk, or arms and legs so that a general strategy selection problem can be identified. This test, therefore, could be useful discriminatively, but due to the lack of test-retest reliability, it cannot be used to evaluate progress.

A limitation of all of the tests discussed is that they cannot be used to determine actual selection, timing, sequencing, and amplitude of muscle activity during the motor response. Tests have been developed that record and process, via computer technology, surface EMG activity and two- or three-dimensional kinematic for the motor coordination of postural responses. Some developmental information has been gathered for children during platform perturbation testing,[28,35] as well as for recording after an auditorily cued arm-pull perturbation during the gait cycle.[32,33] Information on the coordination patterns of small groups of children with cerebral palsy[7] and Down syndrome[8] is available. These studies provide some specific information regarding the differences between "normal" and "aberrant" patterns. Although there may be similarities among children with the same diagnosis, there are wide ranges of responses. Each child's condition, therefore, needs to be evaluated individually. Additionally, the aberrant patterns adopted by children with disabilities may be the most efficient and appropriate patterns for their own individual systems. For example, some preliminary research suggests that when children who are developing typically adopt a crouched posture similar to that of children with spastic diplegia, they exhibit a similar EMG response to a backward movement of a force platform.[73] This finding suggests that the coordination of the motor pattern response may not always be the limiting factor, but rather biomechanical differences of the starting position may determine the response.

Methods of Measuring the Biomechanical System

Two main biomechanical factors have been shown to be related to postural stability in children: force output and range of motion (ROM). Force output has been shown to be related to functional measures of movement that require postural stability, such as running speed,[74] the timed "up and go" mobility test,[75] and the Gross Motor Function Measure,[76] and to measures of ambulation efficiency in children with cerebral palsy.[74,77,78] Force output has also been shown to be related to performance on the gross motor subtest of the Peabody Developmental Motor Scales (PDMS-GM) in children with Down syndrome.[79] Similarly, ROM is related to running speed[80] and the timed "up and go" mobility test[75] in children with cerebral palsy[74] and to PDMS-GM[81] scores in children with Down syndrome.[79]

Although there are relationships, as noted above, of force output and ROM to performance of children's motor activities, simply improving a child's strength or ROM does not guarantee improved postural stability or function. Most daily activities do not demand that the child use a maximal force output or move through a full ROM. The amount of force output or ROM that is required to perform daily activities successfully remains unknown. Because children with motor impairment frequently have ROM limitations and a decreased ability to generate force, assessment and remediation of these biomechanical factors, in our view, should be considered during treatment planning for remediation of all motor activities involving maintenance of postural stability.

Force output has often been evaluated using manual muscle testing (MMT).[82,83] Advantages of MMT include the fact that it requires no special equipment and can be performed in any location. One of the problems with using MMT in children is the variability in different raters' ability to judge the amount of resistance required for a rating of Normal, as this ability varies with the individual's age and with the selected muscle groups.[82] Good intrarater reliability (weighted Kappa=.65–.93 and ICC=.80–96)[84,85] and interrater reliability (ICC=.90),[85] however, have been shown for trained examiners for 18 upper- and lower-extremity muscle groups in children with Duchenne or Becker muscular dystrophy.

Hand-held dynamometry is another clinically feasible method of quantifying force output that uses a strain gauge to record peak torque and is relatively inexpensive. Bohannon[86] has documented standard testing positions for dynamometry, and other therapists have advocated modifications of these positions to improve the specificity of testing (Susan K Effgen, personal communication, 1995). For trained examiners, interrater reliability has been shown to be good for lower-extremity muscles in children with cerebral palsy (ICC[3,1]=.94–.99),[62] children with Down syndrome (ICC[2,1]=.92–.98),[79] and children who were developing typically (ICC[3,1]=.84–1.00).[87] Intrarater reliability was good in children with Duchenne muscular dystrophy (Pearson r=.83–.99).[87] Test-retest reliability was also found to be good in children with meningomyelocele (ICC=.75–.99),[88] children with moderate mental retardation (ICC=.83–.86),[89] children with Duchenne muscular dystrophy (Pearson r=.83–.99),[87] and children who were developing typically (ICC=.79–.93).[90] Dynamometers are advantageous because they are small and portable equipment. One disadvantage is that broad normative data are not available for the pediatric population. Information on small samples has been documented, however, and could be used as a general guide for decision making.[91,92]

Both MMT and dynamometry could aid with the identification of impairments in children. Each test could also be used for evaluative purposes if interrater and test-retest reliability were established by the examiners prior to use. To minimize the chance of examiner error, we suggest that the same rater perform all the measurements.[84,87] A disadvantage of both MMT and dynamometry is that neither test provides information about force generation throughout the ROM during concentric and eccentric contractions or during functional activities.

Isokinetic testing devices have the advantage of generating information through an arc of motion. The machine provides resistance to hold the speed of the motion constant. Disadvantages include the cost of the equipment, lack of portability, difficulty in adapting the devices to small children, and lack of research on children. Another disadvantage is that test results are limited to specific speed selections rather than measuring force output in a functional context.

All three of the force output testing methods discussed involve eliciting a maximal effort. The ability to obtain a maximal effort can be influenced by the child's age or cognitive level. Good test-retest reliability (ICC=.79–.93) of hand-held dynamometry measurements of shoulder and knee flexion and extension has been shown in a small sample of girls as young as 3 years of age.[90] Children with cognitive deficits may have difficulty with the procedures, regardless of their age. Horvat and colleagues,[89] however, have recently demonstrated good test-retest reliability, both within and between sessions (ICC=.83–.86), using hand-held dynamometry for elbow flexion and extension with individuals aged 14 to 24 years who had moderate mental retardation. Examiners should be aware that cooperation and performance can vary with individual children. In young children, force output is similar for boys and girls. As children enter puberty, however, gender differences develop. Clinical judgments for adolescents, therefore, must be made in comparison with same-gender peers.[91]

Children with neurological impairment present additional challenges. Frequently, due to the decreased ROM that can accompany neurologic impairment, the testing positions place the children at the end of their joint ROM. This puts the child at a mechanical disadvantage because the muscle's position is at the end of the length-tension curve. Additionally, children with neurological impairment may have impaired motor control or can only move in synergistic patterns. If a child is unable to push against the testing apparatus, it is difficult to ascertain whether all or a portion of the deficit is due to weakness or to an inability to voluntarily move the extremity in the desired direction on command.

Maintaining postural stability often requires controlled, sustained adjustments rather than maximal bursts of activity. These sustained low-level contractions may not be difficult for children who are developing typically, but they may be impossible in children with neurological dysfunction because of their very low force output ability, poor endurance, and poor biomechanical alignment.[93] Limited data exist about which muscles are important and how much force production is necessary for control of posture. Preliminary data on a small sample of children with cerebral palsy suggest that the ability to generate hip extension, hip abduction, and ankle plantar-flexion force is most important for maintaining postural stability in a standing position.[62] Much research is needed in this area.

Weakness may also force children to use biomechanical alignment for stability. The children may adopt a posture in which they can use gravity and alignment rather than muscle contractions to maintain upright stance. For example, a child may stand with an increased lumbar lordosis to shift the center of gravity farther behind the hip joint, thereby allowing the iliofemoral ligament to provide passive hip extension. Similarly, the child may hyperextend the knees to move the center of gravity farther in front of the knee and provide passive knee extension. By standing in this "knee-locked" position, however, the child assumes a less dynamic posture and is less ready to move to maintain postural stability. These positions may lead to contractures.

Range of motion has been evaluated by standard goniometric techniques.[94] In children with disabilities, interrater and test-retest reliability of goniometric measurements has been problematic because both types of reliability can be influenced by numerous factors such as illness, temperament, medication, and speed of movement.[95–99] The presence of increased reflex activity also may cause inconsistent because muscle length can change based on the duration, intensity, and speed of force exerted to passively move the limb and can provide a more variable end feel than bone or typical soft tissue.[98] Two studies on children with cerebral palsy[95,98] showed the reliability agreement among raters' measurements of ROM may be 10 to 15 degrees apart. In a more recent study,[99] intrarater reliability for standard goniometry in ankle joints of children with juvenile rheumatoid arthritis, children with cerebral palsy, and children who were developing typically has been shown to be moderate to good (standard error of measurement [SEM]=±2.3°–6.7°). The low SEM of 2.3 degrees was for children who were typically developing when the same rater used an average of two measurements. The high SEM of 6.7 degrees was for children with cerebral palsy when different raters measured over time. In children with Duchenne muscular dystrophy, intrarater reliability was higher (ICC=.81–.94) than interrater reliability (ICC=.25–.91).[97] The basic recommendation if using goniometry for evaluative purposes in children is to control the external conditions carefully and always have the same examiner remeasure.[96,99]

Use of videography has been shown to improve goniometric interrater reliability (ICC[2,1]=.84–.99) in children with Down syndrome.[79] Bony landmarks are identified with markers. The child is positioned at a 90-degree angle to the camera, and the ROM procedures are recorded on videotape. The joint angle measurements are then taken from the videotape by freezing a frame and using a goniometer on the screen. Computer methods for measuring kinematic variables can also be used to make the measurements.[100] Although reproducibility and accuracy are generally good (ICC=.99) using computer-scored videography,[100] care must be taken to ensure that the video picture is a valid representation of the child's excursion.[79] Factors such as camera angle and selection of which video frame to analyze could distort the information. This type of ROM measurement allows the therapist to record ROMs that are voluntarily used in functional activities rather than the actual full ROM. Research on these ROMs could provide important information about critical values necessary for maintenance of postural stability.

In addition to providing sufficient range of movement to make postural adjustments, theoretically adequate ROM is necessary to optimize the pull of gravity and to maximize the child's BOS. For example, the common stance of children with spastic diplegia with ankles plantar flexed and hip medially (internally) rotated and adducted considerably narrows the child's BOS. This narrowing of the BOS, in turn, could accentuate the impact of external perturbations, as it becomes more difficult to maintain the center of gravity inside a narrow BOS. Decreased ROM also changes the line of pull of gravity. In typical adult posture, the line of gravity falls slightly behind the hip joint and in front of the knee and ankle joints.[101] This alignment allows the body to use ligamentous and bony alignment to provide some stability rather than using excessive muscle activity. Typically, the plantar flexors are the only muscles that are active when standing still, unless the sway becomes excessive.[101] Introducing even a small knee flexion contracture can disrupt this alignment, shift the line of gravity, and therefore theoretically create a situation in which the child needs to actively contract the quadriceps femoris muscles to maintain a standing position. Research is needed in this area to better define critical values of ROM and the postural alignment necessary for improved postural stability.

Functional Limitation Dimension Measurements Reflecting Postural Stability

Adequate postural stability is necessary to perform basic gross motor skills, and these skills can, in one sense, be defined as the "functional" activity of children. Therefore, assessments that analyze gross motor skill acquisition can provide information regarding a child's postural stability at the level of functional limitations.

There are several developmental assessment instruments designed for infants and young children that are based on the typical sequence of motor skill acquisition. Examples are the Alberta Infant Motor Scale,[102] the Movement Assessment of Infants,[103] the Bayley Scales of Infant Development (2nd edition),[104] and the Peabody Developmental Motor Scales (PDMS).[81] These tests have moderate to good reliability and validity.[21,102–106] (Actual coefficients are detailed in Tab. 2.) Generally, these tests have specific sections related to postural stability. For example, the PDMS is designed for children from birth to 83 months of age and includes a balance subtest as part of the gross motor scale.[81] The balance subtest includes items such as one-foot balance and walking on a balance beam. For older children (aged 4.5–14.5 years), the gross motor section of the Bruininks-Oseretsky Test of Motor Proficiency (BOTMP)[80] provides a reliable balance subtest, with items similar to those of the PDMS, as well as subtests on running speed and agility, bilateral coordination, and strength. Moderate to good reliability and validity have been documented.[80] (Refer to Tab. 2 for the actual coefficients.) The BOTMP was designed for children with mild motor impairment and is very difficult for children with more severe impairment to complete. For children with cerebral palsy, the Gross Motor Function Measure (GMFM)[76] has good interrater and test-retest reliability (Tab. 2).[21,76] Items tested fall under five domains: (1) lying and rolling, (2) crawling and kneeling, (3) sitting, (4) standing, and (5) walking, running, and jumping. All of these domains require postural stability. The GMFM has also been shown to be responsive for evaluation of clinically meaningful change.[21]

Tests such as the Pediatric Evaluation of Disability Inventory (PEDI)[107] and two tests designed for children with juvenile rheumatoid arthritis, the Childhood Health Assessment Questionnaire (CHAQ)[108,109] and the Juvenile Arthritis Status Index (JASI),[110] are examples of tools used to measure children's ability to perform activities of daily living rather than developmental skills. The PEDI uses an interview or observational format and consists of three sections: self-care, mobility, and social function. Studies have shown the PEDI to have good reliability and validity.[107] (Refer to Tab. 2 for actual coefficients.) The CHAQ and JASI are questionnaires that determine the types of activities that children are capable of doing independently in their normal environments. Performance of all mobility and self-care tasks requires adequate postural stability.

These developmental and functionally based tests measure many aspects of movement. By focusing on specific items within the scales, we believe that these tests can be used as discriminative tests to document general problems with postural stability. They are also useful as evaluative measures to document functional movement changes related to treatment of postural stability. Care, however, should be taken regarding the population being evaluated due to problems with responsivity of some of these tests.[21]

Several single-item functional tests related to postural stability were developed for the frail elderly population but have been studied to various extents in a pediatric population. For the Functional Reach Test (FRT),[111] the individual is positioned with the shoulders perpendicular to a wall on which a yardstick has been affixed at shoulder level and is instructed to hold an arm out at 90 degrees of shoulder flexion. The individual is then asked to reach forward as far as possible without touching the wall or moving the feet. The length difference between the starting and ending reach positions is recorded. For children who are developing typically, measurements obtained with the FRT have demonstrated good reliability within a single session ($ICC[2,1]=.98$) and between different days ($ICC[2,1]=.75$) as well as good intrarater and interrater reliability ($ICC[2,1]=.83$).[112] Two studies with small samples of children with balance dysfunction, however, showed poor test-retest reliability ($ICC[2,1]=-.31$[61] and $ICC[1,1]=.34$[113]). Mean reach values and critical reach values (values that are two standard deviations below the mean) have been established for a group of children (N=101) between the ages of 5 and 15 years who are typically developing.[112] Scores below the critical value could indicate a problem with postural stability. Distances that children with disability have been able to reach appear to be different from those of children who are typically developing, demonstrating some construct validity.[61,112,113] Because of the good interrater reliability and the beginning normative data, we contend that the FRT can be used as a discriminative test. It also may be seen as a diagnostic test in terms of documenting, in general, problems with feedforward control of postural stability. At this time, we do not recommend the use of the FRT as an evaluative measure in children due to the poor test-retest reliability with children with disabilities.

Another functionally based test, the timed "up and go" test,[75] consists of recording the amount of time required to rise from a chair, walk 3 m, turn around, return to the chair, and sit down again. Good interrater reliability ($ICC[3,1]=.99$) has been found with testing of children as a part of a study of correlation of balance tests.[62] Beginning data on results of this test in children with cerebral palsy show a correlation (Person $r=.61-.95$) with other assessments related to postural stability (P-CTSIB, FRT, PEDI–mobility, BOTMP–running speed), suggesting some validity to the test as a functional measure of postural stability.[62] This test also shows potential for differentiating between children with and without balance deficits and may, after test-retest examination, prove to be an appropriate evaluative measure.

The Functional Standing Test (FST) was developed to measure "functional standing" in children with spinal cord injury.[114–116] This test requires the child to stand at a station and perform upper-extremity tasks taken from the Jebsen-Taylor Hand Function Test[117] while maintaining postural stability in a standing position. The time it takes to perform each task is recorded. Interrater reliability studies on the FST in both adolescents who are typically developing and those with complete spinal cord injury showed moderate to good reliability (ICC=.60–1.00).[116] This test is a good candidate for an evaluative measure, in our opinion, but further research on test-retest reliability and validity is needed.

Clinical Implications and Suggestions for Future Research

We have discussed the evaluation of postural stability from several perspectives and offered ways to classify current tests of postural stability. We believe that reliable and valid measures should be used to determine the contributing factors of our clients' postural problems so that we can design the most effective treatment possible. Following this, it is equally important to document the effectiveness of our treatment techniques. This is the only way in which we will transform our profession from an "art" to a "science" and be able to help our clients in the most effective and efficient manner.

The impairment dimension assessments of the three primary systems involved in the maintenance of postural stability—the sensory system, the motor system, and the biomechanical system—are administered primarily to identify problematic areas so that specific treatments can be prescribed. Although we have suggested splitting the construct of balancing into these three primary systems, we acknowledge that there are relational effects among these systems. Most children will have a combination of problems in these systems causing their difficulty with postural stability. For example, abnormal motor coordination may cause changes in the biomechanical capabilities of children with neurological deficits. Biomechanical abnormalities, however, may prevent "normal" coordination of postural motor responses and may alter sensory information, especially from the somatosensory system. By minimizing biomechanical abnormalities, the body may have the opportunity to select a more typical motor coordination pattern. To be able to assess these issues, more research is needed on the relationship between changing a child's ROM and force output and subsequent changes in motor coordination and sensory processing.

Therapists should monitor changes in impairments of these three systems over time and with treatment; however, interpretation of these changes needs to be considered carefully because, in general, the impairment dimension tests described have not demonstrated high test-retest reliability. This finding may be due, in part, to behavioral issues in testing children. It also may be due to the fact that children are developing and changing, which when added to the difficulty in controlling the external and internal environmental conditions between testing sessions, makes consistent measurement of postural stability difficult. There is need for further research to examine and improve test-retest reliability of assessments in all three systems. Although current tests can be suggested to have face validity and content validity, and in general have been shown to provide different results in children with and without disabilities, more validity research needs to occur related to the theoretical constructs of the testing and the relationship to other accepted criteria.

Sensory system measurement and test development related to isolating vestibular sensory problems have occurred in two camps: vestibulo-ocular and vestibulospinal. Based on the research to date related to problems with postural stability, we suggest that measurements be focused on postural reactions to altering sensory input rather than on vestibular-ocular testing. The available tests for examining sensory interaction for balancing are limited to either expensive laboratory posturography testing or the P-CTSIB. The P-CTSIB is limited to testing in a standing position and has only shown moderate test-retest reliability. More research to expand testing options of sensory systems and better develop the current methods of testing is needed.

Evaluation of the motor coordination of postural stability has been accomplished in the clinic through use of nonstandardized observations. Although a few tests have been developed, there is a need for more specific, reliable, and comprehensive motor coordination tests related to postural stability. Research using tests of motor coordination offer data on motor coordination during postural control, and these systems are becoming more available to practitioners. This type of testing is expensive, and how the detailed information can be used diagnostically to formulate treatment plans aimed at modifying timing, amplitude, and strategy selection for motor coordination remains unclear. Much research needs to done in this area to understand the findings and to relate them to treatment techniques. Emphasis also needs to be placed on how these tests correlate with more functional tests of balance and on whether more clinically feasible and reliable observational mechanisms can be developed that provide the same information.

The biomechanical system represents the background on which we make our postural adjustments as well as our volitional movements; therefore, the biomechanical system needs to be included in evaluation and treatment of postural instability. Tests developed in this area are limited to measurements of maximal force and ROM and may not reflect the specificity of testing needed for this construct. Research is needed on development of the ability to maintain lower forces and critical values of ROM during tasks requiring postural stability.

When evaluating our clients' progress, we argue that it is not enough to change ROM or the ability to stand in altered sensory conditions in a laboratory or clinical setting. A change in postural stability during functional activities (ie, children's ability to move and interact in their everyday environment) must also occur. Therefore, we recommend also evaluating effectiveness of therapy by assessment at the functional limitation dimension. Because there are only a few single-item functional tests directly related to postural stability and the current developmental and functional tests cover wide ranges of activities, development of more specific functional balance tests needs to occur. These "new" functional balance tests could also be focused on activities to obtain information about the three primary systems. For example, observing children doing a standardized set of activities such as lifting objects of known weight, running a distance, stair climbing, rising up on the toes, and so forth are general indicators of the presence of a minimal level of functional force production and could be scored for motor coordination patterns and adaptation to altered sensory surfaces. Results of this type of combined test development—measures of functional skills combined with impairment dimension measures—may begin to shed light on the critical values of force production, ROM, motor coordination, and sensory integration necessary for postural stability in normal activities.

In summary, there are some available reliable measures for evaluation of postural stability. Therapists need to attend to their theoretical view of the construct of postural stability, their objective of testing, and the qualities of the tool they are using. Research is needed for pediatric test and measurement development in all described areas related to postural stability.

References

1 Horak FB. Clinical measurement of postural control in adults. *Phys Ther.* 1987;67:1881–1884.

2 Shumway-Cook A, Woollacott MH. *Motor Control: Theory and Practical Applications.* Baltimore, Md: Williams & Wilkins; 1995.

3 Shumway-Cook A, McCollum G. Assessment and treatment of balance deficits. In: Montgomery PC, Connolly BH, eds. *Motor Control and Physical Therapy: Theoretical Framework and Practical Applications.* Hixson, Tenn: Chattanooga Group Inc; 1991:123–137.

4 Crowe TK, Horak FB. Motor proficiency associated with vestibular deficits in children with hearing impairments. *Phys Ther.* 1988;68:1493–1499.

5 Horak FB, Shumway-Cook A, Crowe TK, Black O. Vestibular function and motor proficiency of children with impaired hearing, or with learning disability and motor impairment. *Dev Med Child Neurol.* 1988;30:64–79.

6 Shumway-Cook A, Horak FB, Black O. A critical examination of vestibular function in motor-impaired learning disabled children. *Int J Pediatr Otorhinolaryngol.* 1987;14:21–30.

7 Nashner LM, Shumway-Cook A, Marin O. Stance posture control in select groups of children with cerebral palsy: deficits in sensory organization and muscular coordination. *Exp Brain Res.* 1983;49:393–409.

8 Shumway-Cook A, Woollacott M. Dynamics of postural control in the child with Down syndrome. *Phys Ther.* 1985;65:1315–1321.

9 Kowalski K, Di Fabio RP. Gross motor and balance impairments in children and adolescents with epilepsy. *Dev Med Child Neurol.* 1995;37:604–619.

10 Forslund M. Growth and motor performance in preterm children at 8 years of age. *Acta Paediatr.* 1992;81:840–842.

11 Potter CN, Silverman LN. Characteristics of vestibular function and static balance skills in deaf children. *Phys Ther.* 1984;64:1071–1075.

12 Bhattacharya A, Shukla R, Dietrich K, et al. Effect of early lead exposure on children's postural balance. *Dev Med Child Neurol.* 1995;37:861–878.

13 Kohen-Raz R, Volkmar FR, Cohen DJ. Postural control in children with autism. *J Autism Dev Disord.* 1992;22:419–432.

14 Deitz J, Richardson PK, Westcott SL, Crowe TK. Performance of children with learning disabilities on the Pediatric Clinical Test of Sensory Interaction for Balance. *Physical and Occupational Therapy in Pediatrics.* 1996;16:1–21.

15 Kishner B, Guyatt GH. A methodologic framework for assessing health indices. *J Chronic Dis.* 1985;38:27–36.

16 Rosenbaum PL, Russell DJ, Cadman DT, et al. Issues in measuring change in motor function in children with cerebral palsy: a special communication. *Phys Ther.* 1990;70:125–131.

17 National Advisory Board on Medical Rehabilitation Research. *Research Plan for the National Center for Medical Rehabilitation Research.* Bethesda, Md: National Institutes of Health; 1993. NIH Publication No. 93-3509.

18 Horak FB. Assumptions underlying motor control for neurological rehabilitation. In: Lister MJ, ed. *Contemporary Management of Motor Problems: Proceedings of the II Step Conference.* Alexandria, Va: American Physical Therapy Association; 1992:11–28.

19 Portney LG, Watkins MP. *Foundations of Clinical Research: Applications to Practice.* East Norwalk, Conn: Appleton & Lange; 1993:53–67.

20 Guyatt GH, Walter S, Norman G. Measuring change over time: assessing the usefulness of evaluative instruments. *J Chronic Dis.* 1987;40:171–180.

21 Palisano RJ, Kolobe TH, Haley SM, et al. Validity of the Peabody Developmental Gross Motor Scale as an evaluative measure of infants receiving physical therapy. *Phys Ther.* 1995;75:939–948.

22 McGraw M. *Neuromuscular Maturation of the Human Infant.* New York, NY: Hafner Press; 1945.

23 Bradley NS. Motor control: developmental aspects of motor control in skill acquisition. In: Campbell SK, ed. *Physical Therapy for Children.* Philadelphia, Pa: WB Saunders Co; 1994:39–77.

24 Burleigh AL, Horak FB, Malouin F. Modification of postural responses and step initiation: evidence for goal-directed postural interactions. *J Neurophysiol.* 1994;72:2892–2902.

25 Schmidt RA. *Motor Control and Learning.* 2nd ed. Champaign, Ill: Human Kinetics; 1988.

26 Gentile AM. Skill acquisition: action, movement, and neuromotor processes. In: Carr J, Shepherd R, eds. *Movement Science: Foundations for Physical Therapy in Rehabilitation.* Rockville, Md: Aspen Publishers Inc; 1987:93–154.

27 Majsak MJ. Application of motor learning principles to the stroke population. *Topics in Stroke Rehabilitation.* 1996;3:27–59.

28 Shumway-Cook A, Woollacott MH. The growth of stability: postural control from a developmental perspective. *Journal of Motor Behavior.* 1985;17:131–147.

29 Woollacott MH, Shumway-Cook A. Changes in posture control across the life span: a systems approach. *Phys Ther.* 1990;70:799–807.

30 Hayes KC, Riach CL. Preparatory postural adjustments and postural sway in young children. In: Woollacott MH, Shumway-Cook A, eds. *Development of Posture and Gait Across the Life Span*. Columbia, SC: University of South Carolina Press; 1989:97–127.

31 Haas G, Deiner HC, Rapp H, Dichgans J. Development of feedback and feedforward control of upright stance. *Dev Med Child Neurol*. 1989;31:481–488.

32 Hirschfeld H, Forssberg H. Development of anticipatory postural adjustments during locomotion in children. *J Neurophysiol*. 1991;66:12–19.

33 Hirschfeld H, Forssberg H. Phase-dependent modulations of anticipatory postural adjustments during locomotion in children. *J Neurophysiol*. 1992;68:542–550.

34 Riach CL, Hayes KC. Anticipatory postural control in children. *Journal of Motor Behavior*. 1990;22:250–266.

35 Forssberg H, Nashner LM. Ontogenetic development of postural control in man: adaptation to altered support and visual conditions during stance. *J Neuroscience*. 1982;2:545–552.

36 Foudriat BA, Di Fabio RP, Anderson JH. Sensory organization of balance responses in children 3–6 years age: a normative study with diagnostic implications. *Int J Pediatr Otorhinolaryngol*. 1993;27:255–271.

37 Woollacott MH, Shumway-Cook A, Williams HG. The development of posture and balance control in children. In: Woollacott MH, Shumway-Cook A, eds. *Development of Posture and Gait Across the Life Span*. Columbia, SC: University of South Carolina Press; 1989:77–96.

38 Deitz JC, Richardson PK, Atwater SW, Crowe TK. Performance of normal children on the Pediatric Clinical Test of Sensory Interaction for Balance. *Occupational Therapy Journal of Research*. 1991;11:336–356.

39 Richardson PK, Atwater SW, Crowe TK, Deitz JC. Performance of preschoolers on the Pediatric Clinical Test of Sensory Interaction for Balance. *Amer J Occup Ther*. 1992;46:793–800.

40 Sellers JS. Relationship between antigravity control and postural control in young children. *Phys Ther*. 1988;68:486–490.

41 Riach CL, Hayes KC. Maturation of postural sway in young children. *Dev Med Child Neurol*. 1987;29:650–658.

42 Starkes J, Riach CL. The role of vision in the postural control of children. *Clinical Kinesiology*. 1990;44:72–77.

43 Woollacott MH, Debu B, Mowatt M. Neuromuscular control of posture in the infant and child: Is vision dominant? *Journal of Motor Behavior*. 1987;19:167–186.

44 Lee DN, Aronson E. Visual proprioceptive control of standing in human infants. *Perception and Psychophysics*. 1974;15:529–532.

45 Sutherland DH, Olshen RA, Biden EN, et al. *Development of Mature Walking*. London, England: MacKeith Press; 1988.

46 Carpenter MB. Vestibular nuclei: afferent and efferent projections. *Prog Brain Res*. 1988;76:5–15.

47 Diener HC, Dichgans J, Guschlbauer B, Bacher M. Role of visual and static vestibular influences on dynamic posture control. *Human Neurobiology*. 1986;5:105–113.

48 Diener HC, Dichgans J. On the role of vestibular, visual, and somatosensory information for dynamic postural control in humans. *Prog Brain Res*. 1988;76:253–261.

49 Baloh RW. Examination of the vestibular system. In: Baloh RW. *Dizziness, Hearing Loss, and Tinnitus: The Essentials of Neuro-otology*. Philadelphia, Pa: FA Davis Co; 1984:73–96.

50 Horak FB, Shumway-Cook A, Black FO. Are vestibular deficits responsible for developmental disorders in children? *Insights in Otolaryngology*. 1988;3:1–5.

51 Atwater SW, Crowe TK, Deitz JC, Richardson PK. Interrater and test-retest reliability of two pediatric balance tests. *Phys Ther*. 1990;70:79–87.

52 Broadstone BJ, Westcott SL, Deitz JC. Test-retest reliability of two tiltboard tests in children. *Phys Ther*. 1993;73:618–625.

53 Ayres AJ. *Southern California Postrotary Nystagmus Test*. Los Angeles, Calif: Western Psychological Services; 1975.

54 Siegner CB, Crowe TK, Deitz JC. Interrater reliability of the Southern California Postrotary Nystagmus Test. *Physical and Occupational Therapy in Pediatrics*. 1982;2:83–91.

55 Deitz JC, Siegner CB, Crowe TK. The Southern California Postrotary Nystagmus Test: test-retest reliability for preschool children. *Occupational Therapy Journal of Research*. 1981;1:165–177.

56 Polatajko HJ. The Southern California Postrotary Test: a validity study. *Can J Occup Ther*. 1983;50:119–123.

57 Royeen BC, Lesinski G, Ciani S, et al. Relationship of the Southern California Sensory Integration Tests, the Southern California Postrotary Nystagmus Test, and clinical observation accompanying them to evaluate in otolaryngology, opthamology, and audiology: five descriptive case studies. *Am J Occup Ther*. 1981;35:443–450.

58 Shumway-Cook A, Horak FB. Assessing the influence of sensory interaction on balance: suggestion from the field. *Phys Ther*. 1986;66:1548–1550.

59 Crowe TK, Deitz JC, Richardson PK, Atwater SW. Interrater reliability of the Clinical Test of Sensory Interaction for Balance. *Physical and Occupational Therapy in Pediatrics*. 1990;10:1–27.

60 Westcott SL, Crowe TK, Deitz JC, Richardson PK. Test-retest reliability of the Pediatric Clinical Test of Sensory Interaction for Balance (P-CTSIB). *Physical and Occupational Therapy in Pediatrics*. 1994;14:1–22.

61 Pelligrino TT, Buelow B, Krause M, et al. Test-retest reliability of the Pediatric Clinical Test of Sensory Interactions for Balance and the Functional Reach Test in children with standing balance dysfunction. *Pediatric Physical Therapy*. 1995;7:197.

62 Lowes PL. *An Evaluation of the Standing Balance of Children With Cerebral Palsy and the Tools for Assessment*. Philadelphia, Pa: Medical College of Pennsylvania and Hahnemann University; 1996. Unpublished doctoral dissertation.

63 Boyce WF, Gowland C, Rosebaum PL, et al. Measuring quality of movement in cerebral palsy: a review of instruments. *Phys Ther*. 1991;71:813–819.

64 Bernstein A. *The Coordination and Regulation of Movement*. New York, NY: Pergamon Press; 1967.

65 Vereijken B, van Emmerick REA, Whiting HTA, et al. Free(z)ing degrees of freedom in skill acquisition. *Journal of Motor Behavior*. 1992;24:133–142.

66 Nashner LM. Adaptation of human movement to altered environments. *Trends Neurosci*. October 1982:358–361.

67 Luyt L, Bodney S, Keller J, et al. Reliability of determining motor strategy used by children with cerebral palsy during the Pediatric Test of Sensory Interaction for Balance. *Pediatric Physical Therapy*. 1996;8:180.

68 Wilson B, Pollock N, Kaplan BJ, et al. *The Clinical Observations of Motor and Postural Skills*. San Antonio, Tex: Therapy Skill Builders; 1994.

69 Ayres AJ. *Southern California Sensory Integration Tests*. Los Angeles, Calif: Western Psychological Services; 1975.

70 Wilson B, Pollock N, Kaplan BJ, et al. Reliability and construct validity of the Clinical Observation of Motor and Postural Skills. *Am J Occup Ther.* 1992;46:775–783.

71 Fisher AG. *Equilibrium: Development and Clinical Assessment.* Boston, Mass: Boston University; 1984. Unpublished doctoral dissertation.

72 Fisher AG, Bundy AC. Equilibrium reactions in normal children and in boys with sensory integrative dysfunctions. *Occupational Therapy Journal of Research.* 1982;2:171–183.

73 Burtner PA, Woollacott MH, Shumway-Cook A. Muscle activation characteristics for balance control in children with cerebral palsy. *Dev Med Child Neurol.* 1995;37(suppl):27–28. Abstract.

74 Lowes LP, Westcott SL. Relationship of force output and range of motion to functional mobility tests in children with cerebral palsy. *Pediatric Physical Therapy.* 1995;7:200.

75 Podsiadlo D, Richardson S. The timed "up and go": a basic functional mobility test for frail elderly persons. *J Am Geriatr Soc.* 1991;39:142–148.

76 Russell D, Rosenbaum P, Gowland C, et al. *Gross Motor Function Measure.* 2nd ed. Hamilton, Ontario, Canada: Gross Motor Measure Group; 1993.

77 Parker DF, Carriere L, Hebertreit H, et al. Muscle performance and gross motor function of children with spastic cerebral palsy. *Dev Med Child Neurol. 1993;35:17–23.*

78 Damiano DL, Kelly LE, Vaughn CL. Effects of quadriceps femoris muscle strengthening on crouch gait in children with spastic diplegia. *Phys Ther.* 1995;75:658–667.

79 Dichter CG. *Relationship of Muscle Strength and Joint Range of Motion to Gross Motor Abilities in School-aged Children With Down Syndrome.* Philadelphia, Pa: Medical College of Pennsylvania and Hahnemann University; 1994. Unpublished doctoral dissertation.

80 Bruininks R. *Bruininks-Oseretsky Test of Motor Proficiency.* Circle Pines, Minn: American Guidance Service; 1978.

81 Fewell R, Folio R. *Peabody Developmental Motor Scales.* Allen, Tex: Developmental Learning Materials Teaching Resources; 1983.

82 Hislop HJ, Montgomery J. *Daniels and Worthingham's Muscle Testing: Techniques of Manual Examination.* 6th ed. Philadelphia, Pa: WB Saunders Co; 1995.

83 Kendall HO, Kendall FP, Wadsworth GE. *Muscles: Testing and Function.* 2nd ed. Baltimore, Md: Williams & Wilkins; 1971.

84 Florence JM, Pandya S, King WM, et al. Intrarater reliability of manual muscle test (Medical Research Council Scale) grades in Duchenne's muscular dystrophy. *Phys Ther.* 1992;72:115–122.

85 Barr AE, Diamond BE, Wade CK, et al. Reliability of testing measures in Duchenne or Becker muscular dystrophy. *Arch Phys Med Rehabil.* 1991;72:315–319.

86 Bohannon RW. Test-retest reliability of hand-held dynamometry during a single session of strength assessment. *Phys Ther.* 1986;66:206–209.

87 Stuberg WA, Metcalf WK. Reliability of quantitative muscle testing in healthy children and in children with Duchenne muscular dystrophy using hand-held dynamometry. *Phys Ther.* 1988;68:977–982.

88 Effgen SK, Brown DA. Long-term stability of hand-held dynamometric measurements in children who have myelomeningocele. *Phys Ther.* 1992;72:458–465.

89 Horvat M, Croce R, Roswal G. Intratester reliability of the Nicholas Manual Muscle Tester on individuals with intellectual disabilities by a tester having minimal experience. *Arch Phys Med Rehabil.* 1994;76:808–811.

90 Gajdosik CG, Nelson SA, Gleason DK, et al. Reliability of isometric strength measurements of girls ages 3–5 years: a preliminary study. *Pediatric Physical Therapy.* 1994;6:206.

91 Hunt M. *Maximum Voluntary Isometric Contraction of Lower Extremity Muscles in Children.* Philadelphia, Pa: Hahnemann University; 1994. Unpublished master's thesis.

92 Backman E, Odenrick P, Henriksson KG, et al. Isometric muscle force and anthropometric values in normal children aged between 3.5 and 15 years. *Scand J Rehabil Med.* 1989;21:105–114.

93 Beasley WC. Quantitative muscle testing: principles and application to research and clinical services. *Arch Phys Med Rehabil.* 1961;42:398–421.

94 Norkin CC, White DJ. *Measurement of Joint Motion: A Guide to Goniometry.* Philadelphia, Pa: FA Davis Co; 1985.

95 Stuberg WA, Fuchs RH, Miedaner JA. Reliability of goniometric measurements of children with cerebral palsy. *Dev Med Child Neurol.* 1988;30:657–666.

96 Gajdosik RL, Bohannon RW. Clinical measurement of range of motion: review of goniometry emphasizing reliability and validity. *Phys Ther.* 1987;67:1867–1872.

97 Pandya S, Florence JM, King WM, et al. Reliability of goniometric measurements in patients with Duchenne muscular dystrophy. *Phys Ther.* 1985;65:1339–1342.

98 Harris SR, Harthun Smith L, Krukowski L. Goniometric reliability for a child with spastic quadriplegia. *J Pediatr Orthop.* 1985;5:348–351.

99 Watkins B, Darrah J, Pain K. Reliability of passive ankle dorsiflexion measurements in children: comparison of universal and biplane goniometers. *Pediatric Physical Therapy.* 1995;7:3–8.

100 Vander Linden DW, Carlson SJ, Hubbard RL. Reproducibility and accuracy of angle measurements obtained under static conditions with the Motion Analysis Video system. *Phys Ther.* 1992;72:300–305.

101 Pratt NE. *Clinical Musculoskeletal Anatomy.* Philadelphia, Pa: JB Lippincott Co; 1991.

102 Piper M, Darrah J. *Motor Assessment of the Developing Infant.* Philadelphia, Pa: WB Saunders Co; 1994.

103 Chandler L, Andrews M, Swanson M. *Movement Assessment of Infants.* Rolling Bay, Wash: Rolling Bay Press; 1980.

104 Bayley N. *Bayley Scales of Infant Development.* 2nd ed. San Antonio, Tex: Psychological Corporation; 1993.

105 Brander R, Kramer J, Dancsak M, et al. Interrater and test retest reliabilities of the Movement Assessment of Infants. *Pediatric Physical Therapy.* 1993;5:9–15.

106 Harris SR, Haley SM, Tada WL, et al. Reliability of observational measures of the Movement Assessment of Infants. *Phys Ther.* 1984;64:471–475.

107 Haley SM, Coster WJ, Ludlow LH, et al. *Pediatric Evaluation of Disability Inventory.* Boston, Mass: PEDI Research Group; 1992.

108 Singh G, Athreya BH, Fries JF, et al. Measurement of health status in children with juvenile rheumatoid arthritis. *Arthritis Rheum.* 1994;37:1761–1769.

109 Feldman BM, Ayling-Campos A, Luy L, et al. Measuring disability in juvenile dermatomyositis: validity of the Childhood Health Assessment Questionnaire. *J Rheumatol.* 1995;22:326–331.

110 Wright FV, Law M, Crombie V, et al. Development of a self-report functional status index for juvenile rheumatoid arthritis. *J Rheumatol.* 1994;21:536–544.

111 Duncan PW, Weiner DK, Chandler J, Studenski S. Functional reach: a new clinical measure of balance. *J Gerontol.* 1990;45:M192–M197.

112 Donahoe B, Turner D, Worrell T. The use of functional reach as a measurement of balance in boys and girls without disabilities ages 5 to 15 years. *Pediatric Physical Therapy.* 1994;6:189–193.

113 Wheeler A, Shall M, Lewis A, Shepherd J. The reliability of measurements obtained using the Functional Reach Test in children with cerebral palsy. *Pediatric Physical Therapy.* 1996;8:182.

114 Triolo RJ, Reilley B, Freedman W, et al. The functional standing test. *IEEE Eng Med Biol.* December 1992:32–34.

115 Triolo RJ, Reilley B, Freedman W, et al. Development of a clinical evaluation of standing function. *IEEE Trans Rehab Eng.* 1993;1:18–25.

116 Triolo RJ, Bevelheimer T, Eisenhower G, et al. Inter-rater reliability of a clinical test of standing function. *J Spinal Cord Med.* 1995;18:14–22.

117 Jebsen RH, Taylor N, Treischmann RB. An objective standardized test of hand function. *Arch Phys Med Rehabil.* 1969;50:311–319.

Balance Control During Walking in the Older Adult: Research and Its Implications

In this article, we highlight the unique nature of balance control during walking in humans. A control framework, including proactive and reactive balance control, is introduced to lay out age-related changes in different balance control mechanisms during walking. Clinical implications that may be useful for clinicians for assessment and treatment of balance problems that occur during walking are also discussed. [Woollacott MH, Tang P-F. Balance control during walking in the older adult: research and its implications. *Phys Ther.* 1997;77:646–660.]

Key Words: *Assessment, Balance, Older adults, Training, Walking.*

Marjorie H Woollacott

Pei-Fang Tang

Much research has been done on balance control in the older adult population. The ability of healthy and frail older adults to maintain postural stability during quiet standing, perturbed standing, and voluntary movement while standing has been well documented in the literature.[1-7] Research using functional mobility assessments has also helped to identify older adults who are at a high risk of falling during activities of daily living such as rising from a chair, bending over, and turning.[8,9]

Epidemiological studies, however, have shown that 30% to 70% of older adults' falls are due to trips, slips, and missteps; these events mostly take place during walking.[10-15] These statistics convey the important information that walking is the main daily activity in which the majority of the falls of community-dwelling older adults occur. Even though these older adults are capable of independent walking, there could be a substantial decline in their ability to control equilibrium, which does not become evident until a slip or trip happens. Although previous research on balance control has advanced our understanding regarding various aspects of static balance control ability of older adults, there are at least two limitations to generalizing such knowledge to balance control during walking.

First, the task of maintaining in-place balance (ie, "static" balance during standing and sitting) is different from maintaining balance when a person is moving from point A to point B (ie, "dynamic" balance during walking). In static balance, the base of support (BOS) remains stationary and only the body center of mass (COM) moves. The balance task in this case is to maintain the COM within the BOS or the limit of stability (the maximal estimated sway angle of the COM).[16,17] The activity of the ankle muscles is sufficient to maintain static balance during quiet standing.[17] In dynamic balance, however, both the BOS and COM are moving, and the COM is never kept within the BOS during the single-limb support periods. Ankle muscle activity alone has been found to be insufficient to maintain balance of the whole body during walking.[17] Thus, there has to be a different control mechanism for balance during walking. Second, researchers have reported that currently available functional assessment instruments are limited in predicting falls precipitated by slips or trips.[15] Thus, the factors that cause frequent falls during walking in older adults are yet to be identified.

The purpose of this article is threefold. First, we would like to address the nature of the walking task and how this task challenges dynamic balance in humans. Biomechanical analysis of human bipedal locomotion can provide valuable insight into the understanding of the balance demands during human walking. Second, a theoretical framework of the control mechanisms used to achieve balance during walking is introduced. This "proactive and reactive control" framework was originally put forth by Patla.[18] Evidence that relates to this framework is discussed in this article. Studies investigating these two control mechanisms in older adults are introduced. Although research on dynamic balance is

---

MH Woollacott, PhD, is Professor, Department of Exercise and Movement Science and Institute of Neuroscience, University of Oregon, Eugene, OR, 97403 (USA) (mwool@oregon.uoregon.edu). Address all correspondence to Dr Woollacott.

P-F Tang, PhD, PT, is Adjunct Assistant Professor, Department of Exercise and Movement Science and Institute of Neuroscience, University of Oregon.

This work was supported by NIH grant AG05317–06 to Dr Woollacott and a research fellowship from the Geriatrics Section of American Physical Therapy Association to Dr Tang.

just beginning, some valuable information is starting to become available regarding why older adults have a higher tendency to fall during walking. Lastly, the clinical implications of these recent research findings are discussed.

Our discussion will be focused on community-dwelling older adults. These older adults are more likely to be engaged in regular walking activity than frail older adults or nursing home residents. Therefore, they are also more often challenged by walking in various environments.

Biomechanical Challenges to Balance Control in Bipedal Human Locomotion

Locomotion consists of multiple subtasks that have to be fulfilled at the same time for this behavior to be considered successful. The four basic subtasks during locomotion are (1) generation of continuous movement to progress toward a destination, (2) maintenance of equilibrium during progression, (3) adaptability to meet any changes in the environment or other concurrent tasks, and (4) initiation and termination of locomotor movements.[19,20] Although the first subtask involves repetitive lower- and upper-extremity movements to propel the body, the second and third subtasks require a complex integration of locomotor and balance abilities to maintain an upright posture and to properly modify the ongoing locomotor behavior to suit the environmental changes or other task demands.[21,22] The fourth subtask relates to the ability to switch between one status of motion to another. Although this last subtask also involves postural adjustments, it will not be discussed here because of a limitation in space. Readers may refer to recent work by other researchers for in-depth information.[23-26]

In humans, the control of balance during steady-state walking (ie, the second and third subtasks of locomotion) is not an easy task. Compared with other species, humans have two biomechanical disadvantages that make walking an especially challenging task. One disadvantage arises from the use of a bipedal locomotor pattern, which consists of two single-limb support periods. These two periods are relatively long and together take up 75% to 80% of the whole gait cycle duration.[27] During these two periods, the vertical projection of the body's center of mass (COM) travels forward and outside the medial border of the supporting foot.[28] Although this COM and BOS spatial relationship facilitates weight transfer between the two lower extremities, it also inevitably creates potential mediolateral instability during single-limb support periods. That is, the product of the mass of the whole body and the distance between the COM and BOS results in a gravitational moment about the ankle joint that makes the body fall toward the midline. A counterbalancing moment around the hip and lower trunk is required to prevent the whole body from falling toward the midline and at the same time ensure proper weight transfer to the other leg.[29] This counterbalancing moment is largely generated by the hip abductors and trunk lateral flexors, and fine tuned by the ankle evertors and invertors.[29-31]

Foot placement at heel-strike also determines the magnitude of the gravitational moment of the COM about the supporting foot during the single-limb support periods. Winter[17] hypothesized that the foot placement in the mediolateral direction was primarily controlled by the activity of the hip abductors during the swing phase. He tested this hypothesis by asking young adults to walk with wider or narrower step widths than normal. When the young adults widened their step widths, the gluteus medius muscle activity during the swing phase also increased. When they narrowed their step widths, the gluteus medius muscle activity decreased. Thee ankle evertors and invertors, however, did not show concurrent changes in activity level with the widened or narrowed step widths.[17] These findings support Winter's hypothesis that the hip abductors play an important role in regulating step width and balance adjustments associated with different step widths.

Studies on gait patterns of healthy older adults and older adults with recent histories of falls have shown that these older adults have narrower step widths as compared with young adults.[32,33] We believe that older adults may use a narrowed BOS to reduce the gravitational moment of the COM in the mediolateral direction in attempt to minimize lateral instability. It is also possible, however, that the narrowed BOS reflects a decreased control ability of the hip abductors. In addition, Gabell and Nayak[34] noted that the step-to-step variability in step width was greater in healthy older adults during comfortable-speed walking as compared with young adults.[34] The finding of increased within-subject variability in stride width suggests a lack of consistency in the control of lateral stability among older adults.

Traditional gait analysis of older adults has been focused on the sagittal-plane motion; little attention has been paid to lateral stability control. Recent studies on standing balance control of older adults have indicated that the ability to control lateral stability during quiet stance can be used to predict older adults' likelihood of falling when the COM or BOS is disturbed.[15] Moreover, when older adults experience large and rapid perturbations of the support surface in the anteroposterior direction during standing, they more often take steps laterally than do young adults.[4] The more frequent use of lateral steps implies greater lateral instability in older adults when their stance is highly challenged. Whether older adults also have difficulty with regulating lateral stability when their gait is disturbed, however, is unknown. Future research is needed in this area.

A second biomechanical disadvantage of human locomotion has to do with the human body structure—two thirds of the total body weight is centered in the upper body (head-arm-trunk) segment.[35] With this form of weight distribution, the upper body can store a large amount of potential energy. If the upper body is not controlled in an upright position, this potential energy can easily be converted to kinetic energy during a fall and result in a serious injury. Winter and associates[31] noted that at heel-strike and push-off during the gait cycle, it is particularly difficult for a person to maintain the upright posture of the upper body. At heel-strike, a backward hip acceleration is caused by the ground reaction force. Due to this acceleration, the upper body leans forward. Similarly, at push-off, the hip accelerates forward, and as a result, the upper body leans backward. Therefore, during the gait cycle, the upper body continues to oscillate forward and backward because of the changes in the hip acceleration. To overcome this upper-body instability, a counterbalancing torque has to be generated around the hip and trunk. Winter and colleagues[31] found that during normal walking, a hip extensor torque is required at heel-strike to prevent the upper body from falling forward. Similarly, a hip flexor torque is required at push-off to prevent the upper body from falling backward.

During walking, older adults often assume a more rigid and guarded posture than do young adults.[36] Is this how older adults preserve the ability to control the upright posture of the upper body during normal walking? Crowninshield et al[37] found that adults over the age of 60 years showed a decrease in the peak hip joint moments when compared with adults aged 22 to 30 years. This decrease was found to be related to the shorter stride length in the older adults. Therefore, it is possible that because of the decreased ability to control an upright posture of the upper trunk in the sagittal plane, older adults adopt a smaller stride length to reduce the ground reaction force. This reduction in ground reaction force, in turn, decreases the balance challenges to the upright stability of the upper body in the sagittal plane.

The maintenance of the upright posture of the upper body not only prevents a potential fall preceded by an unsteady upper-body movement, it also assists in stabilizing the head and gaze. Pozzo et al[38] found that during

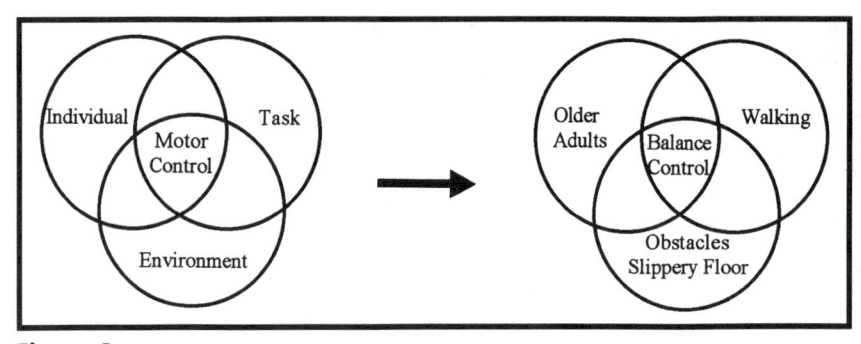

Figure 1.
Adopting a motor control model to the study of balance problems in older adults.

various dynamic tasks, such as free walking, walking in place, running in place, and hopping, the angular displacement of the head from a horizontal plane in line with the semicircular canals was less than 20 degrees, regardless of the large limb movement. They concluded that head stabilization is necessary for gaze orientation. To further understand how head stabilization is achieved during walking, Prince et al[39] examined the activity of paraspinal muscles at nine different spinal levels (C-7, T-2, T-4, T-6, T-8, T-10, T-12, L-2, and L-4) during normal walking. Interestingly, the muscle activation profile revealed that activity of the higher-level paraspinal muscles preceded that of the lower-level paraspinal muscles in a top-down propagation manner. Because the lower-level paraspinal activity coincided well with heel-strike to attenuate the hip posterior acceleration, Prince et al suggested that the paraspinal activity from the higher spinal levels is controlled in an anticipatory fashion to attenuate the expected hip acceleration at heel-strike.

Although similar studies have not been performed on older adults, Winter[40] noted a greater acceleration of the head in older adults during walking as compared with young adults. The impact of this greater acceleration of the head on gaze stabilization in older adults is yet to be studied.

Proactive and Reactive Balance Control During Walking: Theoretical Framework and Research Evidence

Our discussion so far has been centered on balance control during normal walking. Most of the walking-related falls in older adults, however, result from trips, slips, or missteps. How do researchers attack this problem?

Recently, Shumway-Cook and Woollacott[41] pointed out that when studying motor control, it is important to consider the interaction between the individual, the task, and the environment (Fig. 1, graph on the left). According to this point of view, the study of balance control during walking in older adults should take into account the nature of the task (walking) given to an older adult and the environment that puts the older adult at a higher risk of falling. With this perspective in mind, it becomes evident that the investigation of balance control mechanisms during walking in various environments is necessary to understand how older adults perform such a daily task (walking) in a challenging context (such as a slippery surface or a path full of obstacles) (Fig. 1, graph on the right).

This approach is different from research that typically treated balance and gait disorders as two different risk factors for falls or two clinical problems in older adults.[42-44] The approach based on Shumway-Cook and Woollacott's model implies that difficulty with balance and gait abilities are intertwined. Impairments in gait function jeopardize the control of balance during walking. For example, gait disorders resulting from lesions in the central nervous system, such as hyperreflexia of the ankle plantar flexors, could drastically reduce the BOS during walking, which in turn would increase the difficulty of maintaining balance.

Patla[18] suggested two balance control mechanisms for maintaining equilibrium during human walking. The first mechanism, the *proactive* control mechanism, refers to the balance control mechanism that takes place before the body encounters a potential threat to stability. This mechanism functions in two modes. One mode is to activate muscles or generate joint torques to reduce the inherent biomechanical threats to balance during normal walking. The aforementioned control for the upright posture of the upper body belongs to this mode of proactive control. That is, this mode of proactive control is already integrated into the normal walking pattern. A second mode of proactive control involves an early detection of potential environmental hazards and the implementation of postural and locomotion adjustments prior to the actual contact with the hazards. A good example for this mode of proactive control is when a person detours to avoid stepping onto an icy surface in the winter. If the balance threats are not detected in advance, the *reactive* control mechanism is needed. Then, a person has to evoke automatic postural responses to quickly regain balance.

Over the past few years, extensive studies on the second mode of proactive control of balance during walking have been done by Patla and collaborators[18,22,45-47] and Chen and associates.[48-50] The visual system and vigilance, or attention, are the keys to an early detection of potential balance threats.[22,50] Once the type and extent of the balance threats are recognized, complex sensorimotor integration processes are carried out to promptly implement appropriate modifications to the ongoing walking behaviors. For example, Patla and Rietdyk[46] found that the movement of the swing limb was modulated according to the obstacle height, but not the obstacle width, provided that the goal of the person was to step over, rather than around, the obstacle.

Noting the important role of vision in proactive balance control during walking, Patla[18] hypothesized that the high incidence of walking-related falls in older adults might be due to a decrease in the ability to use visual information during walking. To test this hypothesis, he first examined whether young and older adults differed in the ability to visually gather relevant information from their surroundings. In this study, both young adults (undergraduate college students) and older adults (65–85 years of age) were asked to wear opaque liquid-crystal eyeglasses and to press a switch to make the glasses transparent whenever they wanted to sample the environment. The floor across which the subjects walked was either unmarked or had footprints marked at regular intervals on which the subjects were supposed to step. The young and older adults showed no difference in visual sampling frequency or duration when they walked over the unmarked floor. When asked to walk on the footprints, however, the older adults sampled the terrain for longer periods and less often than the young adults, suggesting that they perceived the need for more information to make accurate foot placement in a constrained environment.

In another set of experiments, Patla[18] examined whether older adults required more time than young adults to implement an avoidance strategy when walking. Subjects were asked to walk along a walkway and, when given a visual cue, to either lengthen or shorten their stride to match the position of the cue. He found that both young adults (undergraduate college students) and older adults (65–85 years of age) were able to perform the task when the cue was given two steps in advance. Older adults, however, had more difficulty than young adults in modifying step length when the cue was given only one step in advance. The lengthened visual monitoring in older adults, as previously discovered, or a longer time to implement gait modifications could contribute to older adults' need for longer periods of time to adjust step length. Furthermore, older adults were successful 60% of the time when lengthening the step length and only 38% of the time when shortening the step length, whereas young adults were able to accomplish both tasks 80% of the time. Patla[18] proposed that older adults had more difficulty in shortening the step because of balance problems. He noted that shortening a step requires modulating the forward pitch of the trunk and that older adults have difficulty controlling this aspect of balance when walking.

Similarly, Chen et al[49] investigated whether the minimum response time allowed to modify gait patterns to avoid an obstacle during walking would be different between older and young adults. The obstacle used was a band of light located at a predicted foot placement. This virtual obstacle could be lit up at different times prior to the subject's heel-strike. The time allowed for gait modification before heel-strike ranged between 200 and 450 milliseconds, with increments of 50 milliseconds. The results showed that the rate of success in avoiding the obstacle was higher for young adults than for older adults, regardless whether the time allowed to make a modification to gait was long (96% for young adults, 92% for older adults) or short (21% for young adults, 16% for older adults). These findings are consistent with those of Patla[18] in that older adults need a longer period of time to implement gait modifications to prevent running into an obstacle on the walking path. One question that remains unsolved, however, is whether this longer response time in older adults can be ascribed primarily to a longer time to detect the obstacle, a longer time to execute the avoidance response, or both.

Because visual attention is important for avoiding obstacles, Chen et al[50] hypothesized that older adults may be more affected by a visual distraction presented concurrently with the obstacle as compared with young adults. To test this hypothesis, the subjects were asked to perform a vocal reaction-time task in response to a visual stimulus while performing the same obstacle-avoidance task described above.[50] They found that when the visual distraction was present synchronously with the obstacle appearance, the success rate in avoiding the obstacle decreased to a greater extent in older adults (36%) than in the young adults (20%), as compared with the no-distraction condition. These results indicate that attention demand is greater in older adults than in young adults for successful implementation of a proactive balance control mechanism.

Teasdale and colleagues[51] also reported that attentional demand during normal walking was higher in older adults than young adults, regardless of the phases of the gait cycle. When we consider the findings of Teasdale et al[51] and Chen and colleagues[50] together, it becomes clear that obstacle avoidance is not an easy task for older adults because a large amount of attention has to be allocated not only to the normal gait pattern but also to its modification.

Aside from the differences in the successful rate of implementing the obstacle-avoidance strategy, what are the differences between older and young adults in their actual obstacle-avoidance behaviors? Chen et al[48] investigated whether older adults (mean age=71 years) use different strategies than do young adults (mean age=22 years) in their actual avoidance of obstacles of heights created to simulate natural obstacles in the environment such as a 2.5- to 5.1-cm (1- to 2-in) door threshold or a 15.2-cm (6-in) curb. The control condition was a 0-mm condition in which tape was simply attached on the walkway. The investigators noted no differences between the age groups in foot clearance over the obstacles, but they found that older adults used a more conservative strategy when crossing obstacles, including a slower crossing speed, shorter heel-to-obstacle distance after crossing, and a shorter crossing-step length. They also found that because of the shorter crossing-step length, 4 of the 24 older adults, compared with none of the young adults, accidentally stepped on an obstacle and increased the risk of tripping.

Research by Patla and collaborators[18,45–47] and that by Chen and associates[48–50] have led to more in-depth understanding of proactive balance control during walking in older adults and how this control can be implemented successfully. To date, however, balance responses when an older adult actually trips over an obstacle (ie, the reactive control mechanisms during trips) have not been investigated.

The reactive control mechanism that is different from the proactive control balance mechanism primarily relies on the somatosensory and vestibular systems to determine the extent and type of the stimulus (threat) and to trigger appropriately scaled postural responses.[18] These postural responses are mainly polysynaptic spinal reflexes and supraspinal responses.[52,53]

In 1980, Nashner[53] performed an experiment to examine the reactive balance control mechanisms during perturbed walking. In the study, he perturbed the gait of young adults as they walked across a movable platform incorporated into a 4-m-long walkway. The perturbations were forward or backward translations of the support surface of 8 cm causing an ankle rotation at approximately 40°/s. To examine whether muscle response characteristics changed according to the phase of the step cycle in which the perturbation occurred, he gave perturbations at heel-strike, the beginning of single-limb support phase, mid-stance, and the beginning of double-limb support.

The results showed that in response to perturbations at heel-strike, there were muscle responses in the stretched ankle muscles that began approximately 95 to 110 milliseconds after the onset of platform movement and lasted for about 100 to 400 milliseconds. For example, a forward platform displacement at heel-strike elicited an excitatory response in the tibialis anterior muscle that served to resist the change in the rotational trajectory of the ankle joint. The effects were strongest at heel-strike and the beginning of the single-limb support phase, were weaker at mid-stance, and were absent at the beginning of the double-limb support phase.

Nashner[53] hypothesized that a deviation in the movement of the ankle from its normal stepping trajectory provided a principal source of input to the muscles of the legs. He noted that the responses helped to slow or speed up the body's rate of forward progression to realign the body's COM. He also noted that the leg muscle postural responses during perturbed walking were similar to those observed when equivalent platform movements were given to subjects standing quietly on the platform. Neither response was monosynaptic, and both responses appeared to involve longer-latency response pathways, because the responses were activated at about 90-millisecond latencies.[54,55] Given the similarity in the patterns and onset latencies of the postural responses between perturbed standing and walking, Nashner speculated that the locomotor center uses the same postural synergies that are activated during stance perturbations to respond to perturbations during walking. In particular, he hypothesized that the spinal stepping generators continuously receive input regarding postural instability from both peripheral and central pathways and then incorporate the necessary postural adjustments into the output of the locomotor patterns.

Nashner's hypothesis that the discrepancy between the actual and planned ankle joint trajectories triggers reactive postural responses in platform-perturbed gait has gained additional support from other studies. Dietz and colleagues[56] have examined the ability of young adults to respond to postural perturbations during gait using a treadmill paradigm. In this paradigm, subjects walked on a treadmill that was accelerated (accelerations were 2.5–14 m/s^2 with amplitudes of 3°–6° of ankle angle change) or decelerated at heel-strike at unexpected moments in time. Responses to these perturbations were recorded from the thigh and leg muscles (gastrocnemius, hamstring, tibialis anterior, and quadriceps femoris).

Dietz and associates[56] found that latencies of responses in the gastrocnemius muscle to accelerations of the treadmill ranged from 90 milliseconds for slower accelerations (2.5 m/s^2) down to 70 milliseconds for the fastest accelerations (14 m/s^2). They noted that the duration of the response increased with higher-magnitude perturbations. They also noted that the hamstring muscles were activated about 100 milliseconds after perturbation onset (about 20 milliseconds after onset of gastrocnemius muscle activity). The gastrocnemius muscle's electromyographic response was closely correlated to the duration of the acceleration impulse and ankle joint displacement.

Dietz and colleagues proposed that group II afferents from the ankle muscles were responsible for the activation of the ankle muscle responses because a monosynaptic stretch reflex was not activated, even though stretch velocities were high, and also because previous experiments had shown that the response was preserved after ischemic blockage of group I afferents of the leg and foot.

An important finding in Nashner's study[53] was that postural adjustments were most prominent when the platform movement was imposed at heel-strike and the beginning of single-limb support, and these adjustments became much smaller or absent if the platform perturbation occurred in the later stance phases. This finding suggests that due to the changes in body orientation and support surface, the balance demands differ between the different phases of the gait cycle. Accordingly, postural responses evoked by the same perturbation also differ because of the different times at which the perturbation is imposed. Neurophysiologists have referred to this phenomenon as "phase-dependent modulation of reflexes."[57] The existence of this phenomenon suggests that spinal reflexes are modifiable and are adaptive to task requirements.

This "phase-dependent reflex reversal" phenomenon has an important function in dynamic balance control during locomotion. For instance, Stein[58] used a pneumatic system to apply a mechanical stretch to the gastrocnemius muscle at various times during the stance phase of human walking. He found that the gain of the stretch reflex (as measured by the ratio between the magnitude of gastrocnemius muscle activity in response to the stimulus and the magnitude of the stimulus) was small in early stance, but gradually increased toward late stance. Stein suggested that if the gain of this stretch reflex was set high in early stance by the nervous system, then the reflex would prevent the shank from efficiently rolling over the foot and would impede the continuation of walking. A high stretch reflex gain in late stance is useful, however, because it reinforces the push-off and thus assists in forward progression.

Yang and Stein[59] observed cutaneous reflex reversal in the tibialis anterior muscle when they applied an electrical stimulation to the tibial nerve at the ankle during human walking. In reaction to this stimulus, the medium-latency response (70–120 milliseconds) of the tibialis anterior muscle changed from excitatory, when the stimulus was applied in early swing, to inhibitory, when the stimulus was applied during the transition from swing to stance phase. This inhibitory response of the tibialis anterior muscle during late swing allowed the perturbed leg to fulfill its weight acceptance obligation after the transition to the stance phase. In this study, the most pronounced phasic modulation was in the medium-latency responses, in contrast to the short- and long-latency responses. This finding indicates that this modulation in humans requires supraspinal neural substrates or polysynaptic spinal pathways for control, because medium-latency responses are known to involve these neural substrates.[52]

Thus, the phasic modulation of spinal reflexes is thought to be important for dynamic balance control in human walking. To further understand this contribution, researchers[60,61] have extended the investigation to the reflexive responses of both legs. Eng et al[61] applied a mechanical obstruction to the swing leg during the early and late swing phases of human walking. When the disturbance was imposed in early swing, young adults predominantly presented a flexion pattern of the swing leg (via activation of the biceps femoris and rectus femoris muscles of the perturbed leg) and an enhanced extension of the support leg (by activating the gastrocnemius muscle of the support leg). In contrast, when the swing leg was tripped in late swing, the swing leg showed a lowering response and there was no extension movement of the support leg. Eng et al explained that when the swing leg was perturbed in early swing, the extension of the support leg led to an early heel-off. This action raised the height of the total-body COM and permitted a longer period of time for the perturbed leg to move away from the obstacle. The extension movement of the support leg, however, was unnecessary when the obstacle appeared in late swing. In this case, the subject had already lowered the body's COM to prepare for landing with the perturbed leg. This study provides an illustration that reflexive responses to a realistic trip during human walking are coordinated between both lower extremities.

Because of the risky nature of a tripping task, reactive balance control mechanisms of older adults in response to a trip during walking have not been investigated. Recently, in our laboratory, a study was conducted to explore age-related differences in the reactive balance control mechanisms to slips during walking.[62] A *slip* was defined as a sudden increase in the horizontal velocity of any part of the foot that is in contact with the floor.[62] Healthy young adults (n=33, 20–35 years of age) and older adults (n=32, 70–85 years of age) were tested while walking across a movable platform incorporated into a walkway. A translational platform movement of 10 cm at 40 cm/s, timed to move at one of the three phases of the gait cycle (right heel-strike, mid-stance, or late stance) was used to simulate slips occurring at various times during the gait cycle. This platform movement was chosen because it was compatible with the slips when a person is walking on an icy surface.[62] Subjects were given a total of 48 trials, with the first 12 trials being no-perturbation control trials that were blocked. The rest of the trials were in random order and consisted of 12 forward-perturbation trials, 12 backward-perturbation trials, and 12 no-perturbation trials. Only the right foot was perturbed during the experiment.

The first question being addressed in this research was whether the locus of balance control during slips resides in the leg musculature, as Nashner[53] had suggested, or in the trunk and hip musculature, as had been discovered from nonperturbed normal human walking.[31] To answer this question, we analyzed postural responses from 15 muscles of the bilateral lower legs, thighs, hips, and trunk muscles in the young adults. In responding to the most challenging slip, a forward slip occurring at heel-strike, we found that the postural activity of the tibialis anterior and rectus femoris muscles of the perturbed leg was very important to dynamic balance control. The postural responses from these muscles were not only consistent (occurrence rate of >98%), but also had very short onset latencies ($\bar{X}=91$ milliseconds for the tibialis anterior muscle and 140 milliseconds for the rectus femoris muscle) and long burst durations ($\bar{X}=133$ milliseconds for the tibialis anterior muscle and 203 milliseconds for the rectus femoris muscle). Furthermore, the magnitude of these postural responses were about seven times what would be observed in the muscle activity during normal walking. The activity of the gastrocnemius muscle was suppressed when the tibialis anterior muscle was highly active. This suppression of the gastrocnemius muscle (antagonist) activity indicates an important organizational function of the nervous system to enhance the postural recovery function of the tibialis anterior muscle (agonist) activity in regaining ankle joint trajectory. From the kinematic analysis, it was evident that the tibialis anterior muscle's postural activity served to restore the disrupted ankle joint trajectory and to realign the foot and leg segments of the perturbed lower extremity (Fig. 2). In this process, the knee joint underwent a flexion motion, which indicated eccentric contraction of the rectus femoris muscle to prevent a collapse at the knee (Fig. 3).

Another consistent reactive response was found in the biceps femoris muscle of the perturbed leg. The onset of this postural response ranged between 80 and 130 milliseconds after platform perturbation onset, and its duration lasted about 100 milliseconds (Fig. 3). These findings indicate an important role of this muscle in restoring the normal knee trajectory (knee flexion) after heel-contact. Along with the long burst of the rectus femoris muscle, there was therefore a high prevalence of coactivation between the rectus femoris and biceps femoris muscles to control the knee joint stability. Moreover, the biceps femoris muscle activity during perturbed walking was not reported by previous researchers.

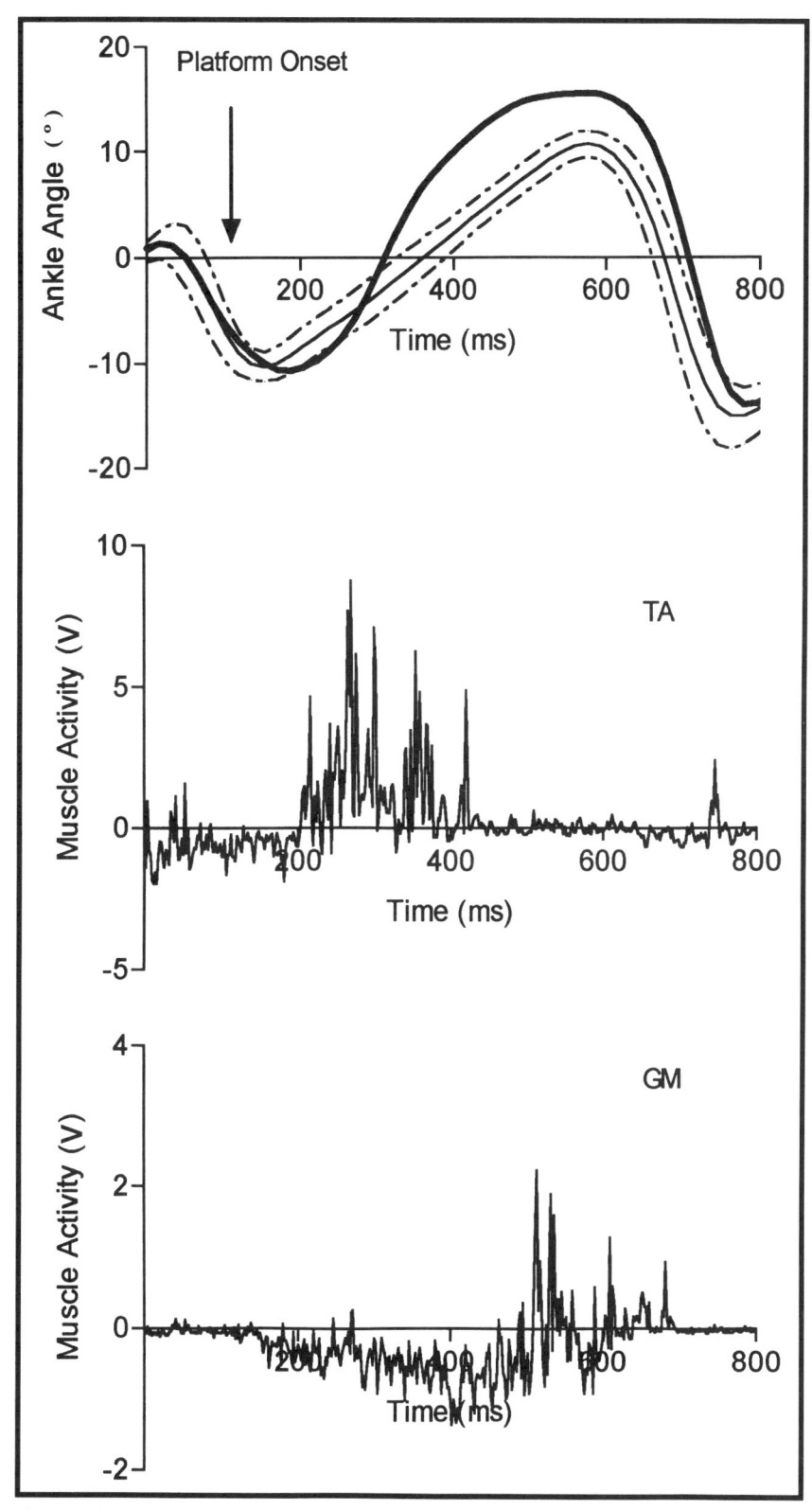

Figure 2.
Ankle joint trajectory and postural muscle activity of the tibialis anterior muscle (TA) and medial head of the gastrocnemius muscle (GM) of the perturbed leg. A positive joint angle represents dorsiflexion, and a negative joint angle represents plantar flexion. The thin solid line represents the mean angle trajectory in the control (normal walking) condition; dotted lines represent one standard deviation above and below the mean; bold line represents perturbed joint angle trace. The electromyographic trace is the difference between the muscle activity in a slip trial and the mean (± 1 SD) muscle activity during the control trials.

Perturbed level walking versus treadmill walking may have had a different influence on the results.

On the nonperturbed side, consistent and early onset of the tibialis anterior, rectus femoris, and biceps femoris muscle responses was also observed after the platform perturbation. Although supplementary kinematic information was not available, it appeared from the video-based analysis that the function of these muscles' activity is to secure the foot lift-off in the early swing phase of the nonperturbed leg. Because the forward platform movement had stretched the right foot forward, the COM of the whole body was likely to drop in the vertical direction after the platform onset. Thus, the activity of the tibialis anterior, rectus femoris, and biceps femoris muscles of the nonperturbed leg may assist directly in ankle dorsiflexion, knee flexion, and hip flexion, respectively, in the early swing phase. These flexion movements in turn prevent the nonperturbed leg from being tripped when the COM drops in the vertical direction. These findings suggest that interlimb coordination is needed in such a dynamic balance task.

Based on the analysis of the frequency at which a muscle became active in response to the platform perturbation, the trunk muscle activity was not needed as frequently as the activity of the above-mentioned six leg muscles (ie, bilateral tibialis anterior, rectus femoris, and biceps femoris). We hypothesized that when the balance threats can be attenuated sufficiently by the lower-extremity muscles during a slip, trunk muscle activity may not be needed.

Next, a comparison of postural responses between the older and young adults was made. Older adults were found to activate the same predominant postural muscles as did the young adults. The primary age-related differences in the postural responses were found to be a combination of a longer onset latency, a longer burst duration, and a smaller burst magnitude in older adults' postural responses as compared with those of young adults (Fig. 4). The combination of these differences resulted in a less effective balance recovery strategy in the older adults. The composite effect of all three factors, rather than a single factor, resulted in the difficulty with dynamic balance in older adults. This composite effect of the postural muscle activity in the older adults probably led to a slower rate in generating postural activity. Age-related losses of fast-twitch muscle fibers or decreased ability in recruiting motoneurons may have contributed to this slower rate of generating postural activity. Furthermore, these insufficient postural responses from the leg muscles often led to a backward lean of the trunk in older adults. As a result, older adults were found to more frequently use arm movement to assist in trunk stabilization and prevent a fall (Fig. 5).

In the analysis of walking speed and stride length, we found that older adults shortened the stride length after the slip, whereas young adults did not shorten their stride length. This shortened stride length could be partially be accounted for by the longer coactivation time between the rectus femoris and biceps femoris muscles of the non-perturbed leg in the older adults as compared with the young adults. Shortening stride length is a common strategy people adopt while walking on icy or slippery surfaces in order to decrease the heel-strike speed and prevent a slip. However, shortening the stride after experiencing a slip, as found in our study, may have a different effect on balance control than shortening the stride while stepping on an icy surface. In particular, in our study, the whole-body COM was passively moved forward by the platform. In this case, a shortened stride length would cause the location of the COM to be closer to the front border of the BOS in the shortened step following the slip. Subsequently, if a subject shortened the step following the slip, he or she would need at least an extra

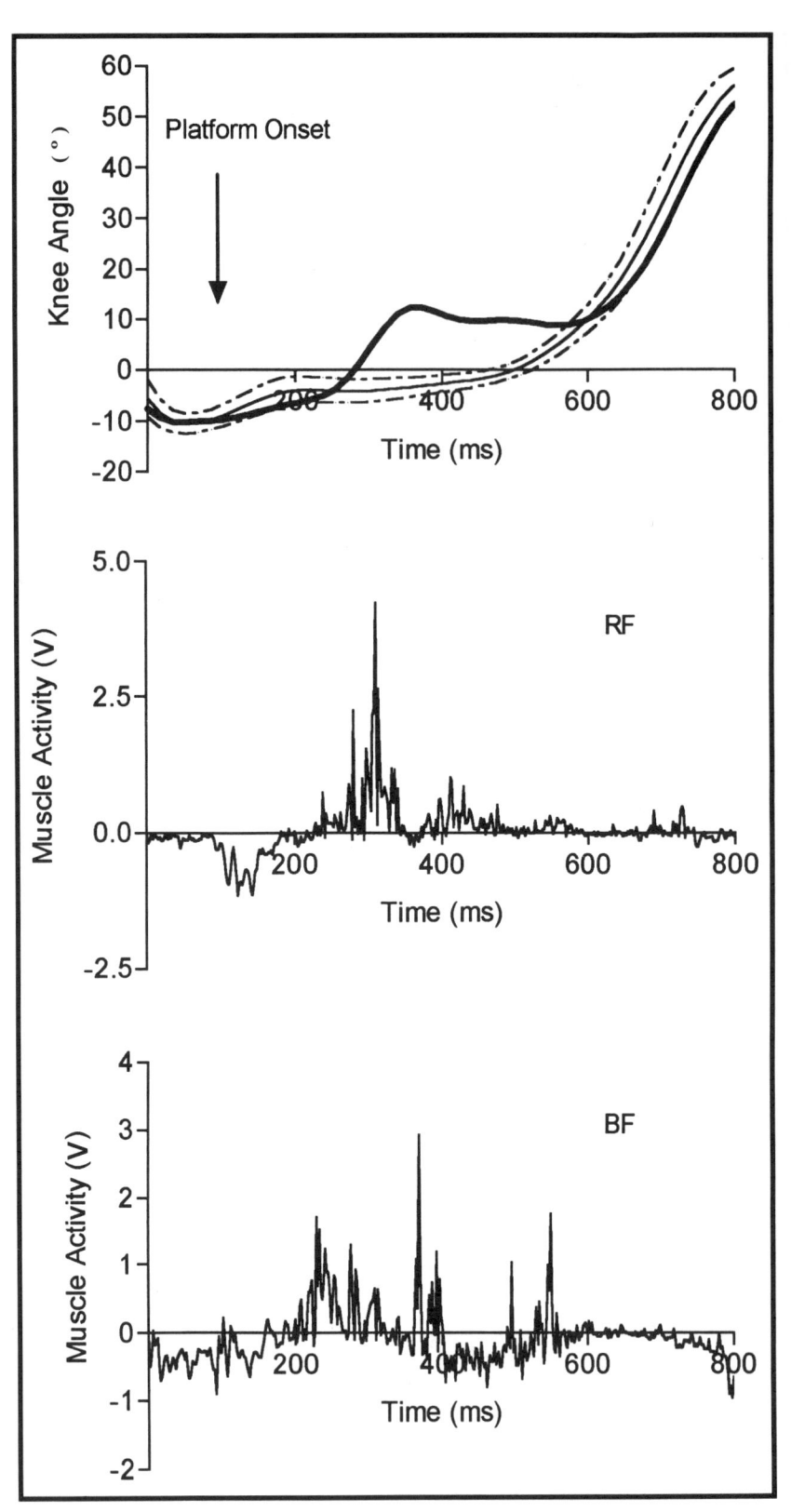

Figure 3.
Knee joint trajectory and postural muscle activity of the rectus femoris muscle (RF) and the biceps femoris muscle (BF) of the perturbed leg. A positive joint angle represents flexion, and a negative joint angle represents extension. The thin solid line represents the mean angle trajectory in the control (normal walking) condition; dotted lines represent one standard deviation above and below the mean; bold line represents perturbed joint angle trace. The electromyographic trace is the difference between the muscle activity in a slip trial and the mean (± 1 SD) activity during the control trials.

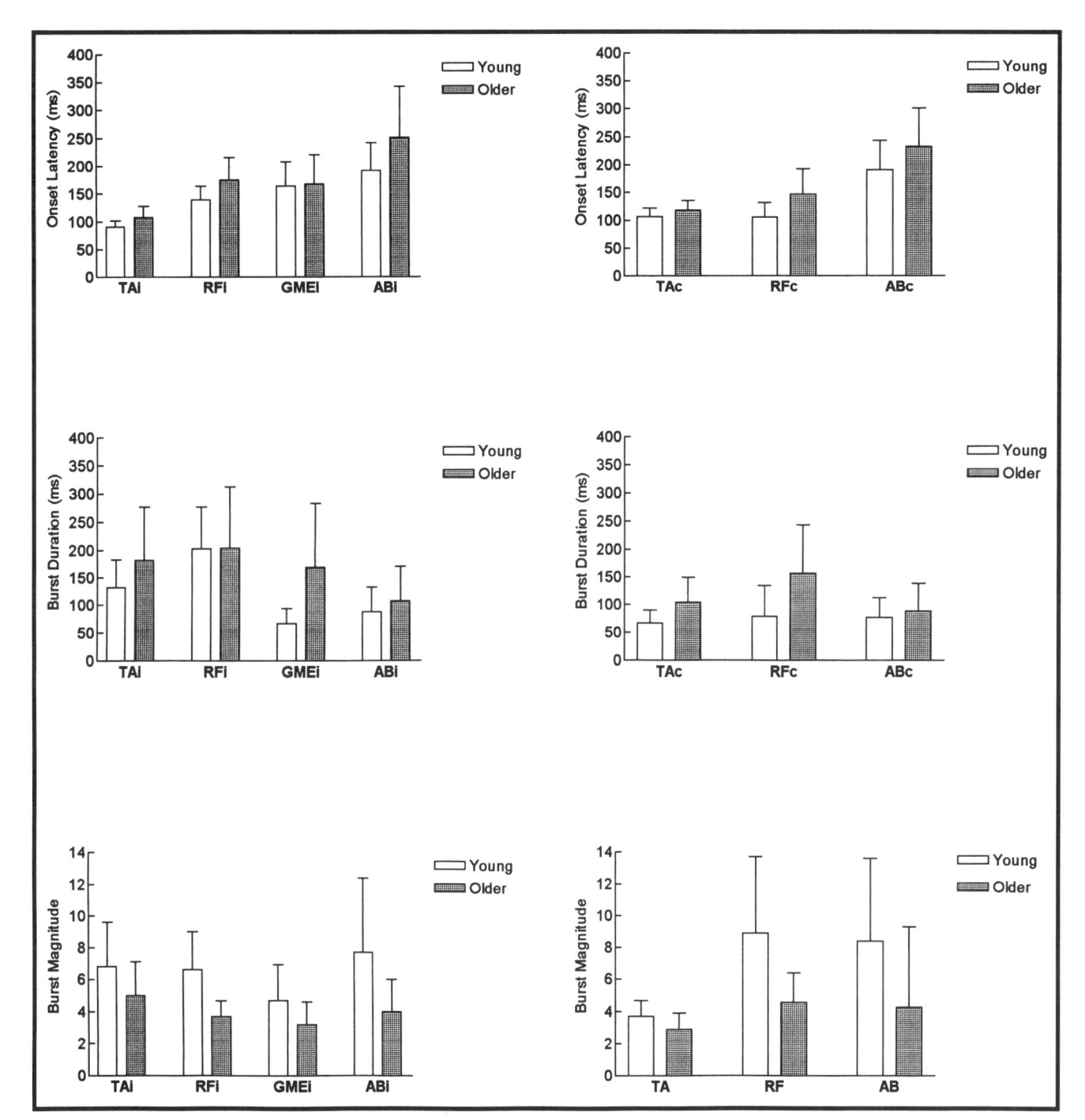

Figure 4.
Differences between young adults (20–35 years of age) and older adults (70–85 years of age) in onset latency, burst duration, and burst magnitude of the anterior muscles on the perturbed and nonperturbed sides. TA=tibialis anterior muscle, RF=rectus femoris muscle, AB=rectus abdominis muscle, GME=gluteus medius muscle. The lower-case "i" stands for ipsilateral (to the perturbed side), and the lower-case "c" stands for contralateral (to the perturbed side). Note that the magnitude of postural activity was calculated as a ratio between the muscle activity in a perturbed trial and the mean of the control trial. Therefore, there is no unit for burst magnitude.

step to regain the normal spatial relationship between the BOS and the COM after the slip. Therefore, stride shortening, as a common conservative balance strategy during walking, may not be an effective strategy for older adults in the current experimental context. Interestingly, as described earlier, Chen et al[48] also found that older adults used a shorter step to cross an obstacle than did young adults. This shortened step length while crossing an obstacle increased the likelihood of tripping for the older adults. Step length regulation appears to be important during both slips and trips. Questions as to why older adults tend to use a smaller step length after a trip or a slip are yet to be answered.

Given the known functional significance of phase-dependent modulation of reflexes, we believed that it would be interesting to examine whether older adults preserve the phase-dependent modulation ability in their postural responses to slips occurring at different times during the stance phase. Therefore, we examined the postural responses from both age groups in reaction to slips occurring at heel-strike and at mid-stance. Because the mid-stance slips were less challenging than the heel-strike slips, both young and older adults showed less frequent postural responses during the mid-stance slips than during the heel-strike slips. The young adults modulated their postural responses by shortening the burst duration and burst magnitude in the mid-stance slips. The older adults, however, showed decreases in burst duration, but not in burst magnitude, of their postural response in the mid-stance slips. We hypothesized that psychological fear, changes in motoneuron recruitment patterns, and changes in muscle physiology may have contributed to the inflexibility of the older adults' postural response.

As a whole, based on this series of experiments, we found that the reactive balance control mechanisms, when encountering an unexpected slip, were less efficient and less flexible in older adults as compared with young adults. More importantly, the less efficient control in the lower extremities often led to upper-trunk instability. Without concurrent arm movements, older adults may be very likely to fall.

Clinical Implications

Assessment of Proactive and Reactive Balance Control Mechanisms During Walking

What might be the appropriate balance tests for the clinicians to use to evaluate balance control during walking? Can gait evaluation predict the likelihood of falls or the type of falls in older adults? We suggest that to glean a complete understanding of a person's ability to control balance during walking, both proactive and reactive control mechanisms have to be assessed. In particular, for the proactive control, the control of upper-body stability in both the sagittal and frontal planes, the ability to stabilize the head, the coordination between the upper and lower extremities, and foot placement are all important features for clinicians to consider in their assessment of a patient's balance control ability during walking. Furthermore, to be able to successfully navigate through various environments, attention and the use of visual information to detect environmental changes are important items to be evaluated. At present, only the gait assessments pertaining to the first form of proactive control are available; assessment tools that evaluate a patient's visual perception during motion or attentional demand during walking

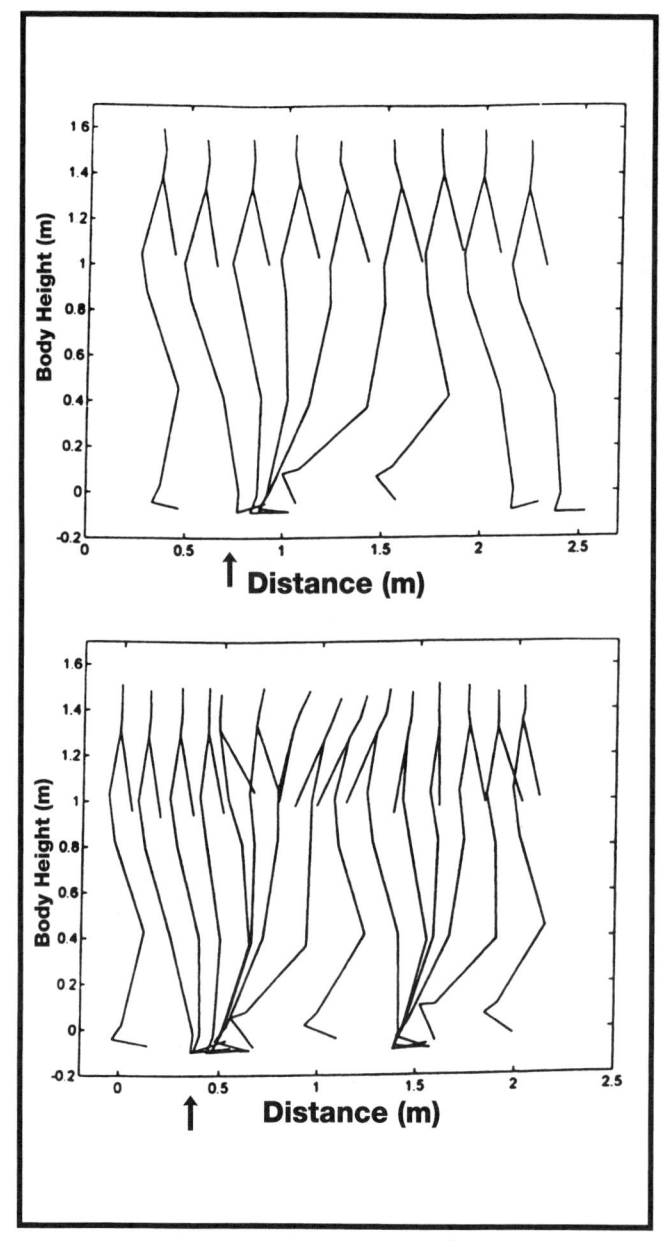

Figure 5.
Reconstructed stick figure of a young adult (top) and an older adult (bottom) during a heel-strike slip. An upward arrow indicates the onset of slip. The horizontal axis is distance (in meters), and the vertical axis is body height (in meters). Note that although the trunk angle of the young adult remained upright after experiencing the slip, the older adult showed a backward lean after the slip. In addition, the older adult's arm first elevated and then unfolded to assist in upper-body balance.

are yet to be developed. Structured evaluation of reactive postural mechanisms in response to trips, slips, missteps, or uneven terrain are also yet to be developed.

Among the existing balance and gait assessment instruments, there are a few that may be particularly useful for clinicians. One such instrument is Wolfson's Gait Abnormality Rating Scale (GARS).[63] This scale consists of observational evaluation of 16 features of gait pattern based on videotaped records. The GARS uses a four-point rating scale: 0=normal, 1=mildly impaired, 2=moderately impaired, and 3=severely impaired. A higher score indicates more impaired gait. All except three items (head forward, shoulder elevation, and upper trunk forward) of the GARS show high interrater reliability ($r=.73-.95$). When the validity of this scale was tested by relating GARS results to fall history in 49 nursing home residents (27 had a history of recent falls) and 22 control subjects, the results showed that the GARS score correlated well with walking speed and stride length, and GARS scores were higher for older fallers than for the control subjects. Among the 16 items of rating, arm-swing amplitude, upper- and lower-extremity synchrony, and guardedness of gait were found to best distinguish the older fallers from the other subjects. Thus, the GARS appeared to be a valid, simple assessment tool for predicting the history of falls. These findings appeared to be congruent with our hypothesis that assessment of the upper-body balance is important for balance control during gait. Unfortunately, the types of falls were not documented in this study, and therefore it is difficult to make an association between performance on the GARS and the type of falls.

Recently, VanSwearingen et al[64] developed a modified version of the GARS (GARS-M). The intent was to simplify the GARS and to predict fall history of community-dwelling, frail older adults. In this study, *frail older adults* were defined as adults over 60 years of age with difficulty in one to three activities of daily living and decreased physiologic reserve. Seven of the 16 GARS items remained in the GARS-M test. These items were variability, guardedness, staggering, foot contact, hip range of motion, shoulder extension, and arm heel-strike synchrony. They found that the GARS-M scores distinguished between these older adults with and without a history of recurrent falls. Similar to the GARS, however, the validity of using this test to predict the types of falls is unknown.

Why should we predict the type of falls? Topper et al[15] classified falls into three categories based on the biomechanical characteristics: (1) falls due to perturbation to the BOS, (2) falls due to perturbation to the COM, and (3) falls with no apparent biomechanical perturbation. Falls due to perturbation of the BOS may indicate an impaired reactive balance control mechanism in an older individual. Falls due to perturbations to the COM can be due to an impairment in the proactive or reactive, or both, mechanisms. Thus, knowledge of the type of fall may assist clinicians in identifying the balance control mechanisms, proactive or reactive, that precipitated the fall. The hypothesis that the type of fall may be highly related to impairment in different balance control mechanisms is supported by the results of the study by Topper and associates.[15] They found that Tinetti's activity-based balance and gait tests were predictive of falls with no obvious biomechanical precipitant and of falls precipitated by a COM perturbation, but not of falls precipitated by a BOS perturbation.

The Berg Balance Scale has been found to be limited in predicting the likelihood of falls among older adults living in independent life care communities in a recent longitudinal study by Thorbahn and Newton.[65] This finding was not surprising because the Berg Balance Scale does not include any items pertaining to gait, and most falls among older adults occur during walking.

Dynamic Balance Training

Winstein[66] documented that balance skills developed through training that involves standing tasks have limited effects on balance control during walking in patients with stroke. Therefore, exercise training focused on improving balance control during walking should include dynamic tasks that involve multisegmental control. Training should also include sensory, motor, and cognition components to improve the acuity and integration ability of the sensory system, effectiveness of the motor system, and vigilance of older adults. Specifically, for the sensory system, visual acuity, depth perception, and motion perception are particularly important for a person to detect an unexpected obstacle in advance. The vestibular system interacts closely with the visual system during walking to stabilize the gaze. An impaired somatosensory system could affect the reactive postural control mechanism. General health, mental status, and certain medications can influence vigilance, attention, or function of the vestibular system.

We suggest that exercise that emphasizes fast and powerful muscle activity generation, such as brisk walking, is necessary for the reactive balance control mechanism to be effective and efficient. Training should include inter-limb coordination as well as the coordination between the lower-extremity and upper-body movements. This multisegmental coordination will ensure better safety in case the early postural responses fail to lead to complete balance recovery. This type of training would increase the number of balance response repertoires that older adults could use to supplement the inefficient early postural responses. For example, Wolf and colleagues[67] reported that tai chi exercise improves balance control in older adults. Although tai chi exercise uses slow movements, the beneficial effect of tai chi exercise on balance control could be due to the dynamic nature of this activity, in that it requires complex whole-body coordination.

References

1 Bohannon RW, Larkin PA, Cook AC, et al. Decrease in timed balance test scores with aging. *Phys Ther.* 1984;64:1067–1070.

2 Duncan PW, Weiner DK, Chandler J, Studenski S. Functional reach: a new clinical measure of balance. *J Gerontol*. 1990;45:M192–M197.

3 Inglin B, Woollacott MH. Age-related changes in anticipatory postural adjustments associated with arm movements. *J Gerontol*. 1988;41: M105–M113.

4 McIlroy WE, Maki BE. Age-related changes in compensatory stepping in response to unpredictable perturbations. *J Geriatr*. 1996;51:M289–M296.

5 Sheldon JH. The effect of age on the control of sway. *Gerontologica Clinica*. 1963;5:129–138.

6 Stelmach GE, Teasdale N, Di Fabio RP, Phillips J. Age-related decline in postural control mechanisms. *Int J Aging Hum Dev*. 1989;29:205–223.

7 Woollacott MH, Shumway-Cook A, Nashner LM. Aging and posture control: changes in sensory organization and muscular coordination. *Int J Aging Hum Dev*. 1986;23:97–114.

8 Berg K, Wood-Dauphinee S, Williams JI, Gayton D. Measuring balance in the elderly: preliminary development of an instrument. *Physiotherapy Canada*. 1989;41:304–311.

9 Tinetti ME. Performance-oriented assessment of mobility problems in elderly patients. *J Am Geriatr Soc*. 1986;34:119–126.

10 Gabell A, Simons MA, Nayak USL. Falls in the healthy elderly: predisposing causes. *Ergonomics*. 1985;28:965–975.

11 Lord SR, Ward JA, Williams P, Anstey KJ. An epidemiological study of falls in older community-dwelling women: the Randwick falls and fractures study. *Aust J Public Health*. 1993;17:240–245.

12 Overstall PW, Exton-Smith AN, Imms FJ, Johnson AL. Falls in the elderly related to postural imbalance. *BMJ*. January 1977:261–264.

13 Sheldon JH. On the natural history of falls in old age. *BMJ*. December 1960:1685–1690.

14 Tinetti ME, Speechley M, Ginter SF. Risk factors for falls among elderly persons living in the community. *N Engl J Med*. 1988;319:1701–1707.

15 Topper AK, Maki BE, Holliday PJ. Are activity-based assessment of balance and gait in the elderly predictive of risk of falling and/or type of fall? *J Am Geriatr Soc*. 1993;41:479–487.

16 Nashner LM. Practical biomechanics and physiology of balance. In: Jacobson GP, Newman CW, Kartush JM, eds. *Handbook of Balance Function Testing*. St Louis, Mo: Mosby-Year Book Inc; 1993:261–279.

17 Winter DA. *A B C (Anatomy, Biomechanics, and Control) of Balance During Standing and Walking*. Waterloo, Ontario, Canada: Waterloo Biomechanics; 1995.

18 Patla AE. Age-related changes in visually guided locomotion over different terrains: major issues. In: Stelmach GE, Homberg V, eds. *Sensorimotor Impairment in the Elderly*. Amsterdam, the Netherlands: Kluwer Academic Publishers; 1993:231–252.

19 Patla AE. Neurobiomechanical bases for the control of human locomotion. In: Bronstein A, Brandt TH, Woollacott MH, eds. *Clinical Aspects of Balance and Gait Disorders*. London, England: Edward Arnold (Publishers) Ltd; 1996:19–40.

20 Shik ML, Orlovsky GN. Neurophysiology of locomotor automatism. *Physiol Rev*. 1976;56:465–501.

21 Mori S, Sakamoto T, Ohta Y, et al. Site-specific postural and locomotor changes evoked in awake, freely moving intact cats by stimulating the brainstem. *Brain Res*. 1989;505:66–74.

22 Patla AE. Visual control of human locomotion. In: Patla AE, ed. *Adaptability of Human Gait*. Amsterdam, the Netherlands: Elsevier Science Publishers BV; 1991:55–95.

23 Burleigh AL, Horak FB, Malouin F. Modification of postural responses and step initiation: evidence for goal-directed postural interactions. *J Neurophysiol*. 1994;72:2892–2902.

24 Burleigh AL, Horak FB. Influence of instruction, prediction, and afferent sensory information on postural organization of step initiation. *J Neurophysiol*. 1996;75:1619–1628.

25 Jian Y, Winter DA, Gilchrist IL. Trajectory of the body COG and COP during initiation and termination of gait. *Gait and Posture*. 1993;1:9–22.

26 Frank JS, Winter DA, Craik RL. Gait disorders and falls in the elderly. In: Bronstein AM, Brandt T, Woollacott MH, eds. *Clinical Disorders of Balance, Posture, and Gait*. London, England: Edward Arnold (Publishers) Ltd; 1996:287–300.

27 Sutherland DA, Kauman KR, Moitoza JR. Kinematics of normal human walking. In: Rose J, Gamble JG, eds. *Human Walking*. Baltimore, Md: Williams & Wilkins; 1995:23–44.

28 Shimba T. An estimation of center of gravity from force platform data. *J Biomech*. 1984;17:53–60.

29 MacKinnon CD, Winter DA. Control of whole body balance in the frontal plane during human walking. *J Biomech*. 1993;26:633–644.

30 Dofferhof ASM, Vink P. The stabilising function of the mm iliocostales and the mm multifidi during walking. *J Anat*. 1985;140:329–336.

31 Winter DA, Ruder GK, MacKinnon CD. Control of balance of upper body during gait. In: Winters JM, Woo S-LY, eds. *Multiple Muscle Systems: Biomechanical and Movement Organization*. New York, NY: Springer-Verlag New York Inc; 1990:534–541.

32 Blanke DJ, Hageman PA. Comparison of gait of young and elderly men. *Phys Ther*. 1989;69:144–148.

33 Guimaraes RM, Issacs B. Characteristics of the gait in old people who fall. *Int Rehabil Med*. 1980;2:177–180.

34 Gabell A, Nakay USL. The effect of age on variability in gait. *J Gerontol*. 1984;39:662–666.

35 Winter DA. *Biomechanics and Motor Control of Human Movement*. New York, NY: John Wiley & Sons Inc; 1991.

36 Murray MP, Kory RC, Clarkson BH. Walking patterns in healthy old men. *J Bone Joint Surg [Am]*. 1969;24:169–178.

37 Crowninshield RD, Brand RA, Johnston RC. The effects of walking velocity and age on hip kinematics and kinetics. *Clin Orthop*. 1978;132:140–144.

38 Pozzo T, Berthoz A, Lefort L. Head stabilization during various locomotor tasks in humans. *Exp Brain Res*. 1990;82:97–106.

39 Prince F, Winter DA, Stergiou P, Walt SE. Anticipatory control of upper body balance during human locomotion. *Gait and Posture*. 1994;2:19–25.

40 Winter DA. *The Biomechanics and Motor Control of Human Gait: Normal, Elderly and Pathological*. Waterloo, Ontario, Canada: University of Waterloo Press; 1991.

41 Shumway-Cook A, Woollacott MH. *Motor Control: Theory and Practical Applications*. Baltimore, Md: Williams & Wilkins; 1995.

42 Alexander NB. Gait disorders in older adults. *J Am Geriatr Soc*. 1996;44:434–451.

43 Nutt JG, Marsden CD, Thompson PD. Human walking and higher-level gait disorders, particularly in the elderly. *Neurology*. 1993;43:268–279.

44 Wolfson LI, Whipple R, Amerman P, et al. Gait and balance in the elderly. *Clin Geriatr Med*. 1985;1:649–659.

45 Patla AE, Prentice S, Robinson C, Neufeld J. Visual control of locomotion: strategies for changing direction and for going over obstacles. *J Exp Psychol Hum Percept Perform.* 1991;17:603–634.

46 Patla AE, Rietdyk S. Visual control of limb trajectory over obstacles during locomotion: effect of obstacle height and width. *Gait and Posture.* 1993;1:45–60.

47 Patla AE, Robinson C, Samways M, Armstrong CJ. Visual control of step length during overground locomotion: task-specific modulation of the locomotor synergy. *J Exp Psychol Hum Percept Perform.* 1989;15:603–617.

48 Chen H-C, Ashton-Miller JA, Alexander NB, Schultz AB. Stepping over obstacles: gait patterns of healthy young and old adults. *J Gerontol.* 1991;46:M196–M203.

49 Chen H-C, Ashton-Miller JA, Alexander NB, Schultz AB. Effects of age and variable response time on ability to step over an obstacle. *J Gerontol.* 1994;49:M227–M233.

50 Chen H-C, Schultz AB, Ashton-Miller JA, et al. Stepping over obstacles: dividing attention impairs performance of old more than young adults. *J Gerontol.* 1996;51:M116–M122.

51 Teasdale N, Lajoie Y, Bard Y, et al. Cognitive processes involved for maintaining postural stability while standing and walking. In: Stelmach GE, Hömberg V, eds. *Sensorimotor Impairment in the Elderly.* Amsterdam, the Netherlands: Kluwer Academic Publishers; 1993:157–168.

52 Dietz V, Quintern J, Berger W. Corrective reactions to stumbling in man: functional significance of spinal and transcortical reflexes. *Neurosci Lett.* 1984;44:131–135.

53 Nashner LM. Balance adjustments of humans perturbed while walking. *J Neurophysiol.* 1980;44:650–664.

54 Nashner LM. Fixed patterns of rapid postural responses among leg muscles during stance. *Exp Brain Res.* 1977;30:13–24.

55 Nashner LM, Woollacott M, Tuma G. Organization of rapid responses to postural and locomotor-like perturbations of standing man. *Exp Brain Res.* 1979;36:463–476.

56 Dietz V, Quintern J, Sillem M. Stumbling reactions in man: significance of proprioceptive and pre-programmed mechanisms. *J Physiol (Lond).* 1987;386:149–163.

57 Forssberg H, Grillner S, Rossignol S. Phase-dependent reflex reversal during walking in chronic spinal cats. *Brain Res.* 1975;85:103–107.

58 Stein RB. Reflex modulation during locomotion: functional significance. In: Patla AE, ed. *Adaptability of Human Gait.* Amsterdam, the Netherlands: Elsevier Science Publishers BV; 1991:21–36.

59 Yang JF, Stein RB. Phase-dependent reflex reversal in human leg muscles during walking. *J Neurophysiol.* 1990;63:1109–1117.

60 Dietz V, Quintern J, Boos G, Berger W. Obstruction of the swing phase during gait: phase-dependent bilateral leg muscle coordination. *Brain Res.* 1986;384:166–169.

61 Eng JJ, Winter DA, Patla AE. Strategies for recovery from a trip in early and late swing during human walking. *Exp Brain Res.* 1994;102:339–349.

62 Tang P-F. *Balance Adjustments in Perturbed Human Walking: Neuromuscular Control Mechanisms and Effects of Aging.* Eugene, Ore: University of Oregon; 1997. Doctoral dissertation.

63 Wolfson L, Whipple R, Amerman P, Tobin JN. Gait assessment in the elderly: a gait abnormality rating scale and its relationship to falls. *J Gerontol.* 1990;45:M12–M19.

64 VanSwearingen JM, Paschal KA, Bonino P, Yang J-F. The modified Gait Abnormality Rating Scale for recognizing the risk of recurrent falls in community-dwelling elderly adults. *Phys Ther.* 1996;76:994–1002.

65 Thorbahn LDB, Newton RA. Use of Berg balance test to predict falls in elderly persons. *Phys Ther.* 1996;76:576–585.

66 Winstein AJ. Standing balance training: effects on balance and locomotion in hemiparetic adults. *Arch Phys Med Rehabil.* 1989;70:755–762.

67 Wolf SL, Barnhart HX, Kutner NG, et al. Reducing frailty and falls in older persons: an investigation of tai chi and computerized balance training. *J Am Geriatr Soc.* 1996;44:489–497.

Additional
Physical Therapy Articles

The Effect of Multidimensional Exercises on Balance, Mobility, and Fall Risk in Community-Dwelling Older Adults

Background and Purpose. This prospective clinical investigation examined the effects of a multidimensional exercise program on balance, mobility, and risk for falls in community-dwelling older adults with a history of falling. Factors used to predict adherence and a successful response to exercise were identified. Subjects. A total of 105 community-dwelling older adults (≥65 years of age) with a history of two or more falls in the previous 6 months (no neurologic diagnosis) participated. They were classified into (1) a control group of fallers (n=21), (2) a fully adherent exercise group (n=52), and (3) a partially adherent exercise group (n=32). Methods. Following evaluation, each patient received an individualized exercise program addressing the impairments and functional disabilities identified during the assessment. The control group received no intervention. Changes in performance on five clinical tests of balance and mobility and fall risk were compared among groups. Results. Both exercise groups scored better than the control group on all measures of balance and mobility. Although both exercise groups showed a reduction in fall risk compared with the control group, the greatest reduction was found in the fully adherent exercise group. Factors associated with successful response to exercise included degree of adherence to exercise program and pretest score on the Tinetti Mobility Assessment. Conclusion and Discussion. Exercise can improve balance and mobility function and reduce the likelihood for falls among community-dwelling older adults with a history of falling. The amount of exercise needed to achieve these results, however, could not be determined from this study. [Shumway-Cook A, Gruber W, Baldwin M, Liao S. The effect of multidimensional exercises on balance, mobility, and fall risk in community-dwelling older adults. Phys Ther. 1997;77:46–57.]

Key Words: *Balance, Exercise, Fall prevention.*

Anne Shumway-Cook
William Gruber
Margaret Baldwin
Shiquan Liao

The risk for falls increases dramatically with age.[1-3] Approximately 25% to 35% of people over the age of 65 years experiences one or more falls each year.[2,4,5] The consequences of falls among older adults are devastating. In people over the age of 65 years, falls are the leading cause of death from injury.[6] Falls also lead to substantial morbidity among older adults. Nearly 70% of all emergency department visits by people over the age of 75 years are related to falls.[6] Forty percent of hospital admissions in this age group are the result of fall-related injuries, resulting in an average length of stay of 11.6 days.[6] Approximately one half of older adults hospitalized for fall-related injuries are discharged to nursing homes.[7]

Because of the devastating effects of falls among older adults, risk factors for predicting falls and fall-related injuries have been studied extensively.[8-11] Factors contributing to increased risk for falls have been categorized into intrinsic factors (those internal to the individual) and extrinsic factors (those associated with environmental features).[12] Intrinsic factors associated with increased likelihood for falls include changes in muscular strength,[13,14] decreased joint flexibility,[15,16] impaired visual sensation,[17] a decline in vestibular function,[18,19] and decreased vibratory sense.[20]

Researchers[10,11,21,22] have shown that among intrinsic factors, impaired stance balance and mobility greatly increase the probability for falls, fractures, and functional dependency among older adults. It has been estimated that between 10% and 25% of all falls are associated with poor balance and gait abnormalities.[23] Deficits within the postural control system controlling stance balance that have been reported include changes in the temporal and spatial sequencing of muscles responding to loss of balance,[24,25] increased dependence on visual cues for postural control,[25,26] and a decreased ability to organize and select sensory information for postural control.[26,27]

Despite the apparent relationship between impaired balance and increased likelihood for falls among elderly individuals, studies examining the effects of exercise on improving balance and reducing risk for falls in this population have had mixed results.[28-35] One possible reason for this inconsistency is the variation in exercise programs utilized in these studies. In addition, many researchers have incorporated exercise into a multifaceted intervention approach, making it difficult to determine the relative contribution of exercise to improving balance and decreasing fall risk.[1]

The purpose of this study was to prospectively examine the effects of a multidimensional exercise program on balance, mobility, and risk for falls among community-dwelling older adults with a history of falls. The research questions were: (1) Does a multidimensional exercise program improve stance balance and mobility and reduce the likelihood for falls in older community-dwelling adults? (2) What factors can be used to predict a successful response to exercise, defined as a reduction in probability for falls? and (3) What factors can be used to predict adherence to an exercise program for elderly persons?

Method

Subjects

The quasi-experimental study involved two groups of community-dwelling older adults, over the age of 65 years, with no known neurologic diagnoses and a self-reported history of two or more falls in the previous 6 months. Subjects involved in the exercise program were selected from among the first 101 patients referred by their physicians to the Safety and Gait Enhancement Program (a fall-intervention program for older adults) of Northwest Hospital (Seattle, Wash) who met the study criteria and agreed to participate. Seventeen participants (14%) in the exercise program dropped out within the first 3 weeks; therefore, the number of exercisers

---

A Shumway-Cook, PhD, PT, is Research Coordinator, Department of Physical Therapy, Northwest Hospital, 10330 Meridian Ave N, Suite 110, Seattle, WA 98133 (USA) (ashumway@nwhsea.org). Address all correspondence to Dr Shumway-Cook.

W Gruber, MD, is Medical Director, Safety and Gait Enhancement Program, Northwest Hospital.

M Baldwin, PT, is Staff Physical Therapist, Department of Physical Therapy, Stevens Memorial Hospital, 21601 76th Ave W, Edmonds, WA 98026.

S Liao, PhD, is Biostatistician, CARE Management Department, Northwest Hospital.

This study was approved by the Institutional Review Board at Northwest Hospital.

Results from this study were presented at the Combined Sections Meeting of the American Physical Therapy Association; February 8–12, 1995; Reno, NV. In addition, they have appeared in abstract form in the June 1995 issue of *Neurology Report*.

This investigation was supported by a grant from Northwest Hospital Foundation, Seattle, WA.

This article was submitted August 29, 1995, and was accepted March 27, 1996.

Table 1.
Baseline Characteristics of Subjects, According to Treatment Group[a]

Characteristic	Control Group (n=21)	Partially Adherent Group (n=32)	Fully Adherent Group (n=52)
Age (y)			
X̄	78	80	79
SD	8	8	8
Range	66–97	65–96	62–97
Gender			
Female	14 (67)	25 (78)	38 (73)
Male	7 (33)	7 (22)	14 (27)
Married	11 (52)	15 (47)	25 (48)
Living situation			
Home	21 (100)	23 (72)	45 (87)
Retirement center (independent)	0 (0)	3 (10)	6 (11)
Retirement center (dependent)	0 (0)	6 (18)	1 (2)
Score on Mini-Mental Test			
No deficit (0–2 errors)	18 (86)	23 (72)	46 (88)
Mild deficit (3–4 errors)	1 (4)	5 (16)	5 (10)
Moderate deficit (5–7 errors)	2 (10)	4 (12)	1 (2)
Severe deficit (8–10 errors)	0 (0)	0 (0)	0 (0)
No. of medications			
0–1	11 (52)	6 (19)	9 (17)
2–3	8 (38)	15 (47)	24 (46)
≥4	2 (10)	11 (34)	19 (37)
No. of comorbidities			
0–1	7 (33)	2 (6)	9 (17)
2–3	12 (57)	21 (66)	22 (42)
≥4	2 (10)	9 (28)	21 (41)
Frequency of imbalance			
None	0 (0)	1 (3)	0 (0)
Monthly	2 (10)	5 (16)	3 (6)
Weekly	8 (38)	3 (9)	7 (13)
Daily	11 (52)	23 (72)	42 (81)
Type of assistive devices			
None	19 (91)	14 (44)	28 (54)
Cane	2 (9)	7 (22)	22 (42)
Walker	0 (0)	11 (34)	2 (4)

[a] Percentages shown in parentheses.

included in this report was 84. Of the 17 participants who left the program, 6 left due to medical complications, 3 died, 3 moved, and 5 left for unknown reasons. Two groups of patients were identified from among the 84 exercisers based on a *post hoc* analysis of adherence to the exercise program. The fully adherent exercise group (n=52) attended outpatient physical therapy sessions two times per week for 8 to 12 weeks and exercised 5 to 7 days per week at home. The partially adherent exercise group (n=32) attended less than 75% of their required therapy sessions and exercised fewer than 4 days per week. A nonequivalent control group of 21 volunteers with a history of falls were recruited from the Seattle area and tested, but received no intervention. This nonequivalent control group design was first described and used in the education literature.[36] Groups are formed on the basis of natural grouping when randomization is not possible.

Table 1 displays the baseline characteristics for each of the three groups. The three groups were comparable with respect to age, gender, marital status, living situation, and mental status. Performance on the Mini Mental Test[37] was used to determine mental status. Frequency of imbalance, defined as near-falls, slips, trips, or stumbles experienced by the subject was determined by self-report.

Procedure

Clinical tests of balance and mobility. After giving informed consent, all subjects underwent an assessment of balance and mobility skills. This assessment included measures for documenting functional abilities related to balance and mobility, assessing underlying sensory and motor strategies critical for these skills, and determining potential sensory and motor impairments contributing to instability and gait impairments.[38] Subjects provided a medical history and a self-report of fall and balance history. Subjects then completed the Mini Mental Test and the Balance Self-Perceptions Test, a short questionnaire in which subjects rate their perceived confidence when performing common activities of daily living. Subjects were asked to rate (on a scale of 1–5, where 1=no confidence and 5=extreme confidence) their degree of confidence in performing 20 basic activities of daily living and instrumental activities of daily living without fear of loss of balance. The questionnaire was a modification of one developed by Tinetti et al[39] in their study examining the relationship between fear of falling and measures of basic and instrumental activities of daily living.

In addition to the self-report measure, the Balance Self-Perceptions Test, performance-based tests were chosen to evaluate functional balance and walking skills. The Berg Balance Scale rates balance during the performance of 14 tasks, including sitting, standing, reaching, leaning over, turning, and stepping.[40] The Three-Minute Walk Test requires subjects to walk at their preferred pace for 3 minutes over a 91.4-m (300-ft) indoor course.[38] The course is carpeted, and involves four different turns. Balance and gait deviations were scored using the Performance-Oriented Mobility Test.[41] The Dynamic Gait Index was used to evaluate the ability to adapt gait to changes in task demands, including changing speeds, head turns in the vertical or horizontal direction, stepping over or around obstacles, and stair ascent and descent.[38] All clinical tools have previously been shown to have good interrater and test-retest reliability.[38–41]

Tests to document sensory and motor impairments included a manual muscle test of strength,[42] range of motion,[43] static postural alignment in sitting and standing positions,[38] presence or absence of coordinated multijoint movements for recovery of perturbed stance balance,[38] cerebellar coordination, sensation-vibration, stereognosis, vision, and presence or absence of dizziness.[44]

All subjects involved in the exercise program were reassessed using the same testing format approximately 8 to 12 weeks following the initial evaluation, just prior to discharge. Control group subjects were reassessed approximately 8 weeks following the initial evaluation.

Reliability testing of assessment protocol. Five physical therapists participated in this study. To ensure reliability and consistency among therapists, all were trained in both the evaluation and treatment procedures. A convenience sample of five community-dwelling older adults (3 female, 2 male, mean age=75 years) with varying balance abilities were used to test reliability of the assessment procedures in a pilot study. Each of the therapists assessed the subjects and was blinded to the results of the other therapists' assessments. Two of the subjects underwent two tests, 1 week apart, in order to determine test-retest reliability.

Interrater reliability was assessed using the ratio of subject variability to the total variability (ie, variability among subjects divided by total variability). A large ratio close to 1.0 would indicate high interrater reliability. There were two components of variability, one contributed by the differences among the subjects and the rest contributed by the multiple raters. Ideally, the proportion of variability contributed by the raters is small relative to the total variability (or equivalently, the subject variability is large proportionally to the total variability). For our study involving five subjects and five raters, the interrater reliability ranged from 0.96 to 1.00 for the assessment procedure of five clinical measures of balance and mobility, indicating excellent interrater reliability.

Intervention. Following evaluation, each patient received an individualized multidimensional exercise program addressing the specific impairments and functional disabilities identified during the assessment. Because each patient presented a different constellation of problems, treatment was not limited to a single form of exercise. However, because all patients participating in the program were referred with balance and mobility problems, they all received a progression of exercises designed to improve balance and mobility skills. Balance exercises focused on improving postural alignment in sitting and standing positions, developing coordinated movement strategies for recovery of balance in sitting and standing, improving the use of senses for postural orientation, improving the ability to make effective anticipatory postural adjustments prior to voluntary movements, and integrating appropriate sensory and motor strategies for controlling posture and balance into functionally related balance and mobility tasks. Mobility retraining focused on improving stability during a variety of gait tasks, including unperturbed gait, perturbed gait, transfers, and stair climbing. In addition, exercises were prescribed in other areas of need, as determined by the evaluating therapist. For example, patients who scored less than 5 on manual muscle testing were given progressive resistive strength training exercises, whereas those who showed a significant impairment in range of motion in the trunk or lower extremities were given flexibility exercises.

In addition to exercises performed twice a week in physical therapy, a home exercise program was established for each patient. All patients maintained a daily log of exercise compliance and kept a record of falls or near-falls for the duration of the program and for 6 months following discharge.

Data Analysis

Scores on the five measures of balance and mobility were obtained before and after participation in the exercise program. *Fall risk*, a surrogated measure defined as the predicted probability for falling, was calculated for each patient based on a logistic regression model that was developed and tested on a different cohort of 44 subjects (22 older adults with a history of falls and 22 older adults without a history of falls) (unpublished research). In the development of the fall-risk model, univariate analyses were first applied to select variables that could potentially be used to identify older adults with a high risk for falling. Potential predictors included demographic variables; variables related to the subjects' medical and balance history; current balance and mobility status as determined by five different clinical tests; and impairments in specific sensory and motor systems such as visual, vibratory or touch/pressure sense, range of motion, strength, and static alignment. Six variables that emerged to be individually and importantly associated with faller and nonfaller status were then used in a stepwise logistic regression analysis. Two variables, self-reported history of imbalance (*IMBALANCE*) and performance on the Berg Balance Scale (*BERG*), were identified by the stepwise logistic regression analysis as highly predictive of falling. The resulting logistic model was

$$log[P/(1-P)] = 10.459 + 2.324\ IMBALANCE - 0.249\ BERG$$

where P = probability of falling and $IMBALANCE$ = 1 if there is a history of instability or 0 if there is no history of instability. Of the 22 fallers, 18 subjects were correctly classified with a predicted probability of ≥0.5 (sensitivity = 82%). Of the 22 nonfallers, 20 subjects were correctly classified using a predicted probability of <0.5 (specificity = 91%).

An analysis of pretest balance and gait scores was done to determine whether differences existed between the control group and the exercise groups. To control for the disparity in initial performance, percentage-of-change scores were used. To assess the effect of exercise on balance, mobility, and fall risk, differences in test scores following intervention were expressed by the percentage of change in test scores: (posttest-pretest)/pretest. Descriptive analyses indicated that outliers existed on the original percentage-of-change scores for all six measures. To reduce the potential influence of outliers on the statistical analysis, a logit transformation was applied: $exp(x)/[1+exp(x)]$. All six measures were transformed into a comparable scale between 0 and 1. Univariate analyses showed that each of the six transformed change scores had an approximately normal distribution, with no outliers. Statistical analyses were then carried out on the transformed scores. For convenience of interpretation, the changes and confidence intervals (CIs) for all measures were then displayed as original percentage of change using inverse transformation (ie, transformed back to the original scales).

Statistical analyses included a multivariate analysis of variance (MANOVA, Wilk's criterion) performed on the five balance and gait measures combined.[45,46] The results of the MANOVA would indicate whether a difference existed among the three groups when the percentages of change in all five clinical measures were considered together. An analysis of variance (ANOVA) was used to assess the difference among the three groups on each of the individual tests. Fall risk was analyzed separately using a univariate analysis of variance. A Tukey's *post hoc* pair-wise comparison was used to examine differences between each pair of the three groups if the overall difference was significant among the three groups. A probability value of less than .05 was considered statistically significant, unless otherwise stated in this report.

For the 84 exercisers, a stepwise regression analysis was used to determine which factors predicted a successful response to exercise, as measured by the reduction in probability for falls. A stepwise logistic regression analysis was used to determine which factors predicted adherence to the prescribed exercise program (ie, fully adherent versus partially adherent, as defined earlier). All statistical analyses were performed using SPSS for Windows, Release 6.0.[47]*

Results

Table 2 displays the pretest and posttest values, percentage of change, and 95% CI for each of the three groups on six dependent measures. Results of the MANOVA showed that a significant difference ($P<.001$) existed among the three groups when the five balance and mobility measures were combined.

Effect of Exercise on Functional Balance Skills

Figure 1 graphs the percentage of change (group mean and 95% CI) of the two balance measures: the Berg Balance Scale and the Balance Self-Perceptions Test. Both exercise groups showed a significant improvement ($P<.001$) compared with the control group on both measures of balance. There was no difference between

---

* SPSS Inc, 444 N Michigan Ave, Chicago, IL 60611.

Table 2.
Group Differences on Balance and Mobility Changes[a]

	Control Group (n=21)	Partially Adherent Group (n=32)	Fully Adherent Group (n=52)
Functional Balance Test			
Pretest	42.2±9.5	32.2±9.7	38.9±7.2
Posttest	40.6±10.7	38.2±9.5	47.8±6.0
% Change	−5%	23%	26%
95% CI	−10% to 1%	14% to 31%	20% to 31%
Balance Self-Perceptions Test			
Pretest	64.1±16.7	54.8±12.6	57.0±12.9
Posttest	59.8±15.7	61.1±14.7	70.4±13.2
% Change	−6%	15%	25%
95% CI	−10% to −1%	6% to 23%	19% to 31%
Dynamic Gait Index			
Pretest	16.0±4.2	10.4±4.0	12.8±3.3
Posttest	13.4±5.3	12.0±4.1	16.9±3.7
% Change	−18%	20%	37%
95% CI	−26% to 9%	8% to 30%	27% to 45%
Tinetti Mobility Test			
Pretest	8.6±2.6	6.2±2.4	7.4±2.6
Posttest	8.1±3.2	7.1±2.6	9.5±2.4
% Change	−7%	25%	38%
95% CI	−16% to 2%	6% to 36%	24% to 46%
Three-Minute Walk Test			
Pretest	692.6±218.9	333.5±179.1	411.6±156.9
Posttest	607.3±223.1	414.1±193.6	617.9±215.8
% Change	−13%	38%	65%
95% CI	−22% to −4%	17% to 49%	39% to 71%
Fall risk (predicted probability)			
Pretest	.77±.27	.91±.21	.90±.12
Posttest	.81±.24	.84±.26	.60±.27
% Change	8%	−33%	−33%
95% CI	1% to 16%	−17% to −4%	−41% to −25%

[a] Pretest and posttest values are means±standard deviation. CI=confidence interval.

the fully adherent and partially adherent exercise groups on either balance measure.

Figure 2 is a scatter plot showing the percentage of change for every individual in each of the three groups on the Functional Balance Scale and the Balance Self-Perceptions Test. The graphs illustrate the differences among individuals within each group and the variability among the groups. Although scores in the control group tended to be more consistent, considerable variability was found in both the fully adherent and partially adherent exercise groups.

Effect of Exercise on Mobility Status

Figure 3 presents the percentage of change (group mean and 95% CI) of the three mobility measures—the Three-Minute Walk Test, the Tinetti Mobility Test, and the Dynamic Gait Index—for each of the three groups. Both exercise groups showed significant improvement ($P<.001$) compared with the control group on all three mobility measures. The only significant difference ($P<.01$) between the fully adherent and partially adherent exercise groups was found on the Dynamic Gait Index.

Figure 4 plots individual percentage-of-change scores for every subject on the three tests of mobility—the Three-Minute Walk Test, the Tinetti Mobility Test, and the Dynamic Gait Index—illustrating the spread of change scores for subjects within each group. Consistent with results from the balance testing, group variability was greater for the two exercise groups than for the control group.

Effect of Exercise on Probability for Falls

Figure 5a shows the percentage of change (group mean and 95% CI) of fall risk in each of the three groups. There was a significant difference ($P<.001$) in fall risk among the three groups. The fully adherent exercise group decreased their fall risk by 33%, and the partially adherent exercise group decreased their fall risk by 11%. In contrast, the control group showed an inverse trend, with an 8% increase in fall risk. Figure 5b is a plot of the change in fall risk for each individual in the three

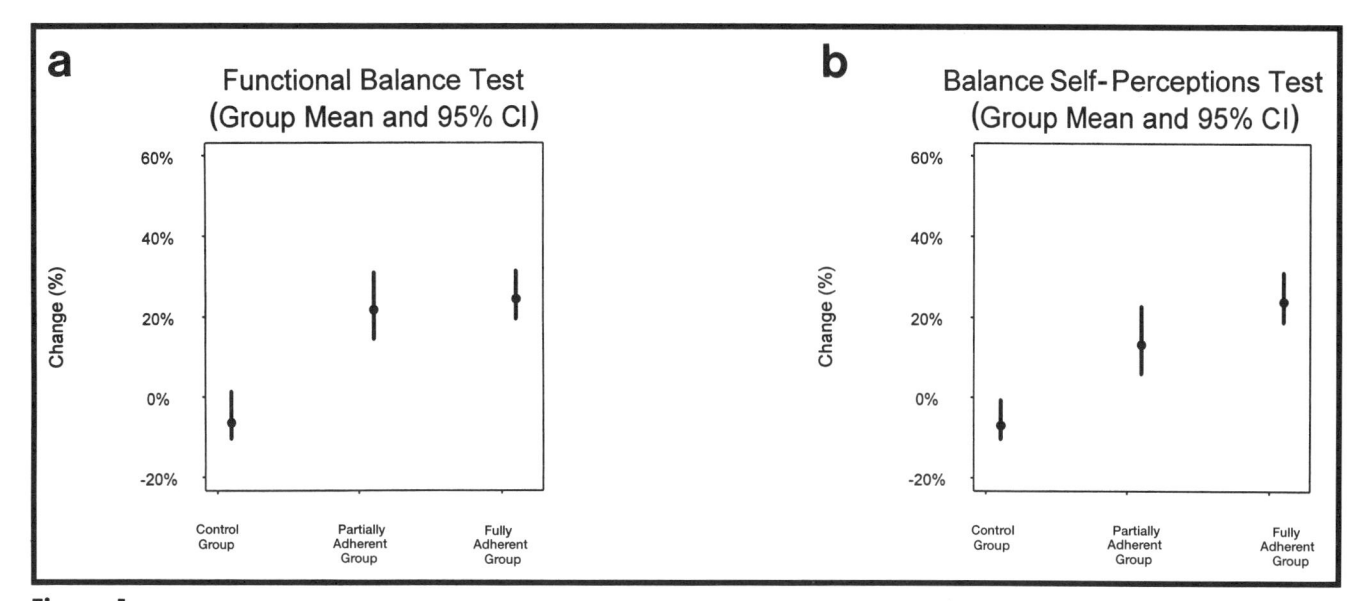

Figure 1.
The effect of exercise on balance skills. Shown are the means and 95% confidence intervals (CIs) for the three groups on (a) the Functional Balance Test and (b) the Balance Self-Perceptions Test.

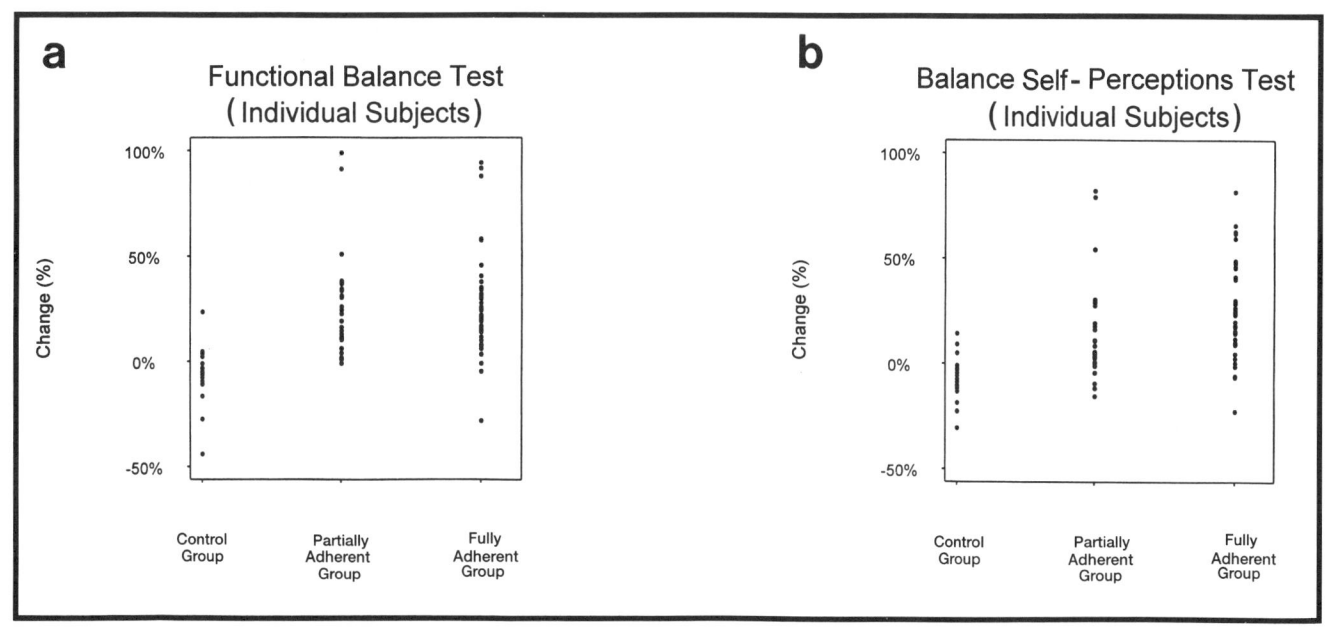

Figure 2.
Intersubject variability on changes in balance skills. Displayed are changes in performance for each individual in each of the three groups on (a) the Functional Balance Test and (b) the Balance Self-Perceptions Test.

groups. The greatest amount of variability was found in the fully adherent exercise group.

Factors Predicting Successful Response to Intervention

For the 84 exercisers, a stepwise regression analysis was done to identify factors that could be used to predict a successful response to exercise, as measured by a reduction in fall risk. The variables identified as predictive included pretest performance on the Tinetti Mobility Assessment and adherence to the prescribed exercise program (full adherence versus partial adherence). Patients who were fully adherent to the exercise program (coded as 1) were more likely to show a reduction in their probability for recurrent falls than those patients who were only partially adherent (coded as 0). The regression coefficient for adherence was −.18 (SE=.06). In addition, patients who scored higher on the Tinetti Mobility Assessment at initial evaluation tended to be more successful in reducing their fall risk. The regression coefficient for the Tinetti Mobility Assessment was −.05 (SE=.01).

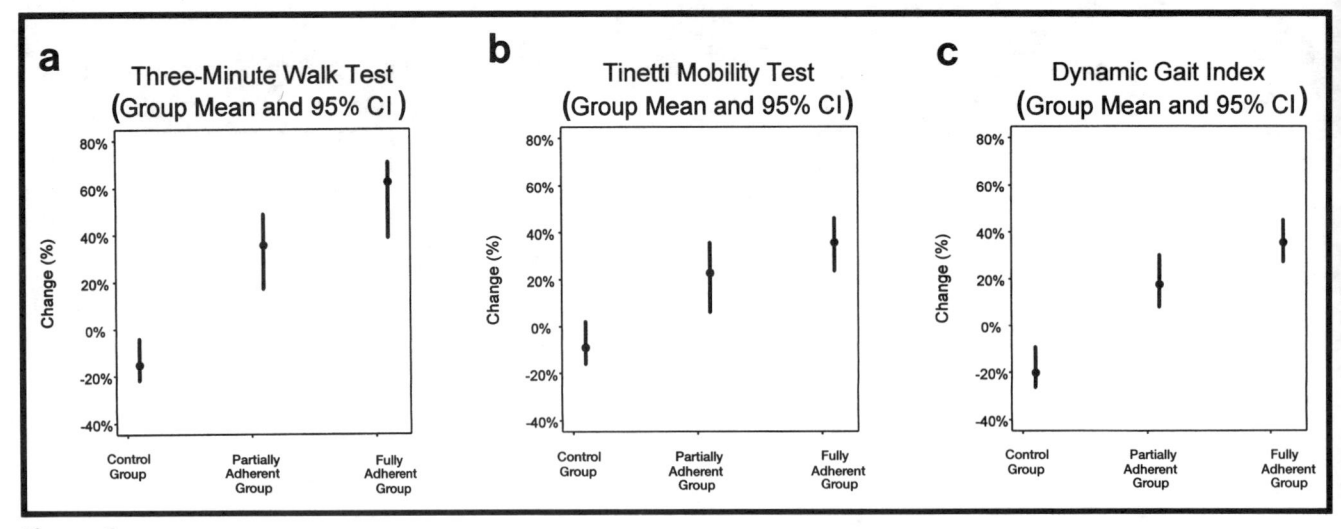

Figure 3.
The effect of exercise on mobility skills. Shown are the means and 95% confidence intervals (CIs) for the three groups on (a) the Three-Minute Walk Test, (b) the Tinetti Mobility Test, and (c) the Dynamic Gait Index.

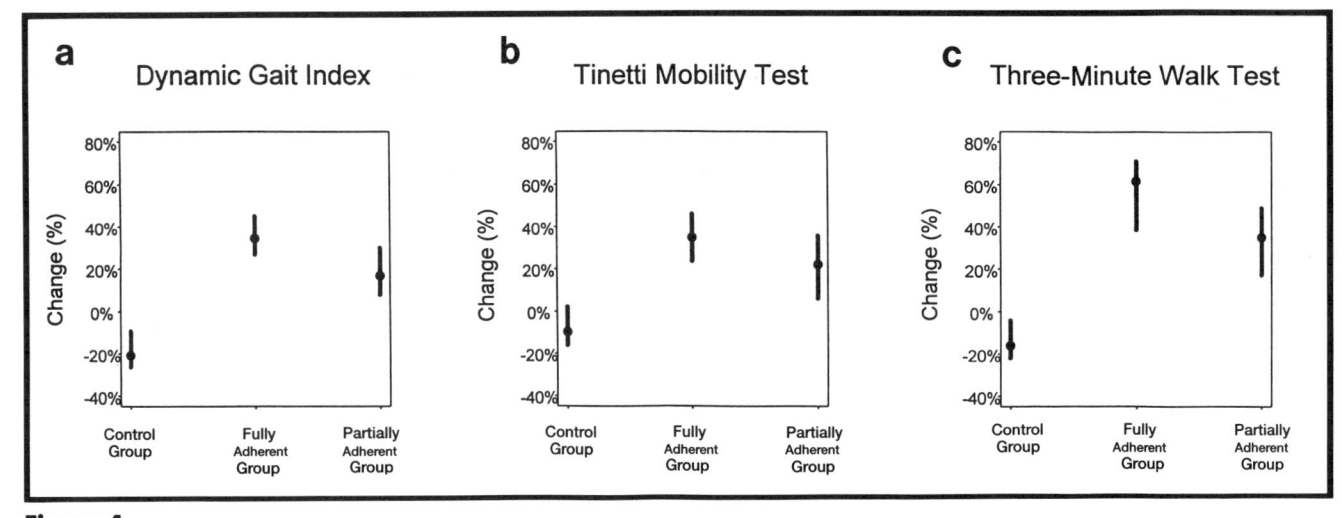

Figure 4.
Intersubject variability on changes in mobility skills. Displayed are changes in performance on (a) the Three-Minute Walk Test, (b) the Tinetti Mobility Test, and (c) the Dynamic Gait Index.

Factors that did not significantly ($P > .05$) predict a patient's ability to successfully reduce probability for falls included age, gender, number of medications, number of comorbidities, living status, performance on clinical measures of balance and mobility (other than the Tinetti Mobility Assessment), frequency of imbalance, and fall history.

Factors Predicting Compliance With Exercise

Results from the stepwise regression analysis indicated that the degree of adherence (total adherence versus partial adherence) was an important predictor of a successful response to exercise (defined as a reduction in fall risk). Patients who were fully adherent to their exercise program had a greater decrease in fall risk than those who were only partially adherent (33% versus 11%, on average). An additional research question we wanted to address was the identification of factor(s) that are potentially predictive of the degree of adherence to an exercise program.

A stepwise logistic regression analysis was used to determine factors that predicted adherence to an exercise program. (Preliminary univariate analyses [t test, chi-square test, or Fisher's Exact Test] indicated that differences existed between the two exercise groups on the following demographic and pretest variables: the type of assistive device used for gait, the Three-Minute Walk Test, the Berg Balance Scale, the Dynamic Gait Index, and the Tinetti Performance-Oriented Mobility Assessment. These five variables were used as candidates in a stepwise logistic regression analysis.) In the final model,

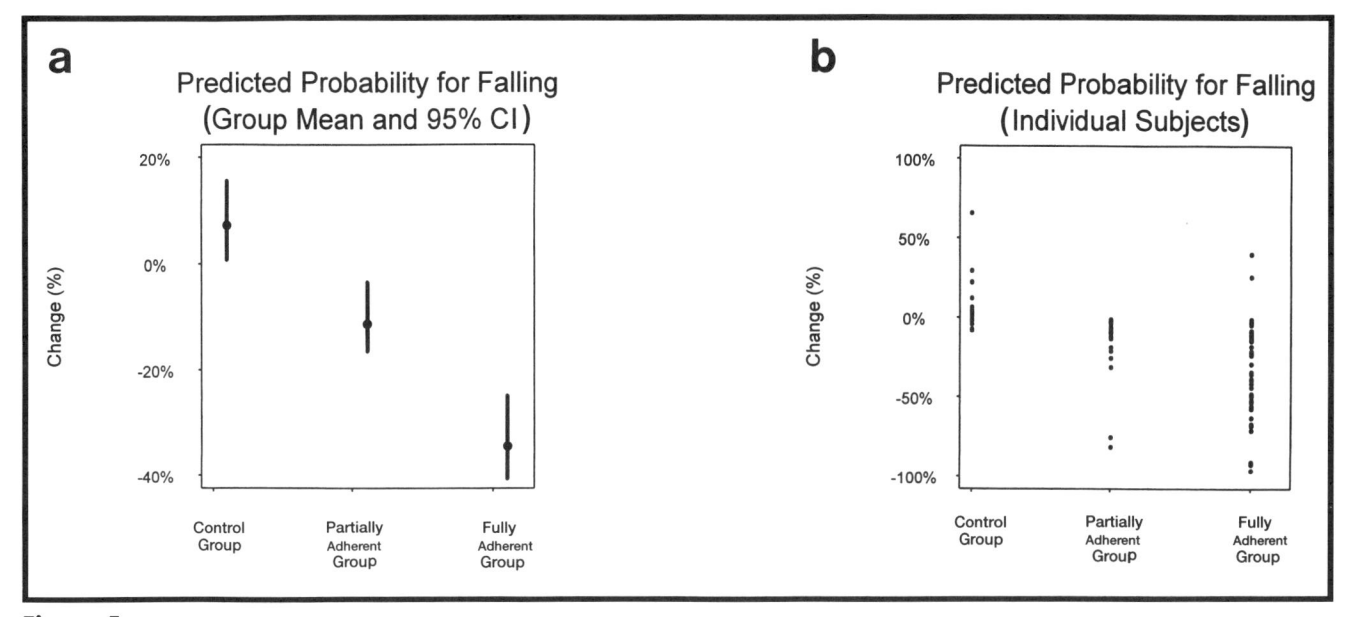

Figure 5.
The effect of exercise on fall risk: (a) mean changes in fall risk and 95% confidence intervals (CIs) for the three groups and (b) scatter plot of the variability of the change in fall risk among the three groups.

type of assistive device used for gait was the only variable that emerged as a predictor of adherence at the .05 level. Patients who used a walker as their primary assistive device were less likely to be adherent to exercise than those who used a cane or no assistive device. The resulting logistic regression model correctly classified 77% of the 83 patients into the two exercise groups (50/51 in the fully adherent group and 21/32 in the partially adherent group).

Factors that did not significantly ($P>.05$) predict adherence to an exercise program in this study included age, gender, marital status, living situation (coded as home versus retirement center), number of prescription medications taken, number of comorbidities, frequency of imbalance, and fall history.

Discussion

Our results show that a multifaceted exercise program improves balance and mobility function in community-dwelling older adults with a history of falls. In addition, adherence to a structured exercise program reduces the risk for falls among older adults.

Our results are consistent with those of two recently published studies that demonstrated that exercise can help to reduce falls, or fall risk, in community-dwelling older adults. Tinetti et al[1] found a reduction in the rate of falls among community-dwelling older adults who participated in a multifocus intervention project that included the use of exercises to improve balance and ability to transfer safely. Province et al[35] used a meta-analysis to examine the effects of exercise on falls and fall-related injuries among seven different facilities participating in the Frailty and Injuries: Cooperative Studies of Intervention Techniques (FICIT) study. Despite the mixed outcomes among the various sites involved in this meta-analysis, Province et al concluded that some form of balance retraining appears to be the most effective type of exercise for reducing fall risk.

Several investigators[28–34,48] have examined the effect of a single form of exercise on balance in older adults, with mixed results. Comparing results from these various studies can be difficult because of the diversity of exercise programs used and the inconsistency in how balance is defined and measured. Lichtenstein et al[33] and Fiatarone et al[34] reported an improvement in balance following high-intensity strength training in older adults. Roberts[28] found that a 6-week program of aerobic walking improved balance among older adults, but changes in falls were not reported. Brown and Holloszy[29] reported improvements in static balance in women over the age of 60 years, but not in men, after 3 months of strength and flexibility training. No change in walking ability was found for either gender.[29] Crilly et al[30] found no improvement in postural sway in 50 older women following a 12-week program of balance retraining. Topp et al[31] found that following a 12-week program of dynamic resistance strength training, older adults showed some improvements in gait speed and balance, although the changes were not different from those of the nonexercising control subjects. Judge et al[48] found no relationship between balance and resistive strength training. Hu and Woollacott[32] reported that exercises focusing on improving the organization of sensory information underlying balance control resulted in a decrease in stance postural sway in older adults. The exercise group had fewer falls during their experimental tests of balance compared with subjects who did not exercise; however, differences in number of falls in a natural environment were not reported.[32]

A Multidimensional Approach to Retraining

The results from our study suggest that a multidimensional exercise program can improve balance, mobility, and fall risk in older adults. Our multifaceted exercise approach was based on a systems model of postural control that suggests that stability emerges from a complex interaction of musculoskeletal and neural systems.[38] A systems approach to understanding balance function in elderly persons examines the extent to which deterioration in specific physiologic and musculoskeletal systems contributes to loss of stability and mobility in this population.[38] Thus, a systems approach to assessment of balance and mobility uses a variety of tests and measurements to document functional abilities and to determine the underlying sensory, motor, and cognitive impairments contributing to functional disabilities.[38] The goals of retraining are (1) to resolve or prevent underlying impairments, (2) to develop effective and efficient task-specific sensory and motor strategies, and (3) to adapt task-specific strategies so that functional tasks can be performed in changing environmental contexts.[38] A multidimensional approach to retraining balance and mobility functions in older adults is intuitively appealing because it is consistent with current research indicating that most falls in older adults involve multiple risk factors and that many of these factors may be remediated.[49] Until now, the effectiveness of this type of approach has not been tested scientifically. Results from our study suggest that a multidimensional approach is successful in improving balance and mobility skills and that these improvements are associated with a reduction in fall risk.

The Importance of Adherence

Although both groups of exercisers showed a reduction in fall risk compared with the control group, who did not exercise, subjects who were completely adherent were more likely to reduce their fall risk than those who were partially adherent. Results showed that both exercise groups showed an improvement in balance and gait skills compared with the control group. Although the fully adherent exercisers performed better as a group on clinical measures of balance and mobility than the partially adherent exercisers, the differences were not statistically significant. Thus, the amount of exercise necessary to show an improvement in balance and mobility skills is not clear from this study.

Results from this study suggest that the type of assistive device used for ambulating was the only factor that predicted the degree of adherence. Patients who walked with no assistive devices or with a cane tended to be more adherent than those who used a walker. This finding suggests that patients with more severe balance problems, as indicated by the use of a walker, do not appear to adhere as well as those patients with less severe balance problems. One reason could be that patients who are severely impaired do not believe that exercise can change their level of function and, therefore, are less likely to adhere.

An important and encouraging finding of this study was that age was not associated with the adherence to exercise and with the reduction of fall risk. Patients who were above the age of 80 years were as likely to be adherent and successful as those in their 60s. This finding suggests that balance and gait retraining programs can be beneficial to very old individuals. Because this study was limited to adults over the age of 65 years who lived in their own homes or in retirement centers, the results may not apply to those under the age of 65 years or to older adults residing in nursing homes.

Limitations of the Study

There were several limitations associated with this study. One limitation was the lack of randomization of subjects to the control group versus the experimental groups. Our study utilized patients who were specifically referred for balance and mobility retraining. It was therefore not possible to randomly assign patients to a nonintervention group. Thus, our study used a quasi-experimental, nonequivalent control group design. This design is reported to be an acceptable alternative to an experimental design when randomization is not possible.[36,50]

A second limitation of the study was that both pretesting and posttesting for each subject were carried out by the therapist responsible for treating that patient, introducing the possibility of evaluator bias. Interrater reliability measurements suggest that all therapists were well trained in the evaluation procedures. In addition, therapists were not given access to pretest scores at the time of posttest evaluation, reducing the probability of evaluator bias.

Finally, our study examined the effects of exercise on fall risk, not on actual frequency of falls. The use of fall risk as a measure of intervention effectiveness has been reported by others as an alternative to reporting actual fall frequency (see Province et al[35] for a review). In addition, our model for predicting fall risk has been shown to be highly related to actual fall frequency (unpublished research).

Conclusion

The effects of falls are devastating, contributing to an increase in mortality and morbidity in adults over the age of 65 years. A multidimensional exercise program is an important factor in improving upright balance and gait function and in reducing the risk for falls in older community-dwelling adults. Both adherence to an exercise program and degree of balance and gait impairment appear to be important factors in determining a successful response to exercise. How much exercise is needed to achieve maximal effects, however, is unclear. Thus, further study is needed to determine the optimal relationship between patient characteristics and exercise frequency and duration.

References

1 Tinetti ME, Baker DI, McAway G, et al. A multifactorial intervention to reduce the risk of falling among elderly people living in the community. *N Engl J Med.* 1994;331:821–827.

2 Hornbrook MC, Stevens J, Wingfield DJ, et al. Preventing falls among community-dwelling older persons: results from a randomized trial. *Gerontologist.* 1994;34:16–23.

3 Blake AJ, Morgan K, Bendall MJ, et al. Falls by elderly people at home: prevalence and associated factors. *Age Ageing.* 1988;17:365–372.

4 Nevitt MC, Cummings SR. Risk factors for recurrent non-syncopoal falls: a prospective study. *JAMA.* 1989;261:2663–2668.

5 Tinetti ME, Ginter SF. Identifying mobility dysfunctions in elderly patients: standard neuromuscular examination or direct assessment? *JAMA.* 1988;259:1190–1193.

6 Sattin RW. Falls among older persons: a public health perspective. *Annu Rev Public Health.* 1992;13:489–508.

7 Sattin RW, Lambert H, Devito CA, et al. The incidence of fall injury events among the elderly in a defined population. *Am J Epidemiol.* 1990;131:1028–1037.

8 Campbell AJ, Borrie MJ, Spears GF. Risk factors for falls in a community-based prospective study of people 70 years and older. *J Gerontol.* 1989;44:M112–M117.

9 Kellogg International Work Group on the Prevention of Falls by the Elderly. The prevention of falls in later life. *Dan Med Bull.* 1987;34:1–24.

10 Tinetti ME, Speechley M, Ginter SF. Risk factors for falls among elderly persons living in the community. *N Engl J Med.* 1988;319:1701–1707.

11 Duncan PW, Studenski S, Chandler J, Prescott B. Functional reach: predictive validity in a sample of elderly male veterans. *J Gerontol.* 1992;47:M93–M98.

12 Nickens H. Intrinsic factors in falling among the elderly. *Arch Intern Med.* 1985;145:1089–1093.

13 Whipple RH, Wolfson LI, Amerman PM. The relationship of knee and ankle weakness to falls in nursing home residents: an isokinetic study. *J Am Geriatr Soc.* 1987;35:13–20.

14 Aniansson A, Grimby F, Gedberg A. Muscle function in old age. *Scand J Rehabil Med.* 1978;6(suppl):43–49.

15 Guralnik JM, Ferrucci L, Simonsick E, et al. Lower-extremity function in persons over the age of 70 years as a predictor of subsequent disability. *N Engl J Med.* 1995;332:556–561.

16 Lewis C, Bottomley J. Musculoskeletal changes with age. In: Lewis C, ed. *Aging: Health Care's Challenge.* 2nd ed. Philadelphia, Pa: FA Davis Co; 1990:145–146.

17 Kosnik W, Winslow L, Kline D, et al. Visual changes in daily life throughout adulthood. *J Gerontol Psych Sci.* 1988;43:63–70.

18 Sloane P, Baloh RW, Honrubia V. The vestibular system in the elderly. *Am J Otolaryngol.* 1989;1:422–429.

19 Ochs AL, Newberry J, Lenhardt ML, Harkins SW. Neural and vestibular aging associated with falls. In: Birren JE, Schaie KW, eds. *Handbook of Psychology of Aging.* New York, NY: Van Nostrand Reinhold; 1985:378–399.

20 Whanger A, Wang HS. Clinical correlates of the vibratory sense in elderly psychiatric patients. *J Gerontol.* 1974;29:39–45.

21 Woollacott MH, Shumway-Cook A. Changes in posture control across the life span: a systems approach. *Phys Ther.* 1990;70:799–807.

22 Maki B, Holliday PJ, Topper AK. Fear of falling and postural performance in the elderly. *J Gerontol.* 1991;46:M123–M131.

23 Nelson RC, Amin MA. Falls in the elderly. *Emerg Med Clin North Am.* 1990;8:309–324.

24 Woollacott MH, Shumway-Cook A, Nashner LM. Aging and posture control: changes in sensory organization and muscular coordination. *Int J Aging Hum Dev.* 1986;23:97–114.

25 Manchester D, Woollacott MH, Zederbauer-Hylton N, Marin O. Visual, vestibular, and somatosensory contributions to balance control in the older adult. *J Gerontol.* 1989;44:M118–M127.

26 Horak F, Shupert C, Mirka A. Components of postural dyscontrol in the elderly: a review. *Neurobiol Aging.* 1989;10:727–745.

27 Peterka RJ, Black FO. Age-related changes in human posture control: sensory organization tests. *Journal of Vestibular Research.* 1990;1:73–85.

28 Roberts B. Effects of walking on balance among elders. *Nurs Res.* 1989;38:180–183.

29 Brown M, Holloszy JO. Effects of a low-intensity exercise program on selected physical performance characteristics of 60- to 70-year-olds. *Aging (Milano).* 1991;3:129–139.

30 Crilly RG, Willems DA, Trenhold KJ, et al. Effect of exercise on postural sway in the elderly. *Gerontology.* 1989;35:137–143.

31 Topp R, Mikesky A, Wigglesworth J, et al. The effect of a 12-week dynamic resistance strength training program on gait velocity and balance of older adults. *Gerontologist.* 1993;33:501–506.

32 Hu M, Woollacott MH. Multisensory training of standing balance in older adults, I: postural stability and one-leg stance balance. *J Gerontol.* 1994;49:M52–M61.

33 Lichtenstein MJ, Shields SL, Shiavi RG, Burger C. Exercise and balance in aged women: a pilot controlled clinical trial. *Arch Phys Med Rehabil.* 1989;70:138–143.

34 Fiatarone MA, Marks EC, Ryan ND, et al. High-intensity strength training in nonagenarians: effects on skeletal muscle. *JAMA.* 1990;263:3029–3034.

35 Province MA, Hadley EC, Hornbrook MC, et al. The effects of exercise on falls in elderly patients. *JAMA.* 1995;272:1341–1347.

36 Campbell D, Stanley J. Experimental and quasi-experimental designs for research on teaching. In: Gage NL, ed. *Handbook of Research on Teaching.* Chicago, Ill: Rand McNally; 1963.

37 Pfeiffer E. Short portable mental status questionnaire. *J Am Geriatr Soc.* 1975;23:433–441.

38 Shumway-Cook A, Woollacott MH. *Motor Control: Theory and Practical Applications.* Baltimore, Md: Williams & Wilkins; 1995.

39 Tinetti ME, Mendes deLeon CF, Doucette JT, Baker DI. Fear of falling and fall-related efficacy in relationship to functioning among community-living elders. *J Gerontol.* 1994;49:140–147.

40 Berg K. *Measuring Balance in the Elderly: Validation of an Instrument.* Montreal, Quebec, Canada: McGill University; 1993. Dissertation.

41 Tinetti ME. Performance-oriented assessment of mobility problems in elderly patients. *J Am Geriatr Soc.* 1986;34:119–126.

42 Kendall F, McCreary EK. *Muscles: Testing and Function.* Baltimore, Md: Williams & Wilkins; 1983.

43 Saunders D. *Evaluation, Treatment, and Prevention of Musculoskeletal Disorders.* Minneapolis, Minn: Viking Press; 1991.

44 Shumway-Cook A, Horak F. Rehabilitation strategies for patients with vestibular deficits. *Neurology Clinics of North America.* 1990;8:441–457.

45 Fisher LD, Van Belle G. *Biostatistics: A Methodology for the Health Sciences.* New York, NY: John Wiley & Sons Inc; 1993.

46 Tabachnick BG, Fidell LS. *Using Multivariate Statistics.* 2nd ed. New York, NY: HarperCollins Publishers; 1989.

47 *SPSS for Windows: Advanced Statistics, Release 6.0.* Chicago, Ill: SPSS Inc; 1993.

48 Judge JO, Whipple RH, Wolfson LI. Effects of resistive and balance exercises on isokinetic strength in older persons. *J Am Geriatr Soc.* 1994;42:937–946.

49 Lipsitz LA, Jonsson PV, Kelley MM, Koestner JS. Causes and correlates of recurrent falls in ambulatory frail elderly. *J Gerontol.* 1991;46:M114–M122.

50 Kenny DA. A quasi-experimental approach to assessing treatment effects in the nonequivalent control group design. *Psychol Bull.* 1975;82:345–362.

The Effect of Tai Chi Quan and Computerized Balance Training on Postural Stability in Older Subjects

Background and Purpose. This study explored whether two exercise programs would affect the ability to minimize postural sway of 72 relatively inactive, older subjects who participated in the Atlanta FICSIT trial. **Subjects.** Subjects were randomly assigned to (1) a computerized balance training group, (2) a tai chi group, or (3) an educational group serving as a control for exercise. Each group consisted of 24 members. **Methods.** All subjects were evaluated under four postural conditions before, immediately after, and 4 months following their respective interventions, each of which was given over 15 weeks. **Results.** Platform balance measures revealed greater stability after training among subjects in the balance training group but little change in stability among subjects in the tai chi and educational group. Subjects in the tai chi group were less afraid of falling after training compared with subjects in other groups with similar covariates. **Conclusion and Discussion.** Unlike computerized balance training, tai chi does not improve measures of postural stability. Because tai chi delayed onset to first or multiple falls in older individuals, this effect does not appear to be associated with measures of enhanced postural stability. Tai chi may gain its success, in part, from promoting confidence without reducing sway rather than primarily facilitating a reduction in sway-based measures. [Wolf SL, Barnhart HX, Ellison GL, et al. The effect of tai chi quan and computerized balance training on postural stability in older subjects. *Phys Ther.* 1997;77:371–381.]

Key Words: *Balance, Exercise, Geriatrics, Movement, Tai chi.*

Steven L Wolf

Huiman X Barnhart

Gary L Ellison

Carol E Coogler

Atlanta FICSIT Group

Many authors[1-4] have noted that exercise is a generic intervention with demonstrated physiological and psychosocial benefits for all age groups, including older individuals with specified chronic conditions. Improvements in muscle strength,[5] muscle mass,[6] cardiovascular status,[7-10] fatigue resistance,[11] and hypertension[12] among older people who exercise are well documented. As facilitators of these improvements, physical therapists seek to regain or maintain maximal independence or prevent dependence for their older clients. These goals are often sought through innovative exercise programs and through precise documentation of physiological changes.

In 1990, the National Institute on Aging initiated the FICSIT (Frailty and Injuries: Cooperative Studies on Intervention Techniques) trials to explore novel interventions designed to have an impact on physiological, behavioral, and environmental dimensions related to frailty or falls in elderly individuals and, in the process, define a common database across sites. The work completed by Fiatarone and colleagues[13] demonstrated that intense strength training improved lower-extremity force by 113% in older nursing home residents compared with a control group with concomitant improvements in gait speed, stair climbing, cross-sectional thigh muscle area, and spontaneous physical activity. Tinetti's group[14] demonstrated that a multifactorial program, including adjustment of medications, home exercise prescription, and behavioral instructions, resulted in a reduction in the numbers of falls among older individuals residing in independent living sites compared with a control group of older people receiving social visits. Wolfson and coworkers[15] showed that a combined strengthening and weight training program had a favorable impact on a variety of balance measures among 110 community-dwelling persons with a mean age of 80 years. When all FICSIT site interventions were grouped into categories by defining the prevailing aspect of each intervention as emphasizing balance, strength, or endurance, those treatments emphasizing a balance component delayed the onset of first falls more than did strength or endurance interventions compared with all control groups across sites.[16] Furthermore, the balance intervention most contributing to this delay was tai chi (TC).

At the Atlanta FICSIT site, the TC intervention for older subjects was compared with computerized balance training (BT) and with a control condition (ED) for subjects who attended weekly educational sessions without changing their exercise routine. We chose to explore these interventions because of our interests in frailty and falls and because of our past interests in using feedback of physiological events to shape movement control.[17,18] These particular interventions present an intriguing contrast. Computerized balance training is an individualized, high-technology procedure, whereas TC is a group activity that promotes socialization and requires no special equipment or space needs.[19] Computerized balance training uses force transducers embedded in platforms that detect and resolve changes in center of mass within three planes.[20-22] Indeed, these devices have been used to train patients with hemiplegia to improve standing balance.[23,24] Our results revealed that TC delayed the onset of first or multiple falls by 47.5% compared with BT or ED and also reduced the subjects' fear of falling.[25]

This finding is relevant because one of the more pervasive objectives of many geriatric therapeutic interventions is to improve or maintain "balance" in order to promote functional independence and eliminate or reduce fall-related events. An important principle underlying this approach is the need to enhance or maintain

---

SL Wolf, PhD, PT, FAPTA, is Professor and Director of Research, Department of Rehabilitation Medicine, Professor of Geriatrics, Department of Medicine, and Associate Professor, Department of Anatomy and Cell Biology, Emory University School of Medicine, Center for Rehabilitation Medicine, 1441 Clifton Rd NE, Atlanta, GA 30322 (USA) (steve@spinal.emory.edu). Address all correspondence to Dr Wolf.

HX Barnhart, PhD, is Assistant Professor, Division of Biostatistics, School of Public Health, Emory University.

GL Ellison is employed by the School of Public Health, Department of Epidemiology and Statistics, University of South Carolina, Columbia, SC 29208.

CE Coogler, ScD, PT, is Assistant Professor, Division of Physical Therapy Education, Department of Rehabilitation Medicine, and Instructor of Geriatrics, Emory University School of Medicine.

The work embodied in this presentation was made possible through Grant No. AG09124 from the National Institute on Aging, National Institutes on Health, US Public Health Service, as part of the FICSIT (Frailty and Injuries: Cooperative Studies on Intervention Techniques) Cooperative Study. All movement forms applied to elderly subjects have been approved by the Human Investigations Committee, Emory University School of Medicine.

This article was submitted August 8, 1996, and was accepted November 14, 1996.

postural stability.[26] Accordingly, the purpose of our study was to explore whether the two training interventions used at the Atlanta FICSIT site actually affected the subjects' ability to minimize postural sway under defined perturbation conditions. This exploration in older individuals is particularly relevant if successful demonstrations of postural stability are viewed as necessary precursors to reductions in falls or diminished fear of falling.

Method

Interventions

Computerized balance training provides feedback to a person who is positioned on a force platform. The resolution of outputs from several force transducers is resolved as a cursor displayed on a monitor placed in front of the subject. Targets can be placed on the screen, and through weight shifts, with or without concurrent movement from the platform on which the individual stands, progressive increases in center of pressure displacement can be explored. In our study, older participants engaged in a 15-week training session, during which they received 1 hour of instruction each week. Training progressed from standing while maintaining a stable center of mass to displacements through greater excursions with targets delineated at appropriate distances. These efforts were undertaken with eyes open and then closed. Training tasks were made more complex by including linear (maximum movement, ±2.54 cm from zero start position; speed, 10–130 seconds per cycle) and angular (maximum movement, 4° toes down and 4° toes up; speed, 4–45 seconds per 4° of tilt) displacements while subjects first maintained a stable center of mass. The subjects would subsequently try to move the cursor into appropriate targets during platform movement. These efforts were made more complex by progressively increasing the range and speed of platform excursions. A more detailed accounting of this intervention is presented elsewhere.[27] Sway data were obtained from the same device with which participants in the BT group were instructed. A device-specific training effect, therefore, could have occurred. At no time, however, did the training regimen include the instruction or task specification used in the evaluation.

Tai chi quan is a martial art that has been used in China for centuries. Within approximately the past 300 years, TC has been adapted as an exercise and practiced in Oriental cultures by people of all age groups, but notably by many older persons. There are 108 "forms" within TC. For the purpose of this study, these forms were synthesized to 10 forms so that the intervention could be successfully completed by cohorts of 12 subjects each over 15 weeks. Each cohort of the TC group met twice a week for 1 hour. The first meeting of the week was to acquaint the group with the form. The second meeting permitted individualized attention to practice and facilitate accurate movement technique. The movement elements contributing to each form became progressively more complex and required gradual increases in head, neck, and trunk rotation, with a simultaneous reduction in base of support.

An ED group was also included as a control for exercise. This group also consisted of two cohorts of 12 members each who met once a week for a 1-hour session over the course of 15 weeks. Meetings were arranged so that a variety of topics were discussed, including polypharmacy, memory loss, bereavement, sleep disturbances, falls, and other issues of importance to each group.

Although the TC group met twice a week in contrast to the weekly meetings of the BT and ED groups, the total contact time with individual participants was the same, that is, approximately 1 hour. At each meeting of the TC group, the instructor would demonstrate and review the movements to be learned. The actual contact time spent explaining and working with subjects in the TC group was comparable to the contact time the clinician experienced with each subject in the BT group each week.

Subjects

To qualify for participation in the Atlanta FICSIT trial, all subjects had to live independently and have access to a central site where all interventions were scheduled. Subjects were at least 70 years of age; free from progressively debilitating processes such as Alzheimer's or Parkinson's disease, metastatic cancer, or severe arthritis; and capable of walking across a room independently or with a cane. All subjects gave informed consent prior to participation.

The Atlanta FICSIT trial consisted of 200 eligible subjects who were randomly assigned to TC, BT, and ED groups. Among these 200 subjects, the last 72 subjects were deliberately recruited from the independent living center at Wesley Woods, a facility about 1.6 km (1 mile) from the Emory University (Atlanta, Ga) campus. For the purposes of this report, we will consider only these 72 subjects, with 24 subjects randomly assigned to each group. The reasons are as follows. First, in contrast to their predecessors in this study, these people tended to be reclusive. They did not participate in activities because of perceived limitations in mobility and were reluctant to leave their rooms other than for meals or some social events. Compared with community-dwelling older subjects who were recruited earlier in the Atlanta FICSIT study and who eagerly sought activities to enhance their lives, these 72 subjects were considerably less active. Second, with few exceptions, complete data sets on force transducer outputs were available for these 72 subjects.

Measurement Equipment

The intent of this study was to examine subtle changes in postural control that might not be detected through the more traditional measures of one-leg or tandem stance times. Accordingly, the Chattecx Balance System™* was selected to acquire postural stability measurements under defined conditions. This device contains two force plates on which an individual stands. Each force plate contains eight transducers that resolve pressure changes into x and y coordinates over 20-second intervals. Several measures can be derived from data storage. The anteroposterior displacement reflects the range of data points gathered in the y axis during efforts at maintaining totally stable posture (COB-Y). Side-to-side displacement reflects the range of data points in the x axis (COB-X). Differences in heel-toe pressure are the differences in voltage values between the posteriorly and anteriorly placed transducers in both planes. The dispersion index reflects the variability or scatter of x and y coordinates and is based on how far the points deviate from the mean center of pressure. For all three measures, the larger the values, the greater will be the displacement, pressure, or sway, respectively. All measures are expressed as voltage resolution of outputs from force transducers that manifest changes in weight distributions.

Measurement Conditions

Subjects were evaluated on the Chattecx Balance System™ before and after interventions as well as at 4-month follow-up. Testing conditions were always sequential and designated as (1) quiet standing, eyes open (condition A), (2) quiet standing, eyes closed (condition B), (3) toes up (angular perturbation of 4° over 4 seconds), eyes open (condition C), and (4) toes up, eyes closed (condition D). In each instance, data were gathered for 20 seconds and each condition was repeated three consecutive times, from which an averaged response was noted.

Data Analysis

Baseline characteristics and preintervention values of balance measures and fear of falling were compared among the three groups. Fisher's Exact chi-square test was used to determine the significance of differences for categorical variables, and the Kruskal-Wallis analysis of variance (F test) was used for continuous variables.[28] For each balance measure (dispersion, COB-X, COB-Y), under each condition, a repeated-measures analysis of covariance (ANCOVA)[29] (two times [postintervention and follow-up] × three groups) was performed to test the overall group effect and the interaction of time and group, where preintervention balance measures and baseline characteristics were used as covariates for

---

* Chattecx Corp, PO Box 489, Chattanooga, TN 37343-0489.

adjustment. In addition to the repeated-measures ANCOVA for each of the 12 balance outcome measures, a factor analysis was also undertaken to reduce the number of outcome variables to a fewer number of factor variables.[29] If the factor variables were intuitively reasonable, that is, if the grouping of factors seemed appropriate to better comprehend and interpret the data, the repeated-measures analyses were performed on the factor variables. The Tukey's method was used for pair-wise comparisons. Probability values less than .05 were considered to be significant in these analyses.

To explore the status of fear of falling in relation to balance measures, scales of the four-scale fear-of-falling questionnaire[14] (1=not at all afraid, 2=somewhat afraid, 3=fairly afraid, 4=very afraid) was combined to form a two-scale measure (1=afraid, 0=not afraid). A logistic regression model was developed to assess the odds ratios for fear-of-falling status in terms of time (preintervention, postintervention, and follow-up), group indicators, balance measures (as time-dependent variables), baseline characteristics, the interaction of time and group indicators, and the interaction of group and balance measures. The generalized estimating equation method[30] was used for parameter estimation. The variables selected for model building were baseline covariates that were significant among the three groups, variables that were known risk factors of fear of falling, and all balance measures. The final model retains all variables with probability values less than .20. The probability value of .20 was chosen because the sample size was relatively small for a dichotomous outcome variable and the goal of this analysis was exploratory. The odds ratios were computed from the final model for interpretation. Standardized residuals were examined for goodness of fit. All analyses were performed on subjects who had complete data at all three time periods for platform or fear-of-falling measurements and who had baseline characteristics used in the modeling.

Results

Baseline Characteristics

More than 40 baseline demographic data, including cognitive and quality-of-life variables, were compared among the three groups. Only a few differences among three intervention groups were observed. Table 1 displays the important baseline variables and some selected baseline variables by group. The BT group engaged in fewer volunteer activities than did the other two groups (6 subjects versus 14 subjects in the ED and TC groups, $P<.028$). The ED group had lower scores for both trails A (34.0 versus 47.3 for the BT group and 48.4 for the TC group, $P<.0003$) and trails B (92.9 versus 121.2 for the BT group and 129.1 for the TC group, $P<.00039$) tests. These tests measure visual conceptual and visuomotor

Table 1.
Baseline Demographic Characteristics[a]

Characteristic	BT (n=24) n (%)	ED (n=24) n (%)	TC (n=24) n (%)	P
Age ($\bar{X}\pm$SD)	77.7±6.5	75.2±4.9	77.7±5.6	.20
Female	19 (79.2)	22 (91.7)	19 (79.2)	.46
Live alone	12 (50.0)	11 (45.8)	13 (54.2)	.846
Volunteer	6 (25.0)	14 (58.3)	14 (58.3)	.028
MMSE score ($\bar{X}\pm$SD)	29.2±1.2	29.3±0.9	29.3±1.0	.90
CES-D score ($\bar{X}\pm$SD)	7.5±5.8	8.4±6.8	7.9±5.8	.97
Raw digit-symbol ($\bar{X}\pm$SD)	38.1±11.4	45.1±12.9	37.5±8.8	.072
Trails A score ($\bar{X}\pm$SD)	47.3±24.9	34.0±12.5	48.8±15.8	.0003
Trails B score ($\bar{X}\pm$SD)	121.2±59.9	92.9±35.5	129.1±38.0	.0039
Weight ($\bar{X}\pm$SD)	153.2±29.9	147.4±21.6	143.5±25.8	.55
Systolic blood pressure ($\bar{X}\pm$SD)	144.5±22.1	141.6±25.9	141.4±21.6	.851
Body mass index ($\bar{X}\pm$SD)	26.3±3.7	25.6±3.9	25.4±3.3	.59
Cancer, malignancy, or tumor	15 (62.5)	6 (25.0)	9 (37.5)	.027
Arthritis	17 (70.8)	15 (62.5)	18 (75.0)	.63
Medication for hypertension	13 (54.2)	11 (45.8)	11 (45.8)	.80
Cataract	13 (54.2)	9 (37.5)	14 (58.3)	.31
Fell last year	6 (25.0)	9 (37.5)	15 (62.5)	.027
Fall self-efficacy scale ($\bar{X}\pm$SD)	14.8±4.6	13.2±2.7	13.4±3.4	.613

[a] Over 23 additional characteristics were not different at baseline. BT=computerized balance training, ED=education (control), TC=tai chi, MMSE=Mini-Mental State Examination, CES-D=Center for Epidemiological Studies Depression Scale.

tracking abilities.[31] Another behavioral test, the Folstein Mini-Mental State Examination,[31] which measures cognitive mental status, and all other behavioral measures did not detect differences at baseline.

More BT group participants had been treated for cancer (15 subjects versus 6 subjects in the ED group and 9 subjects in the TC group, $P<.027$, chi-square test). Although more TC group participants had fallen within the past year (15 subjects versus 6 subjects in the BT group and 9 subjects in the ED group, $P<.027$), these differences were not reflected in baseline responses on the fear-of-falling questionnaire. Additional baseline data among many other variables, including Instrumental Activities of Daily Living Scale[32] score, Sickness Impact Profile[32] score, sleeping patterns, and alcohol intake, were not different among these groups.

Balance Measures

The factor analysis did not result in meaningful factor variables from the 12 balance measures; that is, these balance measures could not be grouped into identifiable and relevant balance variables. Thus, an ANCOVA for repeated measures for each balance measure was used for reporting. There were some differences in preintervention balance measures among the three groups. For consistency, the repeated-measures ANCOVAs (two times [postintervention and follow-up] × three groups) were all adjusted for preintervention balance measures and baseline characteristics. Tables 2 through 4 show the results for balance measures under the four testing conditions at three time points. There were time and group interactions (column 6 in Tabs. 2–4) for dispersion (condition A) and COB-X (condition C). The overall group effects were seen for the dispersion (conditions C and D), COB-X (condition C), and COB-Y (condition A) measures. The Tukey's pair-wise comparisons showed that these group effects were due mostly to the reduction in force values between the BT and TC groups and between the BT and ED groups.

In summary, the dispersions under conditions C and D were reduced substantially between the preintervention and postintervention evaluations for the BT group (condition C, 21.80 to 13.70; condition D, 35.81 to 26.66) compared with the TC group (condition C, 23.78 to 21.17; condition D, 37.81 to 38.49) and the ED group (condition C, 22.13 to 19.59; condition D, 35.03 to 33.82) ($P<.0001$, Tab. 2). Subjects in the BT group also had increased dispersion from the postintervention evaluation to the 4-month follow-up compared with the ED and TC groups for condition A (BT group, 7.44 to 8.14; ED group, 7.22 to 7.43; TC group, 9.57 to 8.30) ($P=.03$). For the COB-X measure in condition C, there was a greater decrease between the preintervention and postintervention evaluations for the BT group (4.50 to 1.07) than for the TC group (3.87 to 3.04) and the ED group (3.08 to 4.07) ($P=.02$, Tab. 3). Subjects in both the BT and TC groups started to increase the COB-X measure at follow-up, but the magnitude was larger for the TC group (3.04 to 5.40, $P=.0184$, Tab. 3). The BT group also had substantially greater reductions in COB-Y measures for conditions A (5.66 to 1.26) and B (10.75 to 5.14) compared with the TC group (condition A, 3.70 to 3.69; condition B, 12.38 to 12.86) and the ED group (condition A, 5.14 to 4.98; condition B, 12.00 to 11.04)

Table 2.
Dispersion Measures by Condition, Time, and Group[a]

Condition/Time[b]	BT Group (n=16) X̄	SD	ED Group (n=19) X̄	SD	TC Group (n=19) X̄	SD	Group P[c]	Interaction P[c]
A							.9891	.0344
Preintervention	9.37	3.35	7.46	2.06	10.50	5.05		
Postintervention	7.44	2.46	7.22	2.72	9.57	3.20		
4-month follow-up	8.14	2.59	7.43	1.86	8.30	3.15		
B							.3118	.0837
Preintervention	15.49	4.17	12.93	4.21	18.15	5.06		
Postintervention	13.97	5.70	14.85	5.40	15.42	4.48		
4-month follow-up	16.27	7.25	14.67	8.70	17.76	8.44		
C							.0001	.2681
Preintervention	21.80	6.09	22.13	5.77	23.78	6.17		
Postintervention	13.70	3.89	19.59	3.86	21.17	4.92		
4-month follow-up	14.81	4.19	18.67	18.67	21.19	6.89		
D							.0001	.4505
Preintervention	35.81	7.78	35.03	6.59	37.81	5.99		
Postintervention	26.66	9.06	33.82	6.62	38.49	6.11		
4-month follow-up	27.62	6.96	33.08	6.98	36.69	6.56		

[a] BT=computerized balance training, ED=education (control), TC=tai chi.
[b] A=quiet standing, eyes open; B=quiet standing, eyes closed; C=toes up, eyes open; D=toes up, eyes closed.
[c] Group and interaction probability values were obtained from 2×3 (two time points×three groups) analysis of covariance using preintervention and baseline characteristics as covariates.

Table 3.
Measures of Center of Balance in the X Axis by Condition, Time, and Group[a]

Condition/Time[b]	BT Group (n=16) X̄	SD	ED Group (n=19) X̄	SD	TC Group (n=19) X̄	SD	Group P[c]	Interaction P[c]
A							.4637	.5596
Preintervention	2.67	2.67	2.01	1.68	2.66	2.28		
Postintervention	1.52	1.12	2.48	2.09	3.42	3.86		
4-month follow-up	1.90	1.85	2.06	1.88	2.69	2.19		
B							.4986	.9323
Preintervention	6.98	6.10	5.08	4.96	7.92	6.18		
Postintervention	3.75	4.16	5.39	4.99	5.40	5.32		
4-month follow-up	5.63	4.27	6.41	5.58	6.78	5.70		
C							.0220	.0184
Preintervention	4.50	3.98	3.08	2.06	3.87	3.28		
Postintervention	1.07	0.62	4.07	3.14	3.04	2.18		
4-month follow-up	1.73	1.95	3.07	2.17	5.40	5.11		
D							.1890	.83619
Preintervention	8.18	5.86	5.39	3.31	6.28	5.42		
Postintervention	6.31	4.63	5.17	3.05	5.34	3.96		
4-month follow-up	7.28	5.88	6.69	3.90	5.64	5.17		

[a] BT=computerized balance training, ED=education (control), TC=tai chi.
[b] A=quiet standing, eyes open; B=quiet standing, eyes closed; C=toes up, eyes open; D=toes up, eyes closed.
[c] Group and interaction probability values were obtained from 2×3 (two time points×three groups) analysis of covariance using preintervention and baseline characteristics as covariates.

(P=.007 and P=.0572, respectively; Tab. 4). Subjects in the TC group tended to show greater dispersion and lateral motion (COB-Y) immediately after the intervention in angular perturbation conditions.

Fear of Falling

Fifty-two subjects had complete data for the fear-of-falling questionnaire and covariate values. Table 5 displays the frequency of fear of falling by group and time. There were no differences in fear-of-falling status

Table 4.
Measures of Center of Balance in the Y Axis by Condition, Time, and Group[a]

Condition/Time[b]	BT Group (n=16) X̄	SD	ED Group (n=19) X̄	SD	TC Group (n=19) X̄	SD	Group P[c]	Interaction P[c]
A							.0070	.6553
Preintervention	5.66	4.56	5.14	5.64	3.70	3.22		
Postintervention	1.26	0.93	4.98	4.07	3.69	4.48		
4-month follow-up	1.86	1.57	4.52	3.36	4.02	3.11		
B							.0572	.1869
Preintervention	10.75	6.72	12.00	12.42	12.38	8.82		
Postintervention	5.14	4.35	11.04	9.79	12.86	7.35		
4-month follow-up	5.70	4.87	6.51	7.22	9.18	7.75		
C							.3244	.3165
Preintervention	6.15	5.59	8.24	7.86	5.37	4.68		
Postintervention	2.29	2.92	6.37	3.62	6.42	6.07		
4-month follow-up	3.71	4.17	4.88	4.74	6.58	8.55		
D							.5858	.6731
Preintervention	12.61	8.60	13.38	10.92	9.13	6.19		
Postintervention	10.87	10.95	12.28	8.26	14.26	7.40		
4-month follow-up	10.91	10.51	10.32	7.41	10.92	6.22		

[a] BT=computerized balance training, ED=education (control), TC=tai chi.
[b] A=quiet standing, eyes open; B=quiet standing, eyes closed; C=toes up, eyes open; D=toes up, eyes closed.
[c] Group and interaction probability values were obtained from 2×3 (two time points×three groups) analysis of covariance using preintervention and baseline characteristics as covariates.

Table 5.
Frequency of Fear of Falling by Group and Time[a]

Time	BT Group (n=17) n (%)	ED Group (n=19) n (%)	TC Group (n=16) n (%)	P
Preintervention	10 (58.8)	11 (57.9)	9 (56.3)	.99
Postintervention	10 (58.8)	13 (68.4)	5 (31.3)	.08
4-month follow-up	10 (58.8)	11 (57.9)	9 (56.3)	.99

[a] BT=computerized balance training, ED=education (control), TC=tai chi.

between the three groups at baseline. Subjects in the TC group appeared to be less afraid immediately after intervention ($P=.08$); specifically, the responses of the subjects in the BT group did not change, two more responses in the ED group showed greater fear (13 versus 11), and four more responses in the TC group showed less fear (5 versus 9). Subjects in all three groups, however, returned toward preintervention levels by the 4-month follow-up. It should be noted that these probability values may not be real, as the correlations from repeated measurements and differences in baseline characteristics were not adjusted. Application of the logistic regression model, using generalized estimating equations, however, addresses this problem. In addition, the same subject may not have reported being "afraid" to fall at all three time points. Seventy-one percent of the subjects in the BT group reported no change in fear-of-falling status at all three time points, compared with 60% in the ED group and 44% in the TC group ($P=.27$).

The logistic regression model for repeated binary outcomes was used to fit these data, adjusting for covariates, using the generalized estimating equation approach. Table 6 presents the results from the final logistic regression model. There was no lack of fit, as determined by small standardized residuals. Living alone was positively associated with fear of falling (odds ratio=3.865, $P=.037$). Systolic blood pressure was negatively associated with fear of falling, but the magnitude was small.

To interpret the variable estimates from time-dependent covariates that interacted with each group, odds ratios were calculated by group for various comparisons in Table 7. Subjects in the TC group were less afraid of falling after the intervention compared with subjects in the BT and ED groups who had similar covariates (odds ratio=0.298 and 1.436, respectively; $P=.13$). The BT and ED groups had increased odds ratios for fear of falling

Table 6.
Logistic Regression Model for Repeated Measures of Fear of Falling Using the Generalized Estimating Equations Approach

Variables[a]	Estimator	Odds Ratio	Z Robust Score	P
Baseline covariates				
Live alone	1.352	3.865	2.09	.037
Systolic blood pressure	−0.027	0.973	−2.45	.014
Fall self-efficacy scale	0.166	1.181	1.32	.187
Time-dependent variables and variables with interaction				
COB-X in condition A	−0.310		−2.76	.006
Time 2 (postintervention) indicator	0.362		0.79	.43
Time 3 (4-month follow-up) indicator	0.091		0.18	.86
BT indicator	0.618		0.86	.39
TC indicator	0.037		0.03	.98
TC indicator×time 2 indicator	−1.574		−1.51	.13
TC indicator×time 3 indicator	−0.156		−0.18	.86
COB-Y in condition A	0.221		2.24	.025
COB-Y in condition A×BT indicator	−0.205		−1.61	.11
COB-Y in condition A×TC indicator	0.011		0.08	.94

[a] BT=computerized balance training; ED=education (control); TC=tai chi; COB-X=center of balance in x axis; COB-Y=center of balance in y axis; condition A=quiet standing, eyes open.

Table 7.
Odds Ratios for Fear of Falling for Time-Dependent Variables That Interact With Group[a]

Variables	BT Group	ED Group	TC Group	P BT Group Versus ED Group	P TC Group Versus ED Group
Preintervention	1.0	1.0	1.0		
Postintervention	1.436	1.436	0.298	NS[b]	.13
4-month follow-up	1.095	1.095	0.937	NS	NS
COB-X in condition A at preintervention	1.0	1.0	1.0		
COB-X in condition A at postintervention (one-unit decrease)	1.958	1.958	0.406	NS	.13
COB-X in condition A at 4-month follow-up (one-unit decrease)	1.493	1.493	1.278	NS	NS
COB-Y in condition A at preintervention	1.0	1.0	1.0		
COB-Y in condition A at postintervention[c] (one-unit decrease)	1.413	1.151	0.236	.11	.11
COB-Y in condition A at 4-month follow-up (one-unit decrease)	1.078	0.878	0.743	NS	NS

[a] BT=computerized balance training; ED=education (control); TC=tai chi; COB-X=center of balance in x axis; COB-Y=center of balance in y axis; condition A=quiet standing, eyes open.
[b] P=.08 for BT group versus TC group.
[c] NS=not significant at .2 level.

between the preintervention and postintervention evaluations for 1 unit of reduction in COB-X for force under condition A, but the odds ratio for fear of falling decreased to 0.406 for the TC group. On average, all subjects showed a small reduction in COB-X under condition A (Tab. 3). There was no interaction between COB-X under condition A and treatment group (Tab. 6). The odds ratio for fear of falling was 1.413 times higher immediately after intervention than before intervention for subjects in the BT group with 1 unit of reduction in COB-Y for force under condition A, but the odds ratio was 0.236 lower for the TC group (P=.08). On average, the BT group had 4.4 units of reduction in COB-Y for force under condition A from the preintervention evaluation to the postintervention evaluation, and the TC group had only 0.01 unit of reduction (Tab. 4). Thus, applying the logistic regression model (Tab. 6) yielded an odds ratio for fear of falling that was 1.34 times higher for the BT group but 0.30 times lower for the TC group, on average.

Discussion

The analyses of data for the 72 inactive older subjects selected from the Atlanta FICSIT randomized trial suggest that the 15-week computerized BT improved postural stability, as reflected in platform data output. The improvement in COB-X or COB-Y in condition A was associated with increased fear-of-falling responses in the

BT and ED groups. The 15-week TC practice did not improve postural stability, but might have reduced fear of falling. Our analyses of fear of falling, however, were based on a small sample size and the possibility of a relatively large Type I error. Further investigations are needed to confirm these exploratory findings.

Evaluation of balance often requires the application of more sophisticated clinical and computer-based tests among older individuals, regardless of whether they are active or inactive. This concern is particularly true if subjects do not have documented histories of falls or definitive pathologies contributing to postural instability. This type of evaluation is also necessary to gain insights into innovative interventions developed to reduce falls or attributes of frailty. In our study, the participants were older, represented varying degrees of independence, and participated in nontraditional treatment forms. The interventions lasted only 15 weeks, and at no time did weekly contact exceed 2 hours. We believe, therefore, that the increased stability demonstrated by the BT group is remarkable.

On first glance, these findings may not be surprising. Subjects in the BT group were trained on the same instrument with which they were tested; thus, a high degree of user familiarity was present. This explanation for improved stability is unlikely for several reasons. First, the testing situation was not included as part of the training, and subjects in the BT group were trained to increase sway. Second, if familiarization with instrumentation had been a primary factor for enhanced postural stability, then we would expect that the other two intervention groups would have shown reduced force platform measurements at repeat test intervals (postintervention and 4-month follow-up).

Coogler and Wolf[33] have reported that among 85 elderly adults, those assigned to the control group tested with the same magnitude of postural stability as subjects engaged in a sensory training balance program measured at 1 week and 4 months after completion of training. Yet, in the present study, the TC group in particular showed increased sway at the postintervention evaluation for several conditions. In contrast, Hu and Woollacott[34] studied 24 older subjects, half of whom were given training for 1 hour a day over 10 to 15 days to enhance stability. Follow-up at 1 and 4 weeks after the completion of training indicated that improved stability persisted in five of eight training conditions, as compared with the control subjects. This improvement was attributed to enhanced integration of sensorimotor function within the nervous system rather than to repetition, selected cognitive processing, or improved endurance. Although the intensity of their intervention was comparable to ours, the robustness of their subjects was probably superior, and the duration of follow-up monitoring was four times shorter. Thus, we would expect decay in their performance by 4-month follow-up as well.

Last, it could be argued that the improved stability might be unique to older people or due to increased muscle strength[34] derived from the BT group. This explanation is also unlikely because there were no baseline differences in strength among the groups[25] and similar magnitudes of stability have been demonstrated on a similar instrument after training of a younger group.[36]

The meaning underlying successful efforts to reduce sway should be viewed in a behavioral context. Therefore, changes in fear of falling responses were examined. These data were evaluated by adjusting for different baseline and time-dependent covariates. Although the impact of these interventions did not affect fear of falling profoundly, only the TC group showed some indication of less fear of falling. In addition, if it can be assumed that a change in a response on a fear-of-falling questionnaire over time indicates a change in attitude toward falls, the BT group showed the least change, with 71% of the subjects always indicating the same response, whereas only 44% of the subjects in the TC group gave the same fear responses over time.

The generalized estimating equation approach was used to fit a logistic regression model so that we might further understand the interrelationship between postural measurements and other key variables. As might be anticipated, living alone increased the odds ratio for fear of falling (odds ratio=3.865, Tab. 6), irrespective of group assignment, whereas lower systolic blood pressure readings were weakly associated with fear of falling. When assessing fear of falling by group and time (Tab. 7) after controlling for all other covariates, the limited impact of BT training became apparent. The BT and ED groups showed an odds ratio for fear of falling of 1.436 at the postintervention evaluation, compared with an odds ratio of 0.298 for the TC group. When trained to improve postural stability, the BT group increased the odds ratio for fear of falling by 1.413 at the postintervention evaluation, compared with an odds ratio of 0.236 for the TC group, for one unit of reduction in sway force in the anteroposterior direction during quiet standing (Tab. 7). Conceivably then, TC training, although promoting less fear of falling and greater sway in specific sagittal or coronal planes, may also allow subjects to feel more confident during quiet standing. Alternatively, increasing postural stability, even during the more basic task of quiet standing, following training with a computerized balance device does not ensure a change in fear of falling when other baseline covariates are controlled. Fear of falling is augmented among these subjects.

From these observations, we conclude that computerized BT, as applied in this study, enhanced postural stability measured from a force platform for participants receiving BT. These changes were not manifest in less fear of falling. These observations, when combined with the fact that BT had no impact on other psychosocial variables such as self-mastery,[25] call into question whether enhanced postural stability in older individuals is a necessary or appropriate condition to influence falling events or acquisition of behaviors that would instill confidence to successfully combat unexpected, real-life perturbations. On the other hand, the increased force transducer values noted after the intervention, which were indicative of less stability, were seen in angular perturbation conditions (dispersion and COB-Y) in the TC group. This observation would only strengthen this difference between the BT and TC groups. This difference between the groups, therefore, may have been caused by the combined enhanced stability of the BT group and the reduced stability of the TC group over time. Neither intervention had enough long-term impact on fear-of-falling responses beyond the intervention, because the odds ratios for fear of falling were virtually identical among all three groups at the 4-month follow-up (Tab. 7).

In light of the fact that TC delays onset time for falling in older individuals,[25] the potential importance of this exercise form warrants more detailed scrutiny. We know that TC emphasizes increased total body movement, particularly in rotational planes, with gradual narrowing of base of support.[35,36] Ostensibly, this movement behavior would encourage greater total body displacement capabilities. If our TC practitioners were incorporating these changes into their postural stances, enhanced sway, especially during angular displacements, would be a very real possibility. This behavior could only be manifest with practice and was seen for angular displacements at postintervention and follow-up evaluations for conditions of dispersion and COB-Y. These observations at the very least raise the intriguing notion that reduced falling events seen in TC practitioners may be associated with training to increase rather than decrease postural instability.

The fact that changes in fear-of-falling responses did not persist to follow-up for the TC group may indicate a need for a more intense or longer intervention to maintain a sense of well-being. Determining the validity of these speculations must await measurements taken from a larger sample of TC practitioners, including those who are more "active" than the subjects from which our platform data were taken.

Last, we do not know the influence that the TC instructor may have had on participant adherence with practice between instructional classes, nor do we know about the intensity of practice efforts of subjects in the TC and BT groups between intervention sessions. Approximately 40% of the subjects in the TC group, however, continued to meet weekly for TC practice after completion of the 4-month follow-up, and 30% of these subjects continued to meet weekly for TC practice 2 years after completion of this study.

Future Directions

Tai chi training may be manifest in less postural stability and more sway to dynamic perturbations. The potential value of TC as an exercise regimen should be explored. This study limited TC sessions to 15 weekly meetings covering 10 "forms." This time interval is remarkably narrow when one considers that TC is practiced among older Chinese individuals on a daily basis and becomes an integral activity much earlier in life than when our older subjects first learned this movement form.[37,38] A more detailed and extended training interval should be studied, particularly among relatively healthy elderly individuals, to assess the extent of psychosocial and physical benefits and the degree to which this exercise form is integrated into routine lifestyles. The influence that both the trainers and the practice intensity between sessions may have on these and other outcome measures also needs to be studied. Future efforts will engage several TC or BT instructors so that physiological changes can be related to the instruction. Efforts to accurately monitor intensity of practice between sessions will also be made. In this study, subjects in the TC group were given an information sheet about each form, whereas subjects in the other groups were not given this information. There is no mechanism to retrieve reliable data on the extent to which this variable affected either the "interest" of the subjects in the BT and ED groups or the intensity with which subjects in the TC group practiced.

Equally as important is the need for future investigations to systematically study the impact of a comprehensive TC intervention on the well-being of more frail, older subjects with a defined diagnosis that has immobilizing consequences.

Analyses of the present data set also suggest that computerized BT can reduce sway at rest or during perturbations with defined displacement and speed characteristics. Whether demonstrating greater postural stability is the most efficacious approach is not yet known, because the outcome did not have a favorable impact on fear of falling or other psychosocial variables.[25] Other avenues of investigation to further assess the benefits of computerized BT can be examined. Among these approaches would be (1) extending the treatment interval to greater than 15 hourly sessions, (2) stressing the limits of stability to the point of near falls as a primary treatment strategy, and (3) engaging in more dynamic movements, including progressively narrowed base of support, during the actual training.

Acknowledgments

We are indebted to Ed Dunlay, PT, of the Chattecx Corporation, who graciously provided software modifications and use of a Chattecx Balance System™ for balance training and stability measurements. The insightful and critical comments of Sandra Clements, RN, coordinator of our FICSIT study, were invaluable, as were the typing and editorial skills of Heidi Limongi, our administrative assistant. We thank Phil Miller, Director of the FICSIT Coordinating Center at Washington University School of Medicine in St Louis, for his constructive suggestions on earlier drafts of the manuscript.

References

1 Stamford BA. Exercise and the elderly. *Exerc Sports Sci Rev.* 1988;16:241–379.

2 Vallbona C, Baker SB. Physical fitness in the elderly. *Arch Phys Med Rehabil.* 1984;65:194–200.

3 Hurley O. *Safe Therapeutic Exercise for the Frail Elderly: An Introduction.* Albany, NY: Center for the Study of Aging; 1988.

4 Fletcher G, ed. *Exercise and the Practice of Medicine.* 2nd ed. Mount Kisco, NY: Futura Publishing Co Inc; 1988.

5 Fiatarone MA, Marks EC, Ryan ND, et al. High-intensity strength training in nonagenarians. *JAMA.* 1990;263:3029–3034.

6 Grimby G. Physical activity and muscle training in the elderly. *Acta Med Scand Suppl.* 1986;711:233–243.

7 Hawker M. *Geriatrics for Physiotherapists and the Allied Professions.* London, United Kingdom: Faber & Faber Ltd; 1974.

8 Harris R, Frankel LJ. *Guide to Fitness After Fifty.* New York, NY: Plenum Press; 1977.

9 Biegel L. *Physical Fitness and the Older Person.* Rockville, Md: Aspen Publishers Inc; 1984.

10 Shephard RJ. *Physical Activity and Aging.* 2nd ed. Rockville, Md: Aspen Publishers Inc; 1987.

11 Gueldner SH, Spradley J. Outdoor walking lowers fatigue. *Journal of Gerontological Nursing.* 1988;14:6–12.

12 Lowenthal DT, Wheat M, Kuffler LA. Coordinating drug use and exercise in elderly hypertensives. *Geriatrics.* 1988;43:69–80.

13 Fiatarone MA, O'Neill EF, Ryan ND, et al. Exercise training and nutritional supplementation for physical frailty in very elderly people. *N Engl J Med.* 1994;330:1769–1775.

14 Tinetti ME, Baker DI, McAvay G, et al. A multifactorial intervention to reduce the risk of falling among elderly living in the community. *N Engl J Med.* 1994;331:821–827.

15 Wolfson L, Whipple R, Derby C, et al. Balance and strength training in older adults: intervention gains and tai chi maintenance. *J Am Geriatr Soc.* 1996;44:498–506.

16 Province MA, Hadley EC, Hornbrook MC, et al. The effects of exercise on falls in elderly patients. *JAMA.* 1995;273:1341–1347.

17 Wolf SL, LeCraw DE, Barton LA, Jann BB. A comparison of motor copy and targeted feedback training techniques for restitution of upper extremity function among neurologic patients. *Phys Ther.* 1989;69:719–735.

18 Wolf SL, Segal RL. Downtraining human biceps-brachii spinal stretch reflexes. *J Neurophysiol.* 1996;75:1637–1645.

19 Wolf SL, Kutner NG, Green RC, McNeely E. The FICSIT Trials, Site 5: Emory University and the Wesley Woods Geriatric Center. *J Am Geriatr Soc.* 1993;41:329–332.

20 Nashner LM, McCollum G. The organization of human postural movements: a formal basis and experimental synthesis. *Behavior and Brain Science.* 1085;8:135–172.

21 Murray MP, Seireg AA, Sepic SB. Normal postural stability and steadiness: quantitative assessment. *J Bone Joint Surg [Am.]* 1975;57:510–516.

22 Wolfson L, Whipple R, Amerman P, Kleinberg A. Stressing the postural response: a quantitative method of teaching balance. *J Am Geriatr Soc.* 1986;34:845–850.

23 Hocherman S, Dickstein R. Platform training and postural stability in hemiplegia. *Arch Phys Med Rehabil.* 1984;65:588–592.

24 Winstein CJ, Gardner ER, McNeal DR, et al. Standing balance training: effect on balance and locomotion in hemiparetic adults. *Arch Phys Med Rehabil.* 1989;70:755–762.

25 Wolf SL, Barnhart HX, Kutner NG, et al. Reducing frailty and falls in older persons: an investigation of tai chi and computerized balance training. *J Am Geriatr Soc.* 1996;44:489–497.

26 Patla AE. A framework for understanding mobility problems in the elderly. In: Craik RL, Oatis C, eds. *Gait Analysis: Theory and Application.* St Louis, Mo: Mosby; 1995:436–449.

27 Wolf SL, Coogler CE, Green RC, Xu T. Novel interventions to prevent falls in the elderly. In: Perry HM III, Morley JE, Coe, RM, eds. *Aging and Musculoskeletal Disorders: Concepts, Diagnosis, and Treatment.* New York, NY: Springer Publishing Co Inc; 1993:178–195.

28 Fisher DL, Van Belle G. *Biostatistics: A Methodology for the Health Sciences.* New York, NY: John Wiley & Sons Inc; 1993.

29 Johnson RA, Wichern DW. *Applied Multivariate Statistical Analysis.* Englewood Cliffs, NJ: Prentice-Hall Inc; 1992.

30 Zeger SL, Liang KY. Longitudinal data analysis for discrete and continuous outcomes. *Biometrics.* 1986;42:121–130.

31 Lezak MD. *Neuropsychological Assessment.* 3rd ed. New York, NY: Oxford University Press Inc; 1995:381–384.

32 Buchner DM, Hornbrook MC, Kutner NG, et al. Development of the common data base for the FICSIT trials. *J Am Geriatr Soc.* 1993;41:297–308.

33 Coogler CE, Wolf SL. Balance training in elderly fallers and non-fallers. *Issues on Aging* (newsletter of the Section on Geriatrics, American Physical Therapy Association). 1996;19:30.

34 Hu M-S, Woollacott MH. Multisensory training of standing balance in older adults, I: postural stability and one-leg stance balance. *J Gerontol.* 1994;49:M52–M61.

35 Wolfson L, Judge J, Whipple R, King M. Strength is a major factor in balance, gait, and the occurrence of falls. *J Gerontol.* 1995;50:M64–M67.

36 Hamman RG, Mekjavic I, Mallinson AI, Longridge NS. Training effects during repeated therapy sessions of balance training using visual feedback. *Arch Phys Med Rehabil.* 1992;73:738–744.

37 Koh TC. Tai chi chaun. *Am J Chin Med.* 1995;9:15–22.

38 *Preliminary Study of Reducing Aging With Taijiquan.* Beijing, People's Republic of China: People's Sports and Exercise Publication; 1983.

Invited Commentary

This study on the effects of tai chi quan and computerized balance training on postural stability raises several important issues for physical therapists who are interested in improving balance in their patients: (1) Sway in stance is not a direct measure of functional postural stability, (2) fear of falling can affect postural strategies, and (3) balance training must be specific for the specific balance problem.

Unfortunately, the authors equate "postural stability" with a measure of sway involving excursion of forces (center of pressure) measured at the surface in stance. Measures of sway, either from surface forces or from body motion, should not be generalized into statements characterizing an individual's postural stability. *Postural stability* refers to the ability to maintain equilibrium by controlling the body's center of mass and to prevent unintentional falls.[1] As shown in this study and in other studies,[2,3] measures of body sway in stance are not accurate indicators of postural instability in daily life and are not always correlated with a tendency to fall or with the perception of instability. Measuring sway as movement of the forces at the surface can also be misleading, because these forces reflect other aspects of the body motion as well as movements of the center of body mass. If a subject sways very slowly as an inverted pendulum, movement of the center-of-pressure forces at the surface is approximately correlated with the position of the body's center of mass.[4] When sway is rapid or when the knees and the hips move, however, the excursion of the center of pressure also reflects kinematics and dynamics of body motion and not just the position of the center of mass.[5]

Standing subjects with large body sway or large body movements are not necessarily unstable. Very large and fast hip and shoulder motions in stance can be associated with very large center-of-pressure excursions but very small center-of-mass motion, and thus excellent equilibrium or stability.[6] Despite large body motions and large force excursions at the surface, people can be very stable if the projection of their center of mass onto the surface remains centered within the boundaries of their base of foot support.[7] Athletes and dancers tend to have larger-than-normal postural sway in response to surface perturbations.[8] Perhaps they have "good balance" because they are able to control their center of body mass very well over a large area of their base of support.

People who stand with very small body sway, small body movements, and small force excursions at the surface are not necessarily stable. Many elderly persons and patients with neurological impairments who have poor postural stability have a high tendency to fall, despite very small body sway in stance. For example, many patients with rigidity and bradykinesia secondary to Parkinson's disease show smaller-than-normal sway in stance and in response to surface displacements, despite their vulnerability to falling.[9,10] Their rigidity makes them stiff, and so they show less-than-normal body motion when perturbed. Their bradykinesia makes them weak and slow, so the forces they exert into the support surface result in smaller-than-normal center-of-pressure excursions in response to surface displacements. Despite their immobility in stance, however, they are quite vulnerable to falls, either spontaneously or when perturbed.

Immobility should not be confused with stability; however, it may be a natural compensation for fear of falling. This study showed that increased fear of falling in the computerized balance training group was associated with decreased sway and that decreased fear of falling in the tai chi group was associated with increased sway. Fear of falling may prevent people from moving and learning to control their center of body mass over the entire extent of their base of support and beyond, and thus reduce their sway but make them more vulnerable for a fall. Perhaps that is why balance training with tai chi quan, which emphasizes control of large center-of-mass motion, is associated with reduced fear of falling and reduced actual falls but with larger center-of-pressure sway. In contrast, computerized balance training in this study, which focused on maintaining the center of pressure within small target positions, resulted in more fear of falling but smaller center-of-pressure sway. There are other differences, however, between the two training approaches, such as the emphasis on proprioceptive and internal sense of body position and motion in tai chi quan versus the focus on visual feedback in computerized balance training. Other types of computerized balance training that emphasize control of large center-of-mass motions and attention to proprioceptive and internal cues about body motion may be as effective as tai chi quan. In any case, therapists should be concerned with fear of falling because it may affect balance performance, although it is not yet clear whether fear of falling could improve balance as well as degrade it, particularly when fear of falling is justified by postural instability.

This study supports other studies that suggest that balance training should be specific for the balance problem.[11–13] Like any other motor skill, the aspects of balance control that are practiced and trained will improve, necessarily carrying over to improvements in other aspects of balance control. It would be helpful for the authors to describe the 10 particular tai chi quan forms practiced by the subjects to try to relate specific aspects of the exercises (weight shifting, rotation, reduced base) to reduced fear of falling, reduced frequency of falls, and larger sway while maintaining stability.

Fay B Horak, PhD, PT
Senior Scientist
RS Dow Neurological Sciences Institute
1120 NW 20th Ave
Portland, OR 97209-1595

References

1 Horak FB, Macpherson JM. Postural orientation and equilibrium. In: Smith JL, ed. *Handbook of Physiology, Section 12: Exercise: Regulation and Integration of Multiple Systems*. New York, NY: Oxford University Press Inc; 1996:255–292.

2 Fernie GR, Gryfe CI, Holliday P, Llewellyn A. The relationship of postural sway in standing to the incidence of falls in geriatric subjects. *Age Ageing*. 1982;11:11–16.

3 Overstall PW, Exton-Smith AN, Imms FJ, Johnson AL. Falls in the elderly related to postural imbalance. *BMJ*. 1977;1:261–264.

4 Murray MP, Seireg A, Scholz RC. Center of gravity, center of pressure, and supportive forces during human activities. *J Appl Physiol*. 1967;23:831–838.

5 Kuo AD, Zajac FE. Human standing posture: multi-joint movement strategies based on biomechanical constraints. *Prog Brain Res*. 1993;97:349–358.

6 Horak FB. Effects of neurological disorders on postural movement strategies in the elderly. In: Vellas B, Toupet M, Rubenstein L, et al, eds. *Falls, Balance, and Gait Disorders in the Elderly*. Paris, France: Elsevier Science Publishers BV; 1992:137–151.

7 Horak FB. Clinical measurement of postural control in adults. *Phys Ther*. 1987;67:1881–1885.

8 Massion J. Movement, posture, and equilibrium: interaction and coordination. *Prog Neurobiol*. 1992;38:35–56.

9 Horak FB, Frank JS, Nutt JG. Effects of dopamine on postural control in parkinsonian subjects: scaling, set, and tone. *J Neurophysiol*. 1995;75:2380–2396.

10 Horak FB, Nutt JG, Nashner LM. Postural inflexibility in parkinsonian subjects. *J Neurol Sci*. 1995;111:46–58.

11 Konrad HR, Tomlinson D, Stockwell CW, et al. Rehabilitation therapy for patients with disequilibrium and balance disorders. *Basic Science Review*. 1994;23:105–108.

12 Shumway-Cook A, Horak FB. Rehabilitation strategies for patients with vestibular deficits. *Neurol Clin*. 1990;8:441–457.

13 Winstein CJ, Gardner ER, McNeal DR, et al. Standing balance training: effect on balance and locomotion in hemiparetic adults. *Arch Phys Med Rehabil*. 1989;70:755–762.

● Author Response

We thank Dr Horak, one of the world's outstanding authorities on posture and movement, for providing such a thoughtful commentary. Given that one important outcome rendered by commentaries and authors' responses is to provoke dialogue and creative thinking among readers, this response is crafted with that perspective in mind.

Dr Horak is most accurate when she states that what we are describing is not postural stability, but rather postural sway. We, too, view sway as a component of posture. Sway can be measured as changes in center of pressure, center of mass, or a combination thereof, and, like kinematic and electromyographic measures, sway contributes to the total picture of biped (or quadruped) stance characteristics. Therefore, sway measures should not be construed as the sole or major component of postural stability.

Where we begin to differ slightly from Horak and Macpherson's definition of postural stability[1] is the inclusion of fall behaviors. Certainly, postural stability and control over the body's center of mass are as vital to the older individual struggling for axial control in a seated reaching task as they are for an individual who has full upright weight-bearing capabilities. We prefer viewing postural stability as the development and execution of a controlled strategy that enables the individual to successfully maintain sitting, biped, and ultimately uniped positions while controlling the environment. We identify balance as the development and execution of a (successful) strategy that prevents a fall from occurring. Thus, balance is called into play during single-limb support or when biped sway becomes so large as to move both center of mass and center of pressure to the fringes of base of support. In such circumstances, the development of a stepping strategy as a protective postural response is mandatory.[2] We believe that most falls, except those associated with orthostatic hypotension on rising from a sitting, supine, or reclined position, rarely occur during biped stance in natural, nonlaboratory environments. Most falls seem to occur as trips or slips, usually in single-limb support, that is, during a step.[3]

Certainly if sway is rapid or hip and knee movements are engaged, kinetics and kinematics come into play, and not just changes in center of mass; however, in our study sway was not rapid, and all subjects were instructed to stand as steady as possible (not sway). We did not observe large truncal or shoulder motions for any of our perturbations. Tai chi involves slow, rhythmic movements with progressively decreasing bases of support with precise truncal rotation.[4] These elements as well as the specific tai chi exercise forms we used are described in detail elsewhere.[5] The tai chi progression minimized the possibility of easily centering the body's mass within a reasonable base of support. We contend that the many step-like movements subjects take in executing advanced tai chi "forms" emphasizing uniped positions are aborted falls. These advanced forms serve the purposes of destabilizing the individual in a controlled fashion, engaging new movement strategies, and facilitating the confidence level of the participant. So stability is not the issue here, but rather learning corrective strategies for instability, or what we define as balance control.

Although none of our subjects were patients, Dr Horak does identify patients, such as those with Parkinson's disease, as having poor stability and a greater tendency to fall even when body sway is minimal. Given our paradigm, we would hypothesize that training these patients to abort falls would require the use of adequate stepping strategies engaged through efforts to scale total sway excursions to the boundaries of the base of support, first in biped and ultimately in uniped fashion.

In our study, the tai chi participants reduced their fear of falling. The computerized balance training strategies did not contribute to a reduction in fear of falling nor did they augment this fear. In the Atlanta FICSIT (Frailty and Falls: Cooperative Studies on Intervention Techniques) trial, balance training did emphasize increased sway and center-of-mass displacement in a biped stance. The reality, however, is that controlled clinical studies have not demonstrated a reduction in fall behaviors or delays in fall occurrences among older individuals using balance machines. Current clinical balance training that emphasizes more pelvic and trunk rotation while manipulating visual representations of force from the platform coupled with push-wall exercises, turns during ambulation, heel-cord stretching, head rotation during ambulation, and rocking on compliant surfaces may improve such results. Therefore, cues that provide kinesthetic awareness and stress the vestibular system while providing feedback about changes in force characteristics during functional weight bearing may prove to be valuable in delaying or reversing fall behaviors.

We do not think that fear of falling could improve balance or degrade it. Rather, the reverse appears to be more appropriate. Fear can be overcome through changes in behaviors, including intrusiveness, confidence, and self-mastery.[6] The factors contributing to these changes reside in the approach, in the strategy used, and in the clinician-client interface. With respect to the last factor, investigations examing the influence of the instructor, whether for tai chi, computerized balance, or more traditional approaches, warrant further exploration.

In summary, what we wish readers and clinicians to ponder is the perception that there is a difference between learning to enhance center-of-mass or center-of-pressure movement of the limits of stability and learning controlled motions as those limits are surpassed. Certainly, cautiously progressing any posturally based intervention toward the latter should engage uniped motions, especially because this position is experienced by most older individuals when encountering falls, whether the modus operandi is a trip or a slip. For individuals with vascular hypersensitivity to sudden postural changes or with defined vestibular disease, this approach might not be as beneficial. In the interim, it is wise to recognize that the ability to control center of pressure during quiet standing or the provision of random but moderate angular perturbations after usual machine-based postural training, without integrating this training into functional activities, is not necessarily associated with an improved fear of falling or a delayed onset of fall events in older, sedentary individuals.

Steven L Wolf, PhD, PT, FAPTA
Huiman X Barnhart, PhD
Gary L Ellison
Carol E Coogler, ScD, PT

References

[1] Horak FB, Macpherson JM. Postural orientation and equilibrium. In: Smith JL, ed. *Handbook of Physiology, Section 12: Exercise: Regulation and Integration of Multiple Systems.* New York, NY: Oxford University Press Inc; 1996:255–292.

[2] McIlroy WE, Maki BE. Age-related changes in compensatory stepping in response to unpredictable perturbations. *J Gerontol.* 1996;51A: M289–M296.

[3] Sattin RW. Falls among older people: a public health perspective. *Ann Rev Public Health.* 1992;13:489–508.

[4] Wolf SL, Coogler CE, Green RC, Xu T. Novel interventions to prevent falls in the elderly. In: Perry HM, Morley JE, Coe RM III, eds. *Aging and Musculoskeletal Disorders: Concepts, Diagnosis, and Treatment.* New York, NY: Springer Publishing Co Inc; 1993:178–195.

[5] Wolf SL, McNeely E, Coogler CE, et al. Exploring the basis for tai chi quan as a therapeutic exercise approach. *Arch Phys Med Rehabil.* In press.

[6] Wolf SL, Barnhart HX, Kutner NG, et al. Reducing frailty and falls in older persons: an investigation of tai chi and computerized balance training. *J Am Geriatric Soc.* 1996;44:489–497.

Predicting the Probability for Falls in Community-Dwelling Older Adults

Background and Purpose. The objective of this retrospective case-control study was to develop a model for predicting the likelihood of falls among community-dwelling older adults. **Subjects.** Forty-four community-dwelling adults (≥65 years of age) with and without a history of falls participated. **Methods.** Subjects completed a health status questionnaire and underwent a clinical evaluation of balance and mobility function. Variables that differed between fallers and nonfallers were identified, using t tests and cross tabulation with chi-square tests. A forward stepwise regression analysis was carried out to identify a combination of variables that effectively predicted fall status. **Results.** Five variables were found to be associated with fall history. These variables were analyzed using logistic regression. The final model combined the score on the Berg Balance Scale with a self-reported history of imbalance to predict fall risk. Sensitivity was 91%, and specificity was 82%. **Conclusion and Discussion.** A simple predictive model based on two risk factors can be used by physical therapists to quantify fall risk in community-dwelling older adults. Identification of patients with a high fall risk can lead to an appropriate referral into a fall prevention program. In addition, fall risk can be used to calculate change resulting from intervention. [Shumway-Cook A, Baldwin M, Polissar NL, Gruber W. Predicting the probability for falls in community-dwelling older adults. *Phys Ther*. 1997;77:812–819.]

Key Words: *Balance, Fall prevention.*

Anne Shumway-Cook

Margaret Baldwin

Nayak L Polissar

William Gruber

Identification of older adults who are at a risk for falling is a vital medical concern. Although falls represent a health hazard to many older adults, there is mounting evidence that suggests that frequency of falls can be reduced through interventions designed to influence factors contributing to increased fall risk among older adults.[1-6]

Approximately 25% to 35% of people over the age of 65 years experience one or more falls each year.[7-9] The consequences of falls among older adults are often devastating. Among people over the age of 65 years, fall-related injuries are the leading cause of death from injury.[10,11] Forty percent of hospital admissions among people over the age of 65 years are reported to be the result of fall-related injuries, resulting in an average length of stay of 11.6 days.[12] Approximately one half of older adults hospitalized for fall-related injuries are discharged to nursing homes.[12] Falls that do not lead to injury often begin a downward spiral of fear that leads to inactivity and decreased strength, agility, and balance and that often results in loss of independence in normal activities of self-care.[4,9,13-15]

Numerous studies[2,4,9,16-20] have investigated the most likely cause or causes of falls, with varying results. Risk factors for falls have been classified as intrinsic (those related to the individual) and extrinsic (those associated with environmental features). Among the intrinsic factors, researchers[2,4,16-18] have identified decreased balance and mobility skills as very strong predictors of the likelihood for falls. Other researchers focusing on intrinsic factors have identified decreased functional skills such as moving from a sitting position to a standing position,[2,19,20] the inability to reach forward in the standing position,[18] the inability to bend over and pick up something from the ground,[4] the inability to descend stairs step over step without using a handrail,[2] and the inability to tandem walk to be important predictors of falls.[2] Lower-extremity weakness has also been reported as an important intrinsic factor found among older adults who have fallen.[3,16,17] Other intrinsic factors, including decreased vibratory sensation in the feet,[20] reduced cognitive function,[16] and prior fall history,[16,21] have also been described as predictors of falls among older adults.

An increased understanding regarding the factors contributing to falls among older adults has led to the development of a variety of fall prevention programs. The goal of fall prevention programs is to modify risk factors and thereby reduce the likelihood for future falls

---

A Shumway-Cook, PhD, PT, is Research Coordinator, Department of Physical Therapy, Northwest Hospital, 1550 N 115 St, MS H020C, Seattle, WA 98133 (USA) (ashumway@nwhsea.org). Address all correspondence to Dr Shumway-Cook.

M Baldwin, PT, is Staff Physical Therapist, Department of Physical Therapy, Providence Hospital, Everett, Wash.

NL Polissar, PhD, is Senior Consultant, Statistics and Epidemiology Research Corp, Seattle, Wash.

W Gruber, MD, is Medical Director, Safety and Gait Enhancement Program, Northwest Hospital.

This study was approved by the Institutional Review Board at Northwest Hospital.

This investigation was supported by a grant from Northwest Hospital Foundation, Seattle, Wash.

This article was submitted June 28, 1996, and was accepted January 15, 1997.

in older adults who are determined to be at high risk. For example, patients with impaired balance and mobility skills can reduce their risk for falls through appropriate exercise.[6,22,23]

A valid and reliable clinical assessment method that identifies relative risk for falls is needed for identifying those individuals who would be appropriate for referral into a fall prevention program. In addition, measures that quantify the risk of falling can potentially be used as a standard for evaluating outcomes following intervention. Thus, the purpose of this research was to develop a model to quantify fall risk among community-dwelling older adults.

Method

Subjects

The first 44 volunteers who met the study criteria were selected from among those people responding to an advertisement in a local newspaper and at local senior centers. Criteria for inclusion in the study were (1) age 65 years or older, (2) living independently in the community, (3) no neurological or musculoskeletal diagnosis that could account for possible imbalance and falls, such as a history of cerebrovascular accident, Parkinson's disease, cardiac problems, transient ischemic attacks, or lower-extremity joint replacements. Subjects were excluded if they reported serious visual or somatosensory impairments.

Subjects were classified as fallers or nonfallers. The criterion for inclusion in the faller category was a self-report of two or more falls within the 6 months prior to the study. A *fall* was defined as any event that led to an unplanned, unexpected contact with a supporting surface. We excluded falls resulting from unavoidable environmental hazards such as a chair collapsing. In addition, we excluded people who had only 1 fall within 6 months, in order to maximize the possibility of selecting a sample of older adults with recurrent falling problems. Twenty-two older adults were classified as fallers, and 22 adults were classified as nonfallers.

Procedure

After giving informed consent, all subjects completed a health status questionnaire, providing information on age, residential status, marital status, medical history, current coexisting medical conditions, self-reported history of imbalance, type of assistive device used for ambulation, and prescription medications used. All subjects completed the Mini Mental Test to determine mental status.[24] In addition, subjects completed the Balance Self-Perceptions Test, a tool used to examine subjects' perceptions regarding the degree to which balance and perceived risk for falls interfere with daily activities.[6] Subjects were asked to rate their degree of confidence (1=no confidence to 5=complete confidence) in performing 12 basic and instrumental activities of daily living without fear of loss of balance. The total score on this self-rating assessment can range from 0 to 60. Higher scores indicate the perception that balance and fear of falls do not limit performance of activities of daily living. The questionnaire is a modification of one developed by Tinetti et al[13] in their study of the relationship between fear of falling and measures of basic and instrumental activities of daily living.

Subjects then underwent a 45-minute performance-based evaluation of balance and mobility function. Balance was evaluated using the Berg Balance Scale, which rates performance from 0 (cannot perform) to 4 (normal performance) on 14 different tasks, including ability to sit, stand, reach, lean over, turn and look over each shoulder, turn in a complete circle, and step.[25] The total possible score on the Berg Balance Scale is 56, indicating excellent balance. The Berg Balance Scale has been shown to have excellent interrater reliability (.96) and relatively good concurrent validity with Tinetti's Performance-Oriented Mobility Index (.91) and Mathias' "Get Up and Go" Test (.76).[25–27]

Mobility was evaluated by asking subjects to walk 15.2 m (50 ft) at their preferred speed and then at their fastest pace. Subjects performed two trials in each condition. Subjects were timed, and mean speed was calculated for both self-paced gait speed and fast-paced gait speed. The Dynamic Gait Index[23] was used to evaluate the ability to adapt gait to changes in task demands. The Dynamic Gait Index rates performance from 0 (poor) to 3 (excellent) on eight different gait tasks, including gait on even surfaces, gait when changing speeds, gait and head turns in a vertical or horizontal direction, stepping over or around obstacles, and gait with pivot turns and steps.[23] Scores on the Dynamic Gait Index range from 0 to 24. The Dynamic Gait Index has been shown to have excellent interrater reliability (.96) and test-retest reliability (.98).[6]

Data Analysis

Histograms and descriptive statistics were calculated, using SPSS version 6 software,* to determine distributions, detect outliers, and consider the need for transformations.[28] There were no unusual distributions or outliers, and no transformations were needed.

We used *t* tests and cross tabulation with chi-square tests to determine which variables differed significantly ($P<.05$) between the fallers and the nonfallers.[29] Results from these analyses allowed the identification of individual variables from the original group of variables that

---
* SPSS Inc, 444 N Michigan Ave, Chicago, IL 60611.

have a strong association with fall history. Spearman correlations among pairs of these variables were calculated to detect similar variables as well as those that had little overlap. Even though some of the variables were dichotomous, the Spearman correlation was judged to be appropriate for assessing the strength of association among these variables. The Spearman correlation coefficient can be used with continuous or ordinal variables. Dichotomous variables are simply a special case of ordinal variables. In addition, the use of Spearman correlations allowed the results to be presented in a consistent format.

The bivariate analysis was used to identify individual variables that were predictive of falling. Because it was probable that a combination of variables would improve the prediction of being a faller, a regression analysis was also carried out to identify any combinations of variables that would be superior to any single variable for predicting fall status. We carried out logistic regression analysis using a forward stepwise procedure, with fall history as the dependent variable (0=no falls, 1=two or more falls).[30] The group of variables with strong associations with fall history were the independent variables. The regression analysis yielded a model for the probability of being in the faller group. Sensitivity and specificity in predicting fall status were calculated for this model. Sensitivity and specificity were also calculated for logistic regression models, with each of several risk factors considered separately. For the purposes of our study, *sensitivity* was defined as the percentage of fallers who were correctly classified and *specificity* was defined as the percentage of nonfallers who were correctly classified.

Results

Association of Risk Factors With Fall Classification

Fallers and nonfallers differed on 5 of 11 risk factors (Tab. 1). Analysis indicated that the two groups showed notable differences on the Berg Balance Scale, use of assistive devices, the Dynamic Gait Index, the Balance Self-Perceptions Test, and history of imbalance. Fallers tended to be more variable in their characteristics, as indicated by larger standard deviations.

Factors that showed nonsignificant differences between the two groups included age, gender, number of medications, self-paced gait speed, and fast-paced gait speed.

Correlation Among Risk Factors

The risk factors that were significantly associated with fall status were also correlated with one another. As shown in Table 2, significant Spearman correlations were found among almost all of the five clinical variables that predicted fall status. The highest correlations ($r=.76$) were found between the Dynamic Gait Index and the Balance Self-Perceptions Test and between the Balance Self-Perceptions Test and the Berg Balance Scale. The weakest and only nonsignificant correlation was found between history of imbalance and the use of an assistive device for ambulation.

Multivariate Model for Falls Classification

To construct a predictive model of fall risk, a forward stepwise logistic regression analysis was used. This procedure produces one model that is likely to be among the best predictive models for fallers, though other

Table 1.
Association of Risk Factors With Fall Classification

Risk Factor	Nonfallers (n=22)	Fallers (n=22)	P (test)
Age (y)			.2 (*t* test)
X̄	74.6	77.6	
SD	5.4	7.8	
Range	65–86	65–94	
Gender (%)			.7 (x^2)
Female	68	77	
Male	32	23	
No. of medications			.2 (*t* test)
X̄	2.2	1.7	
SD	2.9	1.5	
Range	0–11	0–4	
Mini Mental Test (% impaired)	27	45	.2 (x^2)
Assistive device (%)			.05 (x^2)
Any used	0	23	
Cane only	0	14	
Walker only	0	9	
Berg Balance Scale			.0001 (*t* test)
X̄	52.6	39.6	
SD	3.4	11.1	
Range	43–56	4–56	
Dynamic Gait Index			.001 (*t* test)
X̄	20.6	15.6	
SD	2.9	5.7	
Range	5–20	2–20	
Balance Self-Perceptions Test			.01 (*t* test)
X̄	51.4	38.8	
SD	3.4	15.1	
Range	46–60	4–56	
Self-paced gait speed (mph)			.3 (*t* test)
X̄	2.9	2.6	
SD	0.9	0.9	
Range	1.6–5.0	1.1–4.2	
Fast-paced gait speed (mph)			.1 (*t* test)
X̄	4.3	3.7	
SD	1.2	1.4	
Range	2.5–6.8	1.4–5.8	
History of imbalance (%)	41	95	.0002 (x^2)

Table 2.
Spearman Correlation Coefficients Among Risk Factors Significantly Predicting Fall Status

	Berg Balance Scale	Assistive Device	History of Imbalance	Balance Self-Perceptions Test
Assistive device	−.53[a]			
History of imbalance	−.50[b]	.24		
Balance Self-Perceptions Test	.76[a]	−.52[a]	−.60[b]	
Dynamic Gait Index	.67[a]	−.44[b]	−.46[b]	.76[a]

[a] $P \leq .001$.
[b] $P \leq .01$.

Table 3.
Logistic Regression Model for Falls

Risk Factor	Model Coefficient (SE)	P
Berg Balance Scale	−0.25 (0.10)	.01
History of imbalance	2.32 (1.17)	.05
Constant	10.46 (5.33)	.05

Table 4.
Sensitivity and Specificity of Fall Prediction From Individual Risk Factors[a]

Risk Factor	Cutoff Score	Sensitivity (%)	Specificity (%)
Berg Balance Scale	≤49	77	86
Dynamic Gait Index	≤19	59	64
Balance Self-Perceptions Test	≤50	73	82
History of imbalance	Yes	95	59
Assistive device	Yes	23	100
Berg Balance Scale and history of imbalance	++[b]	91	82

[a] Cutoff for all variables is selected to yield a predicted probability of falls of ≥0.5.
[b] ++=history of imbalance was "no" and Berg Balance Scale score was ≤42 or history of imbalance was "yes" and Berg Balance Scale score was ≤51.

models are possible. The variables considered for this model were determined from the analysis of individual risk factors for falls and were the variables shown in Table 1 with probability values of $P<.05$. The variables that were considered were the Berg Balance Scale, the Dynamic Gait Index, the Balance Self-Perceptions Test, history of imbalance, and use of an assistive device.

The final model, shown in Table 3, included both the Berg Balance Scale and history of imbalance (coded as 0 for no history of imbalance and as 1 for a positive history of imbalance within the previous 6 months). The model is related to the probability of falling by the following equation:

Probability = 100% × exp(10.46 − 0.25 × Berg Balance Scale score + 2.32 × history of imbalance score)/[1 + exp(10.46 − 0.25 × Berg Balance Scale score + 2.32 × history of imbalance score)]

This model, for example, would predict that an individual with no history of imbalance (coded as 0) and a score of 54 on the Berg Balance Scale would have a predicted probability of falling of 5%. In contrast, an individual with a history of imbalance (coded as 1) and a Berg Balance Scale score of 42 would have a predicted probability of falling of 91%.

To further evaluate the model, we examined the sensitivity and specificity using the predicted probability of falls compared with the observed fall status of our sample. The cutoff value that jointly maximized both sensitivity and specificity was a predicted probability of 0.5 or larger used to designate a faller. With this cutoff value, sensitivity was 91% (20/22 fallers were correctly classified) and specificity was 82% (18/22 nonfallers were correctly classified).

Choosing a Clinical Test to Identify and Monitor Fall Risk in a Geriatric Population

Several of the risk factors had good sensitivity and specificity for predicting falls. Table 4 illustrates the sensitivity and specificity of fall risk associated with individual clinical measures as well as for the final model developed from stepwise logistic regression. Shown are the four clinical variables that were found to be predictors of fall risk. The cutoff score that corresponds to the probability value of 0.5 is also shown. We used the models for each risk factor to classify subjects as fallers or nonfallers, again choosing a predicted probability of 0.5 or larger to designate fallers. Based on this designation, we calculated sensitivity and specificity for each risk factor and its associated logistic regression model. For example, a score of 49 or less on the Berg Balance Scale corresponded to a predicted probability of 0.5 or larger, and it correctly classified 77% of people with a positive history of falls (sensitivity) and 86% of people who did not have any history of falls (specificity). A score of 19 or less on the Dynamic Gait Index correctly classified 59%

of those with a history of falls, while correctly classifying 64% of those without a positive fall history. As shown in Table 4, the optimal balance between sensitivity and specificity occurs when the Berg Balance Scale score is combined with history of imbalance.

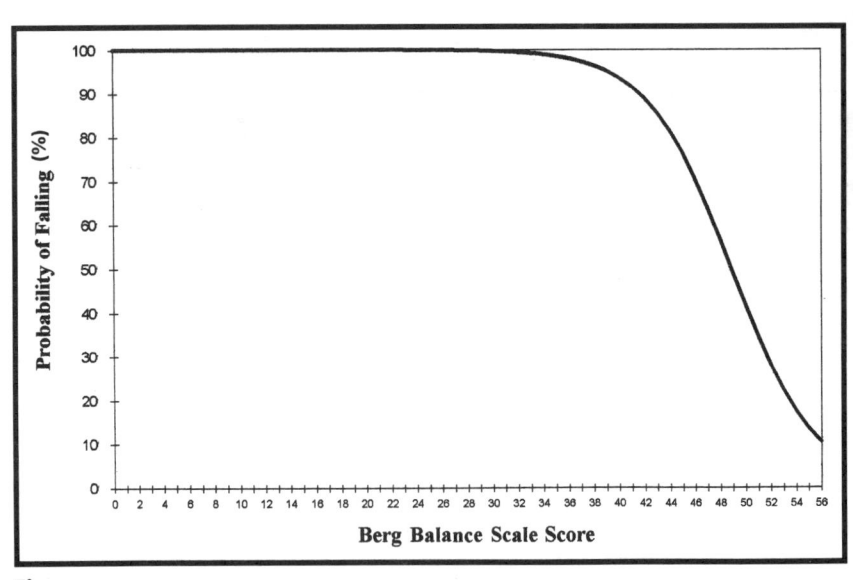

The Berg Balance Scale appears to be the best single predictor of fall status (Tabs. 1 and 4). The predicted probability for falls as a function of the Berg Balance Scale score is plotted in the Figure. The results show that declining Berg Balance Scale scores were associated with increasing fall risk. This relationship, however, was nonlinear. In the range of 56 to 54, each 1-point drop in the Berg Balance Scale scores was associated with a 3% to 4% increase in fall risk. In the range of 54 to 46, a 1-point change in the Berg Balance Scale scores led to a 6% to 8% increase in fall risk. Below the score of 36, fall risk was close to 100%, and further declines in the Berg Balance Scale scores added little to the already extremely high fall risk. Thus, a 1-point change in the Berg Balance Scale score can lead to a very different predicted probability for a fall, depending on where the baseline score is in the scale.

Figure.
Predicted probability for falls as a function of the Berg Balance Scale score.

Discussion

The purpose of this research was to develop a model for quantifying fall risk among community-dwelling older adults. The need to accurately and reliably quantify fall risk is based on the assumption that such a measure is essential to the appropriate referral of individuals at high risk into a fall prevention program. We believe that a valid and reliable measure of fall risk could also be used as an outcome measure for interventions designed to reduce an individual's risk for falls. In this case, the effect of the intervention could be assessed by the decrease in the estimated probability of falling from before to after the intervention.[6]

Eleven factors were originally considered as possible predictors of fall risk, based on a review of the literature. These factors included a range of demographic, medical, self-report, and performance measures related to balance function. An analysis of individual factors identified 5 variables that were significantly related to fall risk: the Berg Balance Scale score, the Dynamic Gait Index score, the Balance Self-Perceptions Test score, history of imbalance, and type of assistive device used for ambulation. Our results did not show that age, gender, or number of medications used predicted fall risk. Thus, our results are not completely consistent with the findings of other researchers who have reported that specific chronic diseases, health-related behaviors, age, and gender are predictive of fall risk in community-dwelling older adults.[4,31,32]

We found strong correlations among the clinical performance-based measures. This finding is not surprising, considering that all of these measures are purported to measure some aspect of balance and mobility function. This finding is consistent with data from other researchers who have reported strong correlations among commonly used clinical tools used to evaluate balance and mobility function in older adults.[33–35] We also found a strong correlation between the performance-based measures and our self-report measure, which is consistent with previous research.[13,33,36] These strong correlations suggest that some assessment measures can be used interchangeably for the purpose of assessing fall risk.

Our analysis demonstrated that the model with the best sensitivity and specificity included two factors: a performance-based measure of balance (the Berg Balance Scale) and a self-report measure of imbalance history (scored as "yes" or "no"). This model had a sensitivity of 91% and a specificity of 82%. Thus, 20 of the 22 fallers were correctly classified, and 18 of the 22 nonfallers were correctly classified. The sensitivity and specificity of this model were superior to any of the clinical variables used in isolation. The single variable that had the next best values of sensitivity and specificity was the Berg Balance Scale. The values of sensitivity and specificity for all models presented here are likely to be higher than those encountered when the predictive models are applied to a new population. This is a general phenomenon that occurs when models are developed on one data set and then applied to new data.

Understanding the meaning of an individual score on a clinical test is greatly enhanced by the ability to relate that score to relevant and meaningful events in a patient's life. The logistic regression model used in our study provides a link between performance on the Berg Balance Scale and risk for falls. Based on this model, the predicted probability for falls increases as the Berg Balance Scale scores decrease in a nonlinear relationship. A score of 56 on the Berg Balance Scale is associated with a 10% predicted probability of falls. As the Berg Balance Scale scores decrease, the predicted probability of falls rapidly increases. A score of 40 or lower is associated with a fall risk of nearly 100%. The model used in our study allows the quantification of relative fall risk. Rather than presenting fall risk as a categorical variable (faller versus nonfaller), the model allows the determination of a gradient of risk from 0 (low risk) to 100 (high risk). This feature of the model increases its value as a measure of change following intervention, because it allows the detection of a relatively small but clinically relevant change in fall risk.

The results of our study suggest that patients who score high on the Berg Balance Scale have a relatively low fall risk and should probably not be referred for further intervention. In contrast, patients who score 40 or less have a high probability for falls and are therefore appropriate for referral into a program designed to improve balance and mobility function and to reduce fall risk. The decision to refer a patient for therapy, however, is complex, often reflecting more factors than just the probability for falls. Individuals who live in their own home without the help and assistance of others and who perceive that their balance and mobility skills are declining may be referred for therapy even though they have a Berg Balance Scale score that is associated with a relatively low probability for falls. The potential consequences of not treating these individuals are great, because a fall leading to a fracture can result in a loss of independence, an extended stay in a skilled nursing facility, and in some cases death.[37–39]

Limitations of the Study
We examined variables that predict probability for falls among a small number of community-dwelling adults aged 65 years and older. The application of this research to individuals living in a skilled nursing facility or to individuals below the age of 65 years would be speculative. In addition, this study was carried out on volunteers. Had subjects been drawn at random from the community, the results might have been different.

Clinical Implications
The growing realization of the personal and economic costs of falls has led to the development of programs designed to reduce the frequency of falls and fall-related injuries among older adults. Because declining balance and mobility function are major factors leading to falls, an important emphasis in physical therapy is the development of interventions that are effective in improving balance and mobility function as a method for decreasing fall risk. As demand for these programs increases, there will be an accompanying need for assessments that effectively identify those individuals who are at risk for falls and that can measure outcomes associated with these programs. This preliminary study has shown a promising method for quantifying fall risk. Results from this initial study need to be confirmed with a larger community-based population.

Conclusions
Falls are a major health problem among elderly people. This research has developed a simple predictive model based on two risk factors that can be used by physical therapists to quantify fall risk in community-dwelling older adults. Assessing fall risk would allow the identification of individuals who would likely benefit from services designed to reduce the risk for further injurious falls. Reducing subsequent frequency of falls and fall-related injuries can result in a significant decrease in health-related costs, an essential consideration in the current managed health care environment.

References
1 Tinetti ME, Baker DI, McAvay G, et al. A multifactorial intervention to reduce the risk of falling among elderly people living in the community. *N Engl J Med.* 1994;331:821–827.

2 Studenski S, Duncan PW, Chandler J, et al. Predicting falls: the role of mobility and nonphysical factors. *J Am Geriatr Soc.* 1994;42:297–302.

3 Guralnik JM, Ferrucci L, Simonsick EM, et al. Lower-extremity function in persons over the age of 70 years as a predictor of subsequent disability. *N Engl J Med.* 1995;332:556–561.

4 O'Loughlin JL, Robitaille Y, Boivin JF, et al. Incidence of and risk factors for falls and injurious falls among the community-dwelling elderly. *Am J Epidemiol.* 1993;137:342–354.

5 Koch M, Gottschalk M, Baker DI, et al. An impairment and disability assessment and treatment protocol for community-living elderly persons. *Phys Ther.* 1994;74:286–298.

6 Shumway-Cook A, Gruber W, Baldwin M, Liao S. The effect of multidimensional exercise on balance, mobility, and fall risk in community-dwelling older adults. *Phys Ther.* 1997;77:46–57.

7 Tinetti ME, Ginter SF. Identifying mobility dysfunctions in elderly patients: standard neuromuscular examination or direct assessment? *JAMA.* 1988;259:1190–1193.

8 Tinetti ME, Speechley M, Ginter SF. Risk factors for falls among elderly persons living in the community. *N Engl J Med.* 1988;319:1701–1707.

9 Nevitt MC, Cummings SR. Risk factors for recurrent non-syncopal falls: a prospective study. *JAMA.* 1989;261:2663–2668.

10 Kanten DN, Mulrow CD, Gerety MB, et al. Falls: an examination of three reporting methods in nursing homes. *J Am Geriatr Soc.* 1993;41:662–666.

11 *Accident Facts and Figures.* Chicago, Ill: National Safety Council; 1987.

12 Sattin RW, Lambert H, Devito CA, et al. The incidence of fall injury events among the elderly in a defined population. *Am J Epidemiol.* 1990;131:1028–1037.

13 Tinetti ME, Mendes de Leon CF, Doucette JT, Baker DI. Fear of falling and fall-related efficacy in relationship to functioning among community-living elders. *J Gerontol.* 1994;49:M140–M147.

14 Tinetti ME, Liu WL, Claus EB. Predictors and prognosis of inability to get up after falls among elderly persons. *JAMA.* 1993;269:65–70.

15 Inouye SK, Wagner DR, Acampora D, et al. A predictive index for functional decline in hospitalized elderly medical patients. *J Gen Intern Med.* 1993;8:645–652.

16 Brians LK, Alexander K, Grota P, et al. The development of the RISK tool for fall prevention. *Rehabilitation Nursing.* 1991;16:67–69.

17 Tinetti ME. Factors associated with serious injury during falls by ambulatory nursing home residents. *J Am Geriatr Soc.* 1987;35:644–648.

18 Duncan PW, Studenski S, Chandler J, et al. Functional reach: predictive validity in a sample of elderly male veterans. *J Gerontol.* 1992;47:M93–M98.

19 Campbell AJ, Borrie MJ, Spears GF. Risk factors of falls in a community-based prospective study of people 70 years and older. *J Gerontol.* 1989;44:M112–M117.

20 Lipsitz LA, Jonsson PV, Kelley MM, et al. Causes and correlates of recurrent falls in ambulatory frail elderly. *J Gerontol.* 1991;46:M114–M122.

21 Schmid MA. Reducing patient falls: a research-based comprehensive fall prevention program. *Mil Med.* 1990;155:202–207.

22 Province MA, Hadley EC, Hornbrook MC, et al. The effects of exercise on falls in elderly patients: a preplanned meta-analysis of the FICSIT trials. *JAMA.* 1995;273:1341–1347.

23 Shumway-Cook A, Woollacott MH. *Motor Control: Theory and Practical Applications.* Baltimore, Md: Williams & Wilkins; 1995.

24 Pfeiffer E. Short portable mental status questionnaire. *J Am Geriatric Soc.* 1975;23:433–441.

25 Berg KO, Wood-Dauphinee SL, Williams JT, et al. Measuring balance in the elderly: validation of an instrument. *Can J Public Health.* 1992;83:S7–S11.

26 Berg KO, Wood-Dauphinee SL, Williams JT, et al. Measuring balance in the elderly: preliminary development of an instrument. *Physiotherapy Canada.* 1989;41:304–311.

27 Berg KO, Maki BE, Williams JI, et al. Clinical and laboratory measures of postural balance in an elderly population. *Arch Phys Med Rehabil.* 1992;73;1073–1080.

28 *SPSS for Windows: Advanced Statistics, Release 6.0.* Chicago, Ill: SPSS Inc; 1993.

29 Fisher LD, Van Belle G. *Biostatistics: A Methodology for the Health Sciences.* New York, NY: John Wiley & Sons; 1993.

30 Tabachnick BG, Fidell LS. *Using Multivariate Statistics.* 2nd ed. New York, NY: HarperCollins Publishers; 1989.

31 Gurlanik JM, Ferrucci L, Simonsick E, et al. Lower-extremity function in persons over the age of 70 years as a predictor of subsequent disability. *N Engl J Med.* 1995;332:556–561.

32 Sager MA, Rudberg MA, Jalaluddin M, et al. Hospital admission risk profile (HARP): identifying older patients at risk for functional decline following acute medical illness and hospitalization. *J Am Geriatr Soc.* 1996;44:251–257.

33 Cress ME, Schechtman KB, Mulrow CD, et al. Relationship between physical performance and self-perceived physical function. *J Am Geriatr Soc.* 1995;43:93–101.

34 Gurlanik J, Simonsick EM, Ferrucci L, et al. A short physical performance battery assessing lower extremity function associated with self-reported disability and prediction of mortality and nursing home admission. *J Gerontol.* 1994;49:M85–M94.

35 Harada N, Chiu V, Damron-Rodriguez JA, et al. Screening for balance and mobility impairment in elderly individuals living in residential care facilities. *Phys Ther.* 1995;75:462–469.

36 Myers AM, Holliday P, Harvey K, et al. Functional performance measures: Are they superior to self-assessments? *J Gerontol.* 1993;48:M196–M206.

37 Sattin RW. Falls among older persons: a public health perspective. *Annu Rev Public Health.* 1992;13:489–508.

38 Murphy J, Isaacs B. The post-fall syndrome: a study of 36 elderly patients. *Gerontology.* 1982;28:265–270.

39 Marottoli RA, Berkman LF, Cooney LM. Decline in physical function following hip fracture. *J Am Geriatr Soc.* 1992;40:861–866.

The Individualized Treatment of a Patient With Benign Paroxysmal Positional Vertigo

The purpose of this case report is to describe the evaluation and treatment of a patient with vertigo. The patient was a 32-year-old male carpenter with a 17-year history of episodic vertigo that occurred when his neck was in the extended position while positioned supine and during walking. His medical and physical therapy evaluative findings were consistent with a diagnosis of benign paroxysmal positional vertigo (BPPV). He was treated with an individualized home exercise program of eye movement exercises, Brandt/Daroff exercises, and general conditioning exercises. Twenty-four days from the start of physical therapy, the patient was free of symptoms even when his neck was in the extended position. [Ford-Smith CD. The individualized treatment of a patient with benign paroxysmal positional vertigo. *Phys Ther.* 1997;77:848–855.]

Key Words: *Benign paroxysmal positional vertigo, Brandt/Daroff exercises, Dizziness, Vertigo.*

Cheryl D Ford-Smith

Vertigo, the false perception of motion,[1] can be a debilitating and annoying impairment, causing patients to seek medical assistance. Patients with vertigo often are referred for physical therapy without a clear differential diagnosis. Therefore, a thorough physical therapy evaluation is essential to designing an effective treatment plan.

One of the most common causes of vertigo in adults is benign paroxysmal positional vertigo (BPPV).[2] *Benign paroxysmal positional vertigo* is defined as vertigo induced by rapid extension of the head or lateral tilt of the head toward the affected ear.[2] One hypothesized cause of BPPV is "cupulolithiasis," a term coined by Schuknecht[3] to describe a labyrinthine disorder that previously had been called "positional vertigo." Schuknecht's description came after postmortem histological studies of the temporal bones of two persons who previously had been diagnosed with unilateral BPPV. The examination revealed basophilic deposits on the cupula of the posterior canal (Figure) of the affected labyrinth. In most cases, the deposits are thought to be disrupted otoconia (calcium carbonate crystals) from the utricular membrane that settle on the cupula of the posterior semicircular canal.[3] The deposits located on the cupula had a higher specific gravity than the specific gravity of the surrounding endolymph, creating an imbalance. Normally, the cupula and the endolymph have the same specific gravity. The deposits on the cupula create an oversensitivity of the posterior canal to angular acceleration in the plane specific to the canal.[4] When the head is placed in the provoking position (eg, head extension), the cupula deflects abnormally, causing nystagmus (nonvoluntary rhythmic oscillation of the eyes[5(pp115–116)]), vertigo, and nausea. The latency of the onset of vertigo and nystagmus is thought to be related to the amount of time required to deflect the cupula.[3] The fatigability (this sensation of vertigo diminishes and stops within 60 seconds) may be due to the dispersement of the deposits into the endolymph and a return of the cupula to its upright position. The patient, therefore, avoids the provoking position to prevent the onset of vertigo and nausea.

This case report describes the decision-making process in the treatment of a patient with a vestibular disorder.

Benign paroxysmal positional vertigo is diagnosed based on the patient's history and the characteristic clinical findings.[3,6] Clinical manifestations of BPPV include (1) vertigo that is induced when the patient is placed in a supine position with the head turned to one side and extended approximately 30 degrees below the horizontal, (2) vertigo that has a delayed onset of 1 to 40 seconds and that eventually stops once the patient is in the provoking position, (3) the presence of torsional nystagmus that coincides with the latency and duration of the complaint of vertigo, and (4) vertigo that rises to a plateau of intensity and then gradually decreases, subsiding within 60 seconds.[6] Seventy percent of individuals experience spontaneous recovery within weeks or months. The condition, however, can persist for years, if untreated, or it can remit and recur after varying periods of time in 20% to 30% of individuals.[2] About 10% of individuals with BPPV can have symptoms bilaterally, but the time of onset, duration, and intensity of symptoms can be different for each side.[2]

CD Ford-Smith, PT, is Assistant Professor, Department of Physical Therapy, School of Allied Health Professions, Medical College of Virginia, Virginia Commonwealth University, PO Box 980224, Richmond, VA 23298-0224 (USA) (cfordsmith@gems.vcu.edu).

This article was submitted September 3, 1996, and was accepted February 24, 1997.

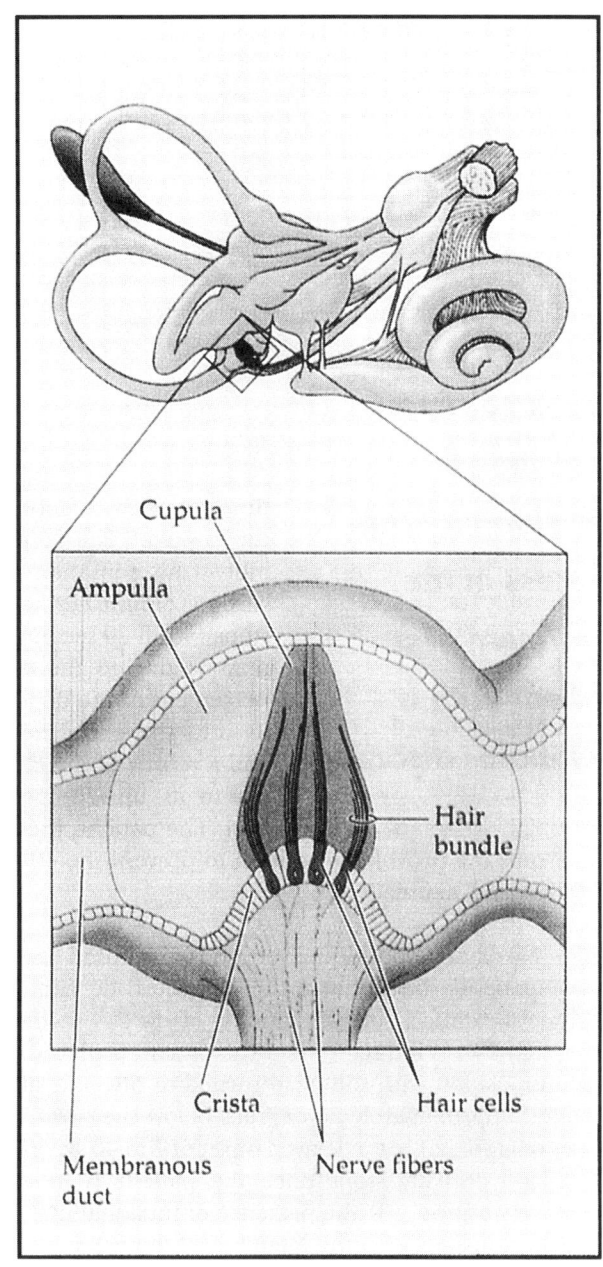

Figure.
The ampulla of the posterior semicircular canal showing the crista, hair bundles, and cupula. (Adapted by permission from Purves D, Augustine GJ, Fitzpatrick D, et al. *Neuroscience*. Sunderland, Mass: Sinauer Associates Inc; 1996.)

Brandt/Daroff exercises[7] often are used for the treatment of BPPV.[8] The exercises are based on the etiology of cupulolithiasis. The goal of this mechanical form of therapy is to dislodge and disperse the otolithic material from the cupula of the posterior canal. In 1980, Brandt and Daroff[7] described the treatment of 67 subjects who demonstrated the classical signs and symptoms of BPPV, as described by Schuknecht.[3] Subjects were 37 to 74 years of age, and symptom duration ranged from 2 days to 8 months. Each subject in the study was seated and assumed a side-lying position on the affected side until the induced vertigo ceased. The subject returned to a sitting position for 30 seconds and then assumed a side-lying position on the opposite side for 30 seconds. Subsequently, each subject repeated the positioning every 3 hours while awake and discontinued the exercises after the subject experienced 2 consecutive days of exercise without vertigo. Sixty-six of the 67 subjects were reported to be completely recovered within 3 to 14 days of initiating treatment, with absence of both vertigo and nystagmus when assuming the provoking head positions. Two of the 66 subjects experienced a recurrence after a few months that responded to a second session of positional therapy. The authors did not describe the characteristics of the reoccurrences or the time frames for each subject's symptoms to once again remit. The subjects were followed at varying intervals over a period of 3 years.

Horak and colleagues[9] examined the effectiveness of three treatment approaches: an individualized vestibular rehabilitation program, a general conditioning exercise program, and a vestibular suppressant medication program. Each treatment program was administered over a period of 6 weeks. Twenty-five subjects with peripheral vestibular disorders and positional or movement-related dizziness and imbalance were randomly assigned to one of the three treatment groups. In the vestibular rehabilitation group, a physical therapist designed individual exercises to deal with each subject's particular combination of problems. The vestibular habituation exercises addressed six domains: (1) position habituation training, (2) sensory or balance retraining, (3) gaze stabilization, (4) general conditioning exercises designed to address dizziness, (5) balance and gaze stability, and (6) therapeutic intervention for secondary impairments. Subjects in all three treatment groups exhibited improvement in symptoms, with the greatest improvement being demonstrated in the vestibular rehabilitation group. The authors concluded that the individualized vestibular rehabilitation approach resulted in both improved balance and reduction in vertigo in patients with chronic peripheral vestibular disorders. The purpose of this case report is to describe the evaluation and individualized treatment, including the use of Brandt/Daroff exercises, of a patient with vertigo who was referred for physical therapy.

Patient Description

The patient was a 32-year-old male carpenter with a complaint of dizziness or heavy-headedness. The patient reported having episodes of dizziness when lying under a cabinet with his neck extended and looking up, reaching overhead with his neck extended, looking up and extending his neck while walking down a store aisle, being awakened at night when turning over in bed, and engaging in physical exercise such as jogging. These episodes of dizziness resulted in poor job performance and occasional nights of interrupted sleep. In his description of an episode, he said that the room seemed to spin around and that he had a feeling of being off balance. He reported having this problem for 17 years, following a motorcycle accident that caused an ankle fracture. He was wearing a helmet at the time of the accident.

The patient previously had used scopolamine ear patches (Transderm Scōp® transdermal therapeutic system[*]) intermittently to relieve the symptoms of dizziness. Scopolamine is used for the prevention of nausea and vomiting related to motion sickness.[10] It is administered via an adhesive disk that is placed behind the ear, over the mastoid process, several hours before a person travels. The patch is reported to be more effective if worn prior to having an episode of dizziness.[9] The patient used this medication as needed, but found it to be relatively ineffective in stopping his episodes of dizziness when his neck was extended. He was taking no medication prior to or during the initial physical therapy evaluation session and had never received physical therapy for his problem. The goals of therapy were (1) for the patient to be free of dizziness when his neck was extended in a supine position or during walking and when turning over in bed and (2) for the patient to be able to resume jogging on a regular basis.

Medical Examination

Prior to being seen for physical therapy, the patient underwent an examination by the audiologist in the Department of Otolaryngology at Virginia Commonwealth University, Medical College of Virginia Campus. The patient received electronystagmography, which is a battery of tests using electrodes around the eyes to quantitatively assess vestibular function. The battery includes ocular motility testing, bithermal caloric testing, and positional testing.[11] The test battery is capable of determining the function of the peripheral vestibular system of the left and right ears separately. Physical therapy is focused on the involved ear.

Ocular motility testing was used to identify neurological lesions. The patient was asked to follow a moving target while quantitative recordings were made of eye movements. Eye velocity and target velocity should demonstrate a 1:1 ratio. The patient demonstrated no spontaneous nystagmus, and his ocular motility was within normal limits. Electronystagmography, however, is considered to be less sensitive than direct visual inspection, so examination of eye movements during the physical therapy evaluation is an important component.[5(p119)]

During caloric testing, each ear is irrigated with warm or cool water. In the normal ear, the stimulus produces nystagmus and may produce vertigo, nausea, and vomiting; the response is absent or diminished in the involved ear. Warm irrigation of the patient's left ear produced a normal response, but there are no comparative data for the right ear. The patient refused to continue with caloric testing following initial irrigation of the left ear because he feared it would provoke his symptoms of vertigo in the right ear. A disadvantage of caloric testing is that because the test simulates only one frequency of head rotation and gives only information about the horizontal canal, the examiner is unable to infer the condition of the entire membranous labyrinth.

Positional testing was performed in five different positions while eye movements were recorded via the electrodes. The positions were sitting, right and left side lying, supine, and supine head-hanging (the patient was rapidly taken from a long sitting position to a supine position with the head rotated to the right or left side and hanging 30°–45° below the horizontal). The patient reported extreme dizziness in the supine position with the head turned to the right and in the head-hanging position with the head rotated to the right. The audiologist reported noting some dizziness in the left side-lying position and in the supine position with the head turned to the left, but no nystagmus occurred and dizziness was not as severe.

In summary, the patient had a normal response to caloric testing of the left ear (which would indicate that the left horizontal canal was not involved), a normal response to ocular motility testing, and an abnormal response to positional testing on the right side, with mild dizziness noted in the left ear-down position. The findings would indicate possible bilateral vestibular system involvement, but the caloric testing was incomplete.

Physical Therapy Examination

A physical therapy evaluation was performed to substantiate the diagnosis of BPPV, to determine vestibular ocular reflex (VOR) function, and to rule out loss of muscle performance or joint range of motion, which could contribute to the patient's feeling being off-balance. Bilateral gross muscle performance testing[12] of the major muscle groups of the shoulders, elbows, wrists, hands, hips, knees, and ankles yielded muscle test grades of greater than fair (ie, normal limb strength). Active range of motion was within normal limits for the shoulders, elbows, wrists, hips, knees, and ankles. Eye movements were visually inspected in the vertical and horizontal directions. Smooth-pursuit eye movements[13(p158)] (characterized by the ability to track a moving target with the eyes while the head is stationary) and saccadic eye movements[13(p110)] (characterized by the ability to rapidly

---

[*] CIBA Consumer Pharmaceuticals, Div of CIBA-GEIGY Corp, 581 Main St, Woodbridge, NJ 07095.

redirect the line vision with the head stationary) exhibited no slowing and no spontaneous nystagmus or provoked symptoms of vertigo. Testing of the VOR in the vertical and horizontal directions produced symptoms of vertigo, with evidence of right-beating horizontal nystagmus (eye movements with a fast component to the right side and a slow component to the left side), implicating right-sided vestibular involvement. The VOR was tested by asking the patient to focus on a stationary target (such as the top of a pen) held at a distance of an arm's length from the eyes while shaking the head side to side, then up and down. The examiner observes the eye movements for accuracy (eye movements equal to head movements), speed, and nystagmus. The VOR enables an individual to maintain a steady stationary image on the retina during head movements.

Positional testing was performed using the Hallpike-Dix maneuver.[14] The patient was placed in a long sitting position on the treatment table with the head turned to one side and the patient's gaze focused on the examiner's forehead. The examiner held the patient's head and rapidly moved the patient into a supine position with the head hanging 30 degrees below the horizontal. The patient was monitored for the onset latency and duration of vertigo, in addition to nystagmus that usually dissipates within 60 seconds. The vertigo and nystagmus usually coincide for both time of onset and duration after the onset. The time of onset and duration of vertigo were not recorded initially because the patient struggled to return to a sitting position immediately after the onset of his symptoms. A modified Hallpike-Dix maneuver was positive with head turning to the right and left, provoking vertigo bilaterally. Nystagmus was difficult to evaluate due to the patient's apprehension and eye blinking. The patient reported that symptoms were more severe on the right side than on the left side. A modified Hallpike-Dix maneuver was used because the patient would not allow his neck to be extended farther than approximately 10 degrees below the horizontal on each side while positioned supine.

As part of the initial evaluation, the patient received dynamic posturography on the Equitest System† in the Physical Therapy Department at the Medical College of Virginia Hospitals. The Equitest System has been extensively described in a previous publication.[15] The Equitest System has two test protocols to examine standing balance: the Sensory Organization Test (SOT) and the Motor Control Test. The SOT protocol has six sensory conditions designed to assess the patient's ability to make effective use of visual, vestibular, and proprioceptive inputs, as well as the patient's ability to suppress inaccurate sensory information required to maintain standing balance. The patient received a computer-generated SOT composite equilibrium score of 82 out of a possible 100 points. Scores near 100 indicate maintenance of upright position with no anterior or posterior excursion. When compared with the performance of age-matched controls, the patient's performance was judged to be normal. The mean composite score for individuals aged 20 to 59 years is 80.[16] The patient was able to maintain a standing position in all six sensory conditions. Patients with BPPV will usually have normal equilibrium scores because their symptoms are caused by neck extension and lateral tilt of the head. During the test, the head is held in midline.

The Motor Control Test consists of a series of linear and rotational platform translations. It assesses the patient's ability to generate force, scale responses to meet the amplitude of the perturbation, and coordinate movement in standing to maintain the center of mass over the base of support. When compared with the performance of age-matched controls, the patient's performance was consistent with normal latency to response and amplitude scaling during forward and backward platform translations. During upward and downward platform rotations, he demonstrated the ability to maintain the upright position. I concluded that the patient's history, medical laboratory test findings, and physical therapy findings of a normal SOT, normal limb strength and active range of motion, abnormal response to VOR testing, and a positive Hallpike-Dix maneuver were consistent with the diagnosis of bilateral BPPV.

Course of Treatment
The patient was given a home exercise program of eye movement exercises to enhance vestibular adaptation and visual-vestibular interaction during movement of the head, along with Brandt/Daroff exercises. The patient was given eye movement exercises because of his decreased VOR response during head movements and his complaint of vertigo with physical activity. Eye movement exercises were used to increase VOR response to head movements and eliminate the onset of vertigo during head movements. The human vestibular system has the capacity to adapt to environmental changes.[17] This attribute can be accentuated to promote recovery after unilateral dysfunction by moving a target across the retina in conjunction with head movements at varied frequencies.[18] Movement of a target across the retina combined with head movements results in an error signal that the brain attempts to rectify by increasing the VOR response. The eye exercises used were similar to those described by Herdman.[19] The patient was asked to hold a business card at arm's length, while sitting and keeping the print in focus. He moved his head from side to side for 2 minutes without stopping and then moved his head up and down for 2 minutes. Next, to facilitate

---
† NeuroCom International Inc, 9570 SE Lawnfield Rd, Clackamas, OR 97015.

visual-vestibular interactions, the patient held a business card at arm's length while sitting and moved the card and his head from side to side in opposite directions. He repeated this activity moving his head and the card up and down in opposite directions. I emphasized to the patient that initially the home exercise program could make the frequency and intensity of his vertigo worse, but that he should not be alarmed because the symptoms would subside with continued performance. Each eye exercise was performed twice daily for 2 minutes. The frequency and duration of the exercises were based on the patient's response to the initial evaluation and his work schedule, and on previous findings that adaptation requires time (more than a few seconds each day).[19]

The Brandt/Daroff exercises were performed as described by Brandt and Daroff.[7] The patient was asked to turn his head to the left about 45 degrees so that the lateral aspect of his occiput would rest on the mat and his chin tilted upward. That position was maintained as he lay on the right side. The position was reversed when he lay on the left side. The Brandt/Daroff exercises were performed for 5 repetitions to each side and increased to 10 repetitions as tolerated by the patient for two to five sessions daily. I decided on the initial number of repetitions in the clinic, where the patient performed repetitions until the perceived intensity of his vertigo and nausea exceeded his tolerance. The frequency and duration of the exercises were based on the patient's work schedule; he was unable to perform sessions every 3 hours while awake, as suggested by Brandt and Daroff.[7]

Three days after the evaluation and initiation of the home exercise program, the patient called the clinic to report that he had experienced a violent attack of vertigo during the Brandt/Daroff exercises and had been seen in the emergency department, where the physician agreed that his treatment was appropriate and prescribed 2.5 mg of Valium®[‡] to be taken as needed. The patient reported that he was too scared to continue therapy, but I encouraged him to continue his home exercise program and suggested that a psychological consultation might help him develop strategies to manage his anxiety. Psychological counseling was not acceptable to the patient. The next day, he discontinued the Valium® and reinitiated his home exercise program.

The patient was seen for two follow-up visits, the first visit 10 days after the initial evaluation and the second visit 14 days later. Follow-up visits consisted of reassessment of eye movements and review of the Brandt/Daroff exercises. On the first follow-up visit, review of eye movements revealed no slowing or nystagmus in the horizontal and vertical directions for smooth-pursuit and saccadic eye movements. Reassessment of the VOR with head movements from side to side and up and down showed right-beating horizontal nystagmus with head movements from side to side. Vestibular ocular reflex performance with head movements up and down demonstrated no deficits. Review of Brandt/Daroff exercises revealed no vertigo in the left side-lying position after 60 seconds. With initiation of exercises in the right side-lying position, the patient had a sensation of vertigo for 1 second. He was told to continue his home exercise program until he experienced 2 consecutive days without vertigo. Eye movement exercises were to be performed in a standing position instead of a sitting position to promote the use of visual and proprioceptive cues with vestibular cues. To meet the patient's goal of jogging again, he began a walking program because he had been sedentary for more than 5 years. The program was to be done on varying surfaces (gravel, concrete, grassy areas, and a track) five times weekly for 15 to 20 minutes. He was instructed to turn his head from left to right and up and down intermittently for 1-minute intervals while walking to enhance visual-vestibular interaction with the environment during dynamic postural responses.

Twenty-four days after the initial evaluation, the patient's complaints, performance of the Hallpike-Dix maneuver, and eye movements were reassessed. He no longer had episodes of vertigo when extending his neck while lying supine or when rolling over in bed. Neck extension to view upper shelves while walking in a store did not provoke vertigo. He also reported being able to perform all aspects of his job without discomfort, such as lying under a sink with his neck extended and gazing overhead.

The Hallpike-Dix maneuver was performed to the right and left sides with no vertigo or nystagmus. The patient assumed the full head-hanging position of 30 degrees below the horizontal, to the right and left while lying supine, without resistance to assuming the position.

Smooth-pursuit, saccadic, and VOR eye movements produced no symptoms of vertigo or nystagmus in a sitting or standing position. The patient was instructed to continue his walking program with head maneuvers for 3 weeks, and then to progress to walking and running five times weekly for 20 to 30 minutes on level surfaces and to discontinue the head maneuvers.

The patient was followed by phone at 1-month intervals for 3 months. One year after the initial evaluation and the start of physical therapy, the patient reported no further episodes of vertigo and a complete return to all activities without symptoms. He reported being anxious

---

[‡] Roche Products Inc, Manati, Puerto Rico 00674.

about the positions that used to make him dizzy, but symptoms were not provoked.

Discussion

After a 17-year history of positional vertigo, this patient's episodes of vertigo with neck extension were resolved after performing an individualized treatment program including Brandt/Daroff exercises. The patient also was able to begin and maintain a regular exercise program of walking and eventually could jog without provoking episodes of vertigo.

During the initial evaluation, the patient described his symptoms as dizziness, but it was clear from his description of the dizziness that he was experiencing vertigo. Dizziness is a complaint that can be associated with many diagnoses. Descriptions can range from light-headedness to a bandlike feeling around the head.[1] Vertigo is the false perception of motion, with a sensation of spinning or of the environment spinning.[1] Vertigo is one of the identifying characteristics of BPPV, so it was important to differentiate vertigo from dizziness.

In general, patients with vertigo are more responsive to rehabilitation if they are treated during the acute onset of symptoms. Patients who are untreated often limit their daily activities, as this patient did with jogging and certain head positions, to prevent the onset of vertigo. In some cases, this limiting of daily activities can result in loss of joint range of motion in the neck, trunk, and legs; decreased job performance; and delayed recovery from vertigo. Studies using animal models suggest that a critical period exists for optimum recovery after a unilateral vestibular lesion.[20] Baboons that were restrained after surgical vestibular neurotomy had prolonged recovery of postural and locomotor function when compared with baboons that were allowed to move freely in their usual environment within hours after surgery. In my experience, patients with chronic or long-standing problems will sometimes have a long rehabilitation or less than full recovery. This patient's recovery could be considered unusual in view of the functional limitations and the 17-year duration of the problem.

There are other approaches to the treatment of persons with BPPV. The single-treatment approaches (one procedure administered one time) described by Epley[21] and Semont et al[22] may have been just as effective in diminishing this patient's vertigo. Herdman and colleagues[8] compared the effectiveness of these single-treatment approaches to determine whether they would be effective alternatives to Brandt/Daroff exercises, which were 98.5% effective in eliminating vertigo and nystagmus.[7] They randomly assigned 30 subjects to each of two groups. One group received a modified Epley maneuver, and the other group received the Semont maneuver. Seventy percent of the subjects who received the modified Epley maneuver experienced remission of their vertigo and nystagmus, and 57% of the subjects who received the Semont maneuver experienced remission of their vertigo and nystagmus. The single-treatment approaches minimize the repeated discomfort of vertigo that is felt when using Brandt/Daroff exercises; however, there are reported cases in which the single-treatment maneuver was repeated a second time to eliminate vertigo.[8,21]

After both the Epley and Semont approaches, the patient is required to remain upright for 48 hours and wear a soft cervical collar. The patient described in this case report was offered the option of a single-treatment approach, but he believed that the Brandt/Daroff exercises would be less offensive because while at work he would not be able to avoid bending over. The Epley approach would have required the patient to take time away from work, which was unacceptable. This approach also would have required him to assume the supine position with his neck extended, which he refused to do early in the initial evaluation. After discussing the options and modifying the frequency of the home exercise program, the patient felt confident that he could be able to carry out the program. A positive treatment outcome of this approach is dependent on the patient's ability to adhere to the program.

In conclusion, this case report illustrates a situation in which, in the presence of BPPV, an individualized treatment program using Brandt/Daroff exercises may promote recovery even after a long-standing history of problems. Theoretically, this mechanical approach is designed to dislodge the debris from the cupula of the posterior canal. If cupulolithiasis is the mechanism for BPPV, then the approach should be effective regardless of the timing of the intervention.

References

1 Jensen JM. Vertigo and dizziness. In: Weiner WJ, Goetz GC, eds. *Neurology for the Non-neurologist*. 3rd ed. Philadelphia, Pa: JB Lippincott Co; 1994:171–172.

2 Brandt TH. *Vertigo: Its Multisensory Syndromes*. London, England: Springer-Verlag; 1991:138–140.

3 Schuknecht HF. Cupulolithiasis. *Arch Otolaryngol*. 1969;90:765–779.

4 Brandt TH. Vertigo and dizziness. In: Asbury AK, McKhann GM, McDonald I, eds. *Diseases of the Nervous System: Clinical Neurobiology*. 2nd ed. Philadelphia, Pa: WB Saunders Co; 1992:561–576.

5 Honrubia V. Quantitative vestibular function tests and the clinical examination. In: Herdman SJ, ed. *Vestibular Rehabilitation*. Philadelphia, Pa: FA Davis Co; 1994:115–116, 119.

6 Herdman SJ. Assessment and management of benign paroxysmal positional vertigo. In: Herdman SJ, ed. *Vestibular Rehabilitation*. Philadelphia, Pa: FA Davis Co; 1994:331.

7 Brandt TH, Daroff RB. Physical therapy for benign paroxysmal positional vertigo. *Arch Otolaryngol*. 1980;106:484–485.

8 Herdman SJ, Tusa RJ, Zee DS, et al. Single treatment approaches to benign paroxysmal positional vertigo. *Arch Otolaryngol Head Neck Surg.* 1993;119:450-454.

9 Horak FB, Jones-Rycewicz C, Black O, Shumway-Cook A. Effects of vestibular rehabilitation on dizziness and imbalance. *Otolaryngol Head Neck Surg.* 1992;106:175-180.

10 *Physicians' Desk Reference.* 47th ed. Montvale, NJ: Medical Economics Co; 1993:881-882.

11 Carl JR. Principles and techniques of electro-oculography. In: Jacobson GP, Newman CW, Kartush JM. *Handbook of Balance Function Testing.* St Louis, Mo: Mosby-Year Book Inc; 1993:69-100.

12 Palmer ML. Gross muscle testing: a review. *Clinical Management in Physical Therapy.* 1985;5(4):18-21.

13 Leigh RJ, Zee DS. *Neurology of Eye Movements.* Philadelphia, Pa: FA Davis Co; 1991:110, 158.

14 Dix MR, Hallpike CS. The pathology, symptomatology, and diagnosis of certain common disorders of the vestibular system. *Ann Otol Rhinol Laryngol.* 1952;6:987-1016.

15 Ford-Smith CD, Wyman JF, Elswick RK, et al. Test-retest reliability of the sensory organization test in noninstitutionalized older adults. *Arch Phys Med Rehabil.* 1995;76:77-81.

16 *Equitest Operator's Manual, Version 4.0.* Clackamas, Ore: NeuroCom International Inc; 1990.

17 Gauthier GM, Robinson DA. Adaptation of the human vestibulo-ocular reflex to magnifying lenses. *Brain Res.* 1975;92:331-335.

18 Herdman SJ. Exercise strategies in vestibular disorders. *Ear Nose Throat J.* 1990;68:961-964.

19 Herdman SJ. Assessment and treatment of balance disorders in the vestibular-deficient patient. In: *Balance Proceedings of the APTA Forum, Nashville, Tenn, June 13-15, 1989.* Alexandria, VA: American Physical Therapy Association; 1990:87-94.

20 Lacour M, Roll JP, Appaix M. Modifications and development of spinal reflexes in the alert baboon following an unilateral vestibular neurotomy. *Brain Res.* 1976;113:255-269.

21 Epley J. The canalith repositioning procedure: for treatment of benign paroxysmal positional vertigo. *Otolaryngol Head Neck Surg.* 1992;107:399-404.

22 Semont A, Freyss G, Vitte E. Curing the BPPV with a liberatory maneuver. *Adv Otorhinolaryngol.* 1988;42:290-293.

Evaluation of Health-Related Quality of Life in Individuals With Vestibular Disease Using Disease-Specific and General Outcome Measures

Background and Purpose. The Dizziness Handicap Inventory (DHI) is a condition-specific health status measure for persons with vestibular disease, and the Medical Outcomes Study 36-Item Short-Form Health Survey (SF-36) is a generic health status assessment. The purposes of this study were (1) to describe the relationship between the DHI and the SF-36, (2) to examine the reliability and responsiveness of these measures for persons in a vestibular rehabilitation program, and (3) to compare health-related quality of life between individuals with vestibular disease and the general population. Subjects. Ninety-five patients, aged 25 to 88 years ($\bar{X}$=57.0, SD=14.9), were assessed. Methods. To determine reliability, 20 subjects completed both questionnaires twice, 24 to 48 hours apart. Thirty-one subjects completed both questionnaires before and after 6 to 8 weeks of vestibular rehabilitation to establish responsiveness. To establish the relationship between the two assessment tools, 95 subjects completed both questionnaires. Results. Each test was moderately to highly reliable (intraclass correlation coefficients [2,1]=.64–.95), but the tests were poorly to moderately correlated to each other (r=.11–.71). The DHI was more responsive to change than the SF-36. The SF-36 scores of individuals were lower than scores of the general population. Conclusion and Discussion. The DHI and the SF-36 provide reliable and responsive measurements, but they appear to provide different information about the health status of patients with vestibular disease. Compared with the general population, patients with vestibular disease had lower scores for health-related quality of life, but these scores improved after 6 to 8 weeks of treatment. Future studies should clarify whether this improved health status is due to vestibular rehabilitation. [Enloe LJ, Shields RK. Evaluation of health-related quality of life in individuals with vestibular disease using disease-specific and general outcome measures. *Phys Ther.* 1997;77:890–903.]

Key Words: *Health-related quality of life, Outcome measures, Psychometric properties, Vestibular disease.*

Lori J Enloe

Richard K Shields

Dizziness accounts for 8 million primary care visits to physicians in the United States annually.[1] Vestibular system disorders are the cause of dizziness in approximately 40% to 50% of patients referred to otolaryngologists[2] and to primary care clinics.[3,4] Individuals with dizziness report a variety of symptoms, including vertigo, nausea, postural instability, blurred vision, and disorientation.[5] These symptoms can result in a variety of emotional and physical problems, including emotional distress, anxiety,[6-8] and an inability to perform activities of daily living or work.[9,10] Vestibular system disorders appear to affect health-related quality of life.

Vestibular rehabilitation includes exercises that are used to manage the symptoms of vertigo and imbalance associated with vestibular disorders. The exercises are designed to improve the individual's quality of life. Exercises may include repetitive eye, head, and body movements to reduce motion intolerance and gaze instability and balance activities to reduce postural instability.[11,12] An individual's progress or lack of progress in vestibular rehabilitation is usually measured by observing changes in motion intolerance, balance, functional abilities, and, more recently, health-related quality of life.[13-15]

The Dizziness Handicap Inventory[16] (DHI) and the Medical Outcomes Study (MOS) 36-Item Short-Form Health Survey[17] (SF-36) are two commonly used health-related quality-of-life survey instruments. The DHI, a disease-specific questionnaire, was developed for individuals with dizziness or balance problems and measures how vertigo and disequilibrium (imbalance) affect an individual's quality of life.[16] Disease-specific questionnaires are thought by some experts to be more responsive to clinical change than generic questionnaires.[17] Generic questionnaires, such as the SF-36, use a global approach to measure health status as it relates to an individual's functional well-being.[18] Generic questionnaires may be used with several populations[17,19] and are less responsive to change than disease-specific questionnaires.[19] Generic questionnaires allow comparisons of health status between disabled and nondisabled individuals as well as comparisons among persons with dissimilar medical conditions. Some researchers[20,21] have found parts of the generic questionnaires to be equally as responsive or more responsive to change than disease-specific questionnaires. Patrick et al[21] found the physical function scale of the SF-36 to be more responsive than either the disease-specific Roland Disability Questionnaire or the Sciatic Frequency Index. Kantz et al[20] reported that the physical function scale of the SF-36 was

---

LJ Enloe, PT, is Physical Therapist, Veterans Administration Medical Center, Iowa City, Iowa. She was a student in the Physical Therapy Graduate Program, The University of Iowa, when this research was completed in partial fulfillment of the requirements for her Master of Arts degree in physical therapy.

RK Shields, PhD, PT, is Assistant Professor, Physical Therapy Graduate Program, College of Medicine, The University of Iowa, 2600 Steindler Bldg, Iowa City, IA 52242-1008 (USA) (richard-shields@uiowa.edu), and Clinical Research Coordinator, University of Iowa Hospitals and Clinics, Iowa City, Iowa. Address all correspondence to Dr Shields at the first address.

This study was approved by The University of Iowa College of Medicine Human Subjects Review Committee.

This study was supported in part by The University of Iowa Physical Therapy Clinical Research Center, which was originally funded by the Foundation for Physical Therapy Inc.

This article was submitted July 3, 1996, and was accepted January 15, 1997.

Table 1.
General Vestibular Diagnostic Classifications for Patient Subsets

General Vestibular Diagnostic Dysfunction	Study Phase		
	Reliability (n=20)	Correlation (N=95)	Responsiveness (n=31)
Unilateral dysfunction	17 (87%)	78 (82.1%)	27 (87.1%)
Bilateral dysfunction	1 (5%)	3 (3.2%)	1 (3.2%)
Central dysfunction	0 (0%)	4 (4.2%)	1 (3.2%)
Mixed (central and peripheral) dysfunction	2 (10%)	4 (4.2%)	1 (3.2%)
Nonspecific dysfunction	0 (0%)	6 (6.3%)	1 (3.2%)

equally responsive as a disease-specific questionnaire for patients with total knee replacements. The more generic SF-36 was developed for general population surveys, clinical practice, research, and health policy assessment.[22] Use of this tool to assess patients with vestibular disease has not been described in the literature. Thus, the health status of individuals with vestibular disease has not previously been compared with the health status of individuals from the general population.

Whether both the DHI and the SF-36 are highly correlated when assessing health-related quality of life in patients with vestibular disorders remains unknown. Whether the DHI and the SF-36 are equally reliable and responsive is also not known. If the questionnaires are highly correlated and are equally reliable and responsive, only one questionnaire may be necessary in clinical practice and research. By understanding the relationship between these questionnaires, practitioners can decide whether either or both questionnaires should be used to assess patients' health status.

Psychometric properties of health-related quality-of-life questionnaires, including reliability and responsiveness, are important in the patient populations for which they are used.[23–25] Reliability of the DHI for patients with vestibular dysfunction was high ($r=.97$) in a study (N=14) by Jacobson et al,[16] but systematic variation was not assessed. The reliability of the SF-36 has been studied extensively,[26,27] but not for individuals with vestibular dysfunction. More importantly, the reliability of the DHI and the SF-36 has not been estimated concurrently for persons with vestibular dysfunction.

Responsiveness is the ability to detect the minimal clinical change in a variable over time.[28] Responsiveness of an instrument may be measured by following a disease through its natural progression or by measuring change following clinical intervention. Measuring change in health-related quality of life of patients with vestibular dysfunction using the DHI and the SF-36 provides an opportunity to compare the responsiveness of these two instruments.

The purposes of this study were (1) to describe the relationship between the DHI and the SF-36 for individuals with vestibular dysfunction, (2) to estimate the reliability and responsiveness of the DHI and the SF-36 for individuals participating in a vestibular rehabilitation program, and (3) to compare the health-related quality of life of individuals before and after vestibular rehabilitation (SF-36, DHI) and to contrast their health status with that of the general population (SF-36).

Method

Subjects

One hundred eight patients with vestibular dysfunction who were referred to the Vestibular Rehabilitation Clinic, University of Iowa Hospitals and Clinics, Iowa City, Iowa, were invited to complete the DHI and the SF-36 over a 15-month period. Five patients (2 men, 3 women) did not participate in the study due to their inability to complete questionnaires independently. Eight additional patients were eliminated because the DHI was incomplete. The patients provided informed consent, were able to read, and met an otolaryngologist's diagnostic criteria for vestibular dysfunction. The otolaryngologist classified patients into five general groups, which were adapted from Baloh.[5] The five general groups were (1) unilateral vestibular dysfunction, (2) bilateral vestibular dysfunction, (3) central vestibular dysfunction, (4) mixed central and peripheral dysfunction, and (5) nonspecific vestibular dysfunction. The distributions of patients by general categories are presented in Table 1.

To estimate reliability, 24 consecutive patients, a subset of the total sample, were tested with both the SF-36 and the DHI. The patients were asked to complete both questionnaires twice, before their physical therapy evaluation and again within a 24- to 48-hour period. Four patients (3 men, 1 woman) did not complete the questionnaires a second time, leaving 20 patients for the final analysis. To describe the relationship between the SF-36 and the DHI, 95 patients completed both questionnaires at their initial physical therapy evaluation. Responsive-

Table 2.
Patient Demographics

Variable	Study Phase								
	Reliability (n=20)			Correlation (N=95)			Responsiveness (n=31)		
	X̄	SD	Range	X̄	SD	Range	X̄	SD	Range
Age (y)	56.45	13.93	36–78	56.99	14.87	25–88	57.77	15.42	34–88
Height (cm)	166.32	10.83	138–183	167.42	9.56	135–190	168.75	8.95	155–190
Weight (kg)	78.65	19.63	54–124	82.28	19.34	46–144	78.08	18.75	49–129
Length of illness[a] (mo)	27.2	35.7	3–120	24.8	32.6	1–120	26.2	37.4	3–120

[a] Length of illness: Any length of illness greater than 10 years was collapsed to 120 months.

ness was estimated using 31 consecutive patients, also a subset of the total sample, who received both the SF-36 and the DHI at two time periods. There were no differences in mean age, height, weight, and length of illness among the three groups. Because the 31 patients in the responsiveness group were a subset of the total sample, additional analysis showed that their demographics were not different from the demographics of the other 64 patients. The diagnoses and demographics for the participating patients are shown in Tables 1 and 2. Sixty patients (67%) were female, and 35 patients (33%) were male.

Instruments

The DHI is a disease-specific questionnaire that was developed to quantify the impact of dizziness on quality of life (Appendix 1).[16] A total possible score of 100 is the result of 36 points from the emotional scale (9 items), 36 points from the functional scale (9 items), and 28 points from the physical scale (7 items). Each question provides a choice of three responses: yes (4 points), sometimes (2 points), or no (0 points). To facilitate the use of the three DHI scales separately in all calculations, each scale's score was calculated as the percentage of the total possible points for each scale. For example, 24 points on the emotional scale received a score of 67% (24/36×100). Next, the total score and the three scale scores were transformed by subtracting each score from 100 so that 0 represented poor function due to dizziness or unsteadiness and 100 represented no problems due to dizziness or unsteadiness. The DHI does not focus its questions on any particular time interval.

The SF-36, which consists of eight health scales, was used to measure generic health-related quality of life (Appendix 2).[27] The eight health scales of the SF-36 are (1) physical function (10 items), (2) role limitation due to physical problems (4 items), (3) bodily pain (2 items), (4) general health (5 items), (5) social function (2 items), (6) vitality/energy (4 items), (7) role limitation due to emotional problems (4 items), and (8) mental health (5 items). The standard SF-36 form asks questions regarding the past 4 weeks.

The eight health concepts of the SF-36 are summarized in two summary scales: the physical component summary scale (PCS-36) and the mental component summary scale (MCS-36). Although both scales are calculated from weighted aggregates of all eight SF-36 domains, the PCS-36 and the MCS-36 are heavily weighted with respective SF-36 scores. The PCS-36 is weighted more heavily with physical function, bodily pain, and role limitation (physical) scores. The MCS-36 is weighted more heavily with mental health, role limitation (emotional), social function, and vitality/energy scores.[27]

The SF-36 data were analyzed using a Statistical Analysis Software* code developed by the Medical Outcomes Trust at the New England Medical Center.[27,29] For missing data, a computer algorithm substituted the average score of one scale if greater than 50% of the items were present.[27] The eight scales were scored individually and transformed, resulting in a scale ranging from 0 to 100, with 0 denoting poor health. The SF-36 summary scores were calculated according to methods described by Ware et al.[29] Specifically, each of the eight SF-36 scores was standardized using a Z transformation. The mean score of the US population was subtracted from the score of the respective SF-36 scale, then the difference was divided by the respective scale's standard deviation. In the next step, aggregate scores were calculated for the PCS-36 and the MCS-36 using weights for each SF-36 scale determined by factor analysis. Finally, the PCS-36 and the MCS-36 received a linear T-score transformation by multiplying each score by the standard deviation of the general US population (±10) and adding 50 (mean score of the general US population). That is, the PCS-36 and MCS-36 scores were referenced to normative values.

Procedure

Three different procedures were completed for estimating the test-retest reliability of the SF-36 and the DHI, measuring the relationship between the SF-36 and the

---

* SAS Institute Inc, PO Box 8000, Cary, NC 27511-8000.

DHI, and comparing the responsiveness of the SF-36 and the DHI. To estimate the test-retest reliability of the SF-36 and the DHI, 20 patients completed both questionnaires twice over a 24- to 48-hour period. This short time was chosen due to the unpredictable nature of symptoms in patients with vestibular problems.[7,30] The patients completed the two surveys before their physical therapy evaluation and once at home 24 to 48 hours later. The patients completed the SF-36 first, followed by the DHI, for both occasions. The SF-36 survey was completed first to allow the patients to focus first on their general quality of life, and then to focus on the disease-specific factors affecting their quality of life. The patients were contacted by the investigator (LJE) between 24 and 48 hours after their physical therapy appointment to verify completion of the surveys. If a patient had not completed the surveys, he or she was asked to complete them during the telephone call. Two patients completed the surveys during the telephone interview by reading their responses to the investigator.

The relationship between the SF-36 and the DHI was determined with the 95 patients who completed the SF-36 and the DHI prior to their initial physical therapy evaluation. To determine the responsiveness of the SF-36 and the DHI, a subset of 31 patients completed both questionnaires twice. The patients completed the SF-36 and the DHI once at their initial physical therapy visit and once at follow-up to physical therapy ($\bar{X}$=6.9 weeks, SD=2.7). Six to eight weeks was chosen to assess responsiveness because this time was associated with improvement in patients receiving vestibular rehabilitation.[13,14]

Data Analysis
Descriptive statistics for the DHI scores and the SF-36 scores were calculated for the patients in each group. The percentage floor and ceiling effects for both the DHI and the SF-36 were computed for the total sample. Floor effects are present when individuals score poorly, at the bottom of the scale, so that no further decrement may occur. The opposite is true for ceiling effects.

The relationship between the SF-36 and the DHI was described using the Pearson product-moment correlation coefficient (r). Correlations between the scales within each questionnaire were also computed. The test-retest reliability of the SF-36 and the DHI was estimated using the intraclass correlation coefficient (ICC[2,1]) and the Pearson product-moment correlation coefficient. Test-retest reliability was determined for the total DHI score, the three DHI scales, the eight SF-36 scales, and the SF-36 summary scales. The standard error of the measurement (SEM) for the 95% confidence interval was also calculated.

Dependent t tests were completed to determine whether the DHI and the SF-36 changed for the subset of 31 patients before and after 6 to 8 weeks of vestibular rehabilitation. Responsiveness was determined by calculating the mean change as a percentage of the full scale range of all DHI and SF-36 scales over the 6- to 8-week period. The mean change as a percentage of the full scale range was equal to the absolute change of all DHI and SF-36 variables because the possible scores range from 0 to 100 for each questionnaire. For example, a change of 10 points on either questionnaire represents a 10% change with respect to the range (0–100) of the total scale. Unlike the scoring of the DHI and the SF-36 scales, however, the SF-36 component summary scores (PCS-36 and MCS-36 scores) do not range from 0 to 100. Therefore, the SF-36 component summary score range was determined by inputting maximum and minimum values into the formulas for calculating the summary scores.[29] The resulting ranges of 74.55 (1.73–76.28) and 70.73 (3.11—76.28) were determined for the PCS-36 and MCS-36 scores, respectively. Normalizing the SF-36 component summary scores to the total range of the scale enabled comparisons between the DHI summary score and the SF-36 component summary score.

Dependent t tests were used to compare the mean change (as a percentage of full scale range) of the SF-36 scales and DHI scales related to physical health. Comparisons were also made between the mean change of the SF-36 scales and DHI scales related to mental health. Dependent t tests were used based on the assumption that both the SF-36 and the DHI are health-related quality-of-life measures and thus measure similar concepts. Bonferroni adjustments were made for multiple comparisons.

The responsiveness of the DHI and SF-36 scores was also estimated using Guyatt's statistic.[28] Guyatt's responsiveness formula is: clinical change/square root (2 × mean square error). Deyo et al[23] have shown that the denominator of this equation is equivalent to the standard deviation of the score changes across a 24-hour test-retest period; therefore, this calculation was used for the denominator. The values for the denominator were taken from the baseline assessments of the 20 patients participating in the reliability component of the study. The numerator represented the change for the DHI and SF-36 scores and was obtained before and after 6 to 8 weeks of vestibular rehabilitation. The number of patients required to detect this change was calculated according to the procedure described by Guyatt et al,[28] using an alpha level of .05 and beta level of .10 and assuming that independent groups would be selected in a randomized clinical trial.

Table 3.
Dizziness Handicap Inventory[16] (DHI) and Medical Outcomes Study 36-Item Short-Form Health Survey[27,29] (SF-36) Scores (N=95)

Variable	X̄	SD	Minimum	Maximum	Percentage of Floor Effects	Percentage of Ceiling Effects
DHI						
Total	53.57	20.82	6.00	96.00	0	0
Functional	51.11	26.01	0	100.00	4.20	1.00
Physical	45.34	23.32	0	100.00	5.30	1.00
Emotional	62.45	21.45	5.56	100.00	0	2.10
SF-36						
Physical function	51.59	26.17	0	100.00	1.00	2.10
Role limitation (physical)	22.10	31.76	0	100.00	55.80	8.40
Bodily pain	57.37	28.97	0	100.00	3.20	18.90
General health	58.07	21.95	0	97.00	1.00	1.00
Vitality/energy	37.79	23.55	0	100.00	4.20	1.00
Social function	55.92	28.88	0	100.00	2.10	14.70
Role limitation (emotional)	45.61	38.91	0	100.00	30.50	25.30
Mental health	65.77	18.51	16.00	96.00	1.00	0
Physical component summary	36.53	10.25	16.30	56.20	0	0
Mental component summary	43.24	10.42	23.03	64.55	0	0

Results

Completion rates for the SF-36 and the DHI were similar to previously reported completion rates for the SF-36.[26] Ninety-five percent (n=98) of the SF-36 questionnaires were complete. Three percent, 2%, and 1% of the patients did not complete 1, 2, and 4 items, respectively. Ninety-two percent (n=95) of the DHI questionnaires were complete, with 8% of the patients missing 1 item.

Descriptive statistics, including the percentage of scores that could not go lower (floor) and the percentage of scores that could not go higher (ceiling), for the DHI and SF-36 scores of the 95 patients are presented in Table 3. The scales with the greatest floor effects were the SF-36 scales role limitation (physical) and role limitation (emotional). The scales with the greatest ceiling effect were the SF-36 scales bodily pain, social function, and role limitation (emotional). The DHI scales exhibited minimal floor and ceiling effects.

The correlation matrix for the DHI and SF-36 scores is shown in Table 4. The reported probability values signify that the Pearson product-moment correlations were significantly different from zero. The correlations between the DHI and the SF-36 ranged from .11 to .71. The highest correlation was between the social function score of the SF-36 and the DHI emotional score ($r=.71$). The three scales of the SF-36 that were most related to mental health (role limitation due to emotional problems, mental health, vitality/energy) had correlations between .40 and .50 with the DHI emotional score. The correlation between the PCS-36 score and the DHI functional score was .54. The MCS-36 score and the DHI emotional score also had a correlation of .54.

The test-retest correlation coefficients and the SEMs for the DHI and the SF-36 for the 20 patients in the reliability component of the study are shown in Table 5. The ICCs ranged from .79 to .95 for the DHI and from .64 to .92 for the SF-36. For the DHI, the emotional scale had the lowest SEM. For the SF-36, the PCS-36 and MCS-36 had the lowest SEMs and the role limitation (physical) and role limitation (emotional) scales had the highest SEMs.

Scores for all DHI scales and for the PCS-36 and the physical function, role limitation (physical), bodily pain, vitality/energy, social function scales of the SF-36 were changed after an average of 7 weeks of rehabilitation ($P<.01$). The absolute mean changes (as a percentage of full scale) for the DHI scales and the SF-36 scales are shown in Table 6. The total DHI score changed 11.94%, while the PCS-36 and MCS-36 scores changed 6.67% and 4.35%, respectively.

Results of the dependent t tests comparing the changes in DHI scores with changes in SF-36 scores are presented in Table 6. The change in the DHI functional score (15.59%) was greater than the change in the PCS-36 score (6.67%) ($P=.006$). The change in the mental health score (0.71%), which was lower than the change in the DHI emotional score (8.06%) ($P=.016$), was the only individual SF-36 score that was different from the DHI scores.

The numbers of patients required to detect the measured change for the DHI and SF-36 are presented in Table 7. The DHI functional scale was the most responsive scale, requiring only 7.24 patients to detect the measured clinical change. Physical function was the

Table 4.
Correlation Matrix for Dizziness Handicap Inventory[16] (DHI) and Medical Outcomes Study 36-Item Short-Form Health Survey[27,29] (SF-36) Scores (N=95)[a]

	SF-36											DHI			
Variable	Physical Function	Role Limitation (Physical)	Bodily Pain	General Health	Vitality/ Energy	Social Function	Role Limitation (Emotional)	Mental Health	Physical Component Summary	Mental Component Summary		Functional	Physical	Emotional	Total
SF-36															
Physical function	1.00														
Role limitation (physical)	.56	1.00													
Bodily pain	.52	.40	1.00												
General health	.33[b]	.23[c]	.37[d]	1.00											
Vitality/energy	.48	.37[d]	.39	.41	1.00										
Social function	.60	.54	.41	.39	.47	1.00									
Role limitation (emotional)	.24[c]	.50	.27[e]	.11[f]	.33[d]	.37[d]	1.00								
Mental health	.23	.34[g]	.28[e]	.29[b]	.48	.40	.48	1.00							
Physical component summary	.84	.62	.74	.56	.46	.56	.09[f]	.09[f]	1.00						
Mental component summary	.17[f]	.38	.21[c]	.26[c]	.59	.56	.78	.83	.01[f]	1.00					
DHI															
Functional	.65	.50	.41	.16[f]	.42	.63	.33[c]	.26[d]	.54	.33[g]		1.00			
Physical	.48	.38[d]	.35[d]	.13[f]	.27[e]	.44	.11[f]	.27[e]	.44	.19[f]		.67	1.00		
Emotional	.55	.50	.28[e]	.22[c]	.41	.71	.42	.48	.39	.54		.74	.54	1.00	
Total	.65	.53	.39	.20[f]	.43	.68	.34[g]	.38[d]	.53	.41		.94	.81	.87	1.00

[a] All probability values=.0001, except as noted.
[b] $P<.005$.
[c] $P<.05$.
[d] $P<.0005$.
[e] $P<.01$.
[f] Not significant.
[g] $P<.001$.

Table 5.
Dizziness Handicap Inventory[16] (DHI) and Medical Outcomes Study 36-Item Short-Form Health Survey[27,29] (SF-36) Test-Retest Reliability Correlation Coefficients

Variable	Test X̄	Test SD	Retest X̄	Retest SD	ICC[a] (2,1)	Pearson r	±2×SEM[b]
DHI							
Total	47.70	23.30	52.20	25.54	.94	.96	9.32
Functional	43.61	29.25	47.78	27.71	.95	.94	11.70
Emotional	59.44	24.19	62.78	25.81	.95	.95	9.68
Physical	37.86	24.32	44.29	28.44	.79	.82	20.64
SF-36							
Physical function	48.81	28.06	54.25	28.20	.90	.91	16.84
Role limitation (physical)	25.00	40.56	25.00	38.28	.64	.64	48.67
Bodily pain	63.70	28.43	66.75	27.88	.90	.90	17.98
General health	57.45	21.10	61.70	23.38	.79	.79	21.16
Vitality/energy	46.00	23.93	48.25	24.13	.91	.91	14.36
Social function	54.37	31.49	55.00	32.55	.90	.90	19.92
Role limitation (emotional)	48.33	48.33	36.37	41.75	.81	.83	36.20
Mental health	68.10	68.10	69.00	22.62	.91	.92	11.96
Physical component summary	36.76	10.12	38.92	8.93	.85	.87	7.28
Mental component summary	44.88	12.40	43.35	11.01	.92	.94	6.06

[a] ICC=intraclass correlation coefficient.
[b] ±2×SEM=standard error of the measurement for 95% confidence interval=2×[(SD)×(square root (1-r)]. Test SD was used for SEM calculation.

Table 6.
Mean Percentage of Change in Dizziness Handicap Inventory[16] (DHI) and Medical Outcomes Study 36-Item Short-Form Health Survey[27,29] (SF-36) Scores Between Test and Retest[a]

Variable (Possible Range)	X̄	SD	Minimum	Maximum
DHI				
1. Total (100)	11.94	15.60	−18.00	54.00
2. Functional (100)	15.59	19.79	−22.22	66.67
3. Physical (100)	12.21	18.46	−21.43	57.14
4. Emotional (100)	8.06	16.34	−22.22	44.44
SF-36				
Physical function (100)[1-3b]	12.74	19.36	−20.00	75.00
Role limitation (physical) (100)[1-3b]	23.39	48.71	−75.00	100.00
Bodily pain (100)	10.13	20.46	−22.00	80.00
General health (100)	−1.90	15.41	−30.00	40.00
Vitality/energy (100)[4]	10.00	18.79	−20.00	55.00
Social function (100)[1-4c]	18.14	25.99	−25.00	75.00
Role limitation (emotional) (100)[4]	16.13	52.26	−66.67	100.00
Mental health (100)[4*]	0.71	14.13	−32.00	32.00
Physical component summary (74.55)[1-3b*]	6.67	9.44	−13.26	30.31
Mental component summary (70.73)[1,4d]	4.35	15.02	−20.84	33.76

[a] Mean change (% of full scale)=absolute change/total possible range × 100. Superscript numbers show which SF-36 variables were compared with respective DHI variables. Asterisk (*) indicates significant difference with specified variables at specified probability value.
[b] Probability value for multiple comparisons=.0167=(.05/3).
[c] Probability value for multiple comparisons=.0125=(.05/4).
[d] Probability value for multiple comparisons=.025=(.05/2).

most responsive SF-36 scale, requiring 22.07 patients to detect the measured change. The total DHI and PCS-36 required 9.43 and 25.87 patients, respectively, to detect measured changes. Overall, the DHI appeared to be more responsive than the SF-36.

The SF-36 scores for the patients with vestibular dysfunction before entering the vestibular rehabilitation program and after 6 to 8 weeks of vestibular rehabilitation (n=31) are shown with the SF-36 normative general population data[27] in the Figure (upper and lower panels). The SF-36 scores for the 31 patients prior to vestibular rehabilitation were not different from the SF-36 scores for the larger group of 95 patients seen before vestibular rehabilitation. Because the 31 patients were a subset of the 95 patients evaluated before vestib-

Table 7.
Responsiveness (Guyatt's) for the Dizziness Handicap Inventory[16] (DHI) and Medical Outcomes Study 36-Item Short-Form Health Survey[27,29] (SF-36) Scores

Variable	Mean Change (Retest-Test) (n=31)	Variability in Stable Patients[a] (n=20)	Guyatt's Responsiveness Statistic[28]	Sample Size[b]
DHI				
Total	11.94	7.19	1.66	9.43
Functional	15.59	8.23	1.89	7.24
Physical	12.21	16.37	0.75	46.71
Emotional	8.06	7.07	1.14	19.97
SF-36				
Physical function	12.74	11.74	1.08	22.07
Role limitation (physical)	23.39	33.71	0.69	54.00
Bodily pain	10.12	12.36	0.82	38.70
General health	−1.90	14.96	−0.13	16.06
Vitality/energy	10.00	10.19	0.98	26.99
Social function	18.14	14.32	1.27	16.19
Role limitation (emotional)	16.13	24.84	0.65	61.64
Mental health	0.71	9.00	0.08	41.80
Physical component summary	4.97	4.96	1.002	25.87
Mental component summary	3.08	4.43	0.70	53.72

[a] Stable patient variability was calculated from the variability of the patients in the reliability phase of the study.
[b] Sample size=2×[(3.605)×(variability/clinical change)^2]. Sample size calculated for independent groups (α=.05, β=.10).

ular rehabilitation, an additional analysis comparing the 31 patients and the other 64 patients indicated that there was no difference in their SF-36 scores. The general population data were taken from the National Survey of Functional Health Status,[27] a mail and telephone survey that include the SF-36. The 2,474 patients in that survey varied in age from 18 to 94 years; 57% were female and 71% were under the age of 65 years.[27] The 31 patients with vestibular disease in the responsiveness component of our study varied in age from 34 to 88 years; 58% were female and 61% were under the age of 65 years. As depicted in the Figure, patients entering a vestibular rehabilitation program had lower scores on the SF-36 scales than did the general population (P<.05). At follow-up, however, the patients receiving vestibular rehabilitation had scores that were generally closer to those of the normative general population. In particular, role limitation (physical) and social function scales of the SF-36 were greatly improved (P=.012 and P=.0005, respectively).

Discussion

Ceiling and floor effects interfere with a tests ability to provide clinically useful information about function of patients at a single point in time and over time. A test should have little to no ceiling and floor effects to be useful. Increasing the range of health status improves the precision of the instrument.[26] The DHI had minimal ceiling and floor effects, whereas the SF-36 scores showed ceiling or floor effects for some scales (Tab. 1). Floor effects were present for the role limitation (physical) and role limitation (emotional) scales and were greater than the 15% recommended by McHorney and Tarlov[31] for use with individual patients. Ceiling effects were present in the bodily pain scale (18.9%), the social function scale (14.7%), and the role limitation (emotional) scale (25.3%) in this study.

The relationship between the DHI and the SF-36 was similar to other comparisons between disease-specific and generic quality-of-life measures.[20,32] The DHI and the SF-36 were not highly correlated. The highest correlation between the two questionnaires (ie, between the DHI emotional scale and SF-36 social function scale) was .71. Similarities between these two scales are more obvious after reviewing the questions. The DHI emotional scale questions include "Because of your problem, are you afraid to leave home without someone accompanying you?" and "Has your problem placed stress on your relationship with members of your family or friends?" The SF-36 social function scale includes the question "During the past 4 weeks, how much of the time has your physical or mental health interfered with social activities?" Thus, the DHI and the SF-36 may reflect different concepts, which may be complementary.

Our investigation, as well as other studies,[20,32] demonstrated that correlations between disease-specific and generic instruments vary, depending on the instruments. Scales such as the physical function scale may be highly correlated with disease-specific instruments.[20] In our study, the SF-36 physical function scale showed one of the highest correlations to the DHI functional scale (r=.65). Additional studies are needed to validate this

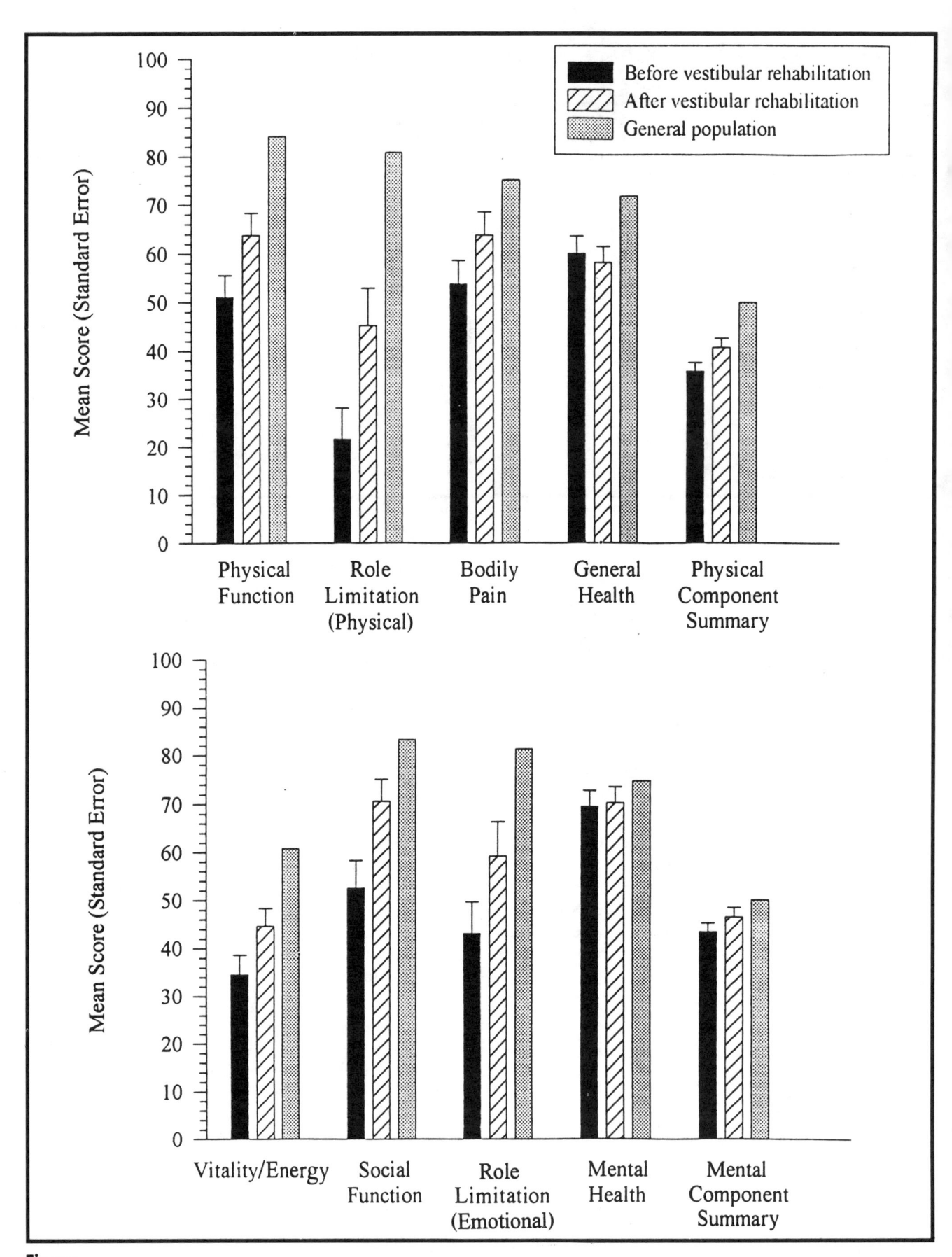

Figure.
Medical Outcomes Study 36-Item Short-Form Health Survey[27,29] (SF-36) scores for patients with vestibular disease (n=31) prior to and following 6 to 8 weeks of vestibular rehabilitation and for the general population (N=2,474).[27] The upper panel shows the physical health domains of the SF-36 and the physical health summary score. The lower panel shows the mental health domains of the SF-36 and the mental health summary score.

finding by comparing both measures with impairment or performance tests.

Another issue that may have affected the relationship between the DHI and the SF-36 is the construct of the DHI. Further analysis of the correlations of the individual DHI scales indicated that the individual DHI scales may be cross correlated and not measure one particular health concept. Fifty-five percent of the variability in the scores for the DHI functional scale was accounted for by the DHI emotional scale. Forty-five percent of the variability in the DHI functional scale was accounted for by the DHI physical scale. Rasch analysis,[33] which was beyond the scope of this study, may be used to determine the unidimensionality and reproducibility of each item's position along a scale. Thus, the scaling properties of the DHI warrant further investigation.

The test-retest reliability of the self-administered DHI was similar to the reliability reported by Jacobson and Newman[16] for their face-to-face interview with 14 patients. Jacobson and Newman reported that same-day test-retest reliability varied from .92 for the DHI physical scale scores to .97 for the DHI emotional and total scale scores. In our study, the DHI showed a similar level of reliability, suggesting that the DHI physical, emotional, and total scores may be important measurements in clinical practice.

Examination of the data showed that the low ICC for the SF-36 role limitation (physical) scale may have been related to how the patients interpreted the single question making up this health concept. Two patients had opposite scores on the test and the retest. The patients may have misread the question or may have changed their response due to education and increased awareness of their conditions after their physical therapy evaluation. In addition, the distribution of the SF-36 role limitation (physical) scores was not normal. Twelve patients had a score of 0. Although the distribution was skewed, Streiner and Norman[34] noted that the ICC statistic is robust even for unequal distributions. The Spearman rank correlation ($r=.65$) was similar to the Pearson product-moment correlation ($r=.64$) for the SF-36 role limitation (physical) scale.

The test-retest reliability of the SF-36 for patients with vestibular dysfunction was similar to the test-retest reliability found for other patient populations,[35–37] further verifying the generalized reproducibility of the SF-36. Direct comparisons were difficult because other studies did not provide the range of scores for the test-retest reliability sample and the time interval for administering the test varied. The SEMs calculated in our study also provided additional information regarding the degree of error in the SF-36 and the DHI. Although both the DHI and the SF-36 had reliable measurements, the variability in the SF-36 and DHI scores requires relatively large changes before a therapist could be sure that true change has occurred.

The purpose of testing responsiveness was for us to determine whether the DHI and SF-36 scores changed equally over time. All the DHI variables and most of the SF-36 variables, except for the MCS-36 and the general health, role limitation (emotional), mental health scales, showed changes between the baseline assessment and the assessment done after approximately 6 to 8 weeks of rehabilitation. Because there was no control group, we do not know whether this change was due to physical therapy, medical intervention, or spontaneous remission. Randomized controlled clinical trials are under way in an attempt to understand the effect of specific vestibular rehabilitation protocols on this change in health status. For our study, vestibular rehabilitation was not precisely defined. In general, the treatments were home programs consisting of exercises to assist with balance and reduce motion sensitivity. There is a wide array of treatments routinely recommended for each of the diagnostic groups comprising vestibular pathology.

Two factors may have affected the use of the dependent t test in determining whether the two questionnaires were equally responsive. First, an assumption was made that each questionnaire had similar scaling properties when the absolute raw score taken as a percentage of full scale was used for analysis. For example, a 10-point change in scores on the SF-36 was equivalent to a 10-point change in scores on the DHI, given that the scores for each scale ranged from 0 to 100. Further studies are needed to determine whether this scaling assumption is true. The method of adjusting the PCS-36 and MCS-36 scores, however, appears to be more valid than taking a true percentage change (pretest score − posttest score/pretest score × 100) where an identical absolute change in scores is highly influenced by the baseline (pretest) score. Second, the total score range for the PCS-36 and MCS-36 is not from 0 to 100. The true range was estimated by entering the highest possible and lowest possible SF-36 scores into the formulas used to calculate the component summary scores. This normalization was needed so that absolute changes in the PCS-36 and MCS-36 scores could be compared with the changes in scores for the DHI (0–100). An alternate method would be to use the range of scores for the patients in our study instead of using the highest and lowest possible scores. A separate analysis using the range of scores from our study showed no differences in changes in scores between the DHI and the SF-36; thus, the SF-36 and DHI would be considered equally responsive. We contend, therefore, that the method of defining the range for the PCS-36 and MCS-36 scores contributed to the findings of our study.

Responsiveness has not been previously determined for the DHI and the SF-36 in patients with vestibular dysfunction. Comparisons between generic and disease-specific instruments, however, have shown similar results. In a study comparing the Roland Disability Questionnaire with the SF-36, Guyatt's responsiveness statistic was compared in 318 patients who had an improvement in their sciatic pain symptoms over 3 months.[21] The SF-36 physical function scale (2.3) and bodily pain scale (2.0) were more responsive than the Sciatic Frequency Index (−1.6). The SF-36 physical function scale (2.3) was more responsive than the modified Roland disease-specific scale (−2.0). The responsiveness was negative because a decrease in scores represented an improvement in symptoms. Like our vestibular study, this study showed that some of the SF-36 scales were more responsive than the disease-specific scales.

An interesting finding was the similarity in responsiveness between the SF-36 component summary scores and the SF-36 individual scores. The responsiveness of the PCS-36 scores (1.00) was similar to that of the SF-36 physical function scores (1.08). The use of the PCS-36 is supported by this finding because its sensitivity to change was good, even though it factors in several aspects of physical health. Thus, a global representation of the physical health domain may be obtained without losing test score sensitivity. McHorney and Tarlov[31] suggested that an additional advantage of the PCS-36 was standard deviations of the scores were smaller, resulting in a better likelihood that the scale may be used with individuals. A disadvantage, however, is that clinically relevant information about the patients' function and well being may be lost.[31] All of these issues should be considered when using the component score to monitor clinical outcomes.

A minimal change should be used for the numerator of the Guyatt statistic when calculating responsiveness.[28] The time interval for change used for Guyatt's responsiveness statistic was an estimate based on previous clinical studies[13,14] and may vary based on the severity of an individual's dysfunction and diagnosis. Thus, the responsiveness in our study is only a preliminary indication of responsiveness of the DHI and the SF-36 for patients receiving vestibular rehabilitation.

Patients with vestibular dysfunction who are referred for vestibular rehabilitation have lower SF-36 scores than does the general population.[27] The population of individuals with vestibular disease represents many diagnoses, so these measurements were restricted to the case mix making up our study (Tab. 1). Analysis of the data of the 31 patients evaluated before and after 6 to 8 weeks of rehabilitation showed that their SF-36 scores were similar to those of the other 64 patients, who were evaluated only once. Six to 8 weeks after the baseline evaluation, however, the scores of the 31 patients were improved but remained lower than the general population means (Figure). Direct comparison with general population data is limited because the age range varies and other confounding variables such as weight, height, other comorbid conditions could not be compared. The length of illness in the patients in our study ranged from 1 to 120 months, with a mean of about 26 months. Although this group represents a broad spectrum of individuals with vestibular dysfunction, these SF-36 scores suggest that individuals referred for vestibular rehabilitation have an extremely poor perception of their health-related quality of life.

Because normative descriptive data have not been developed for the DHI, comparisons between our subjects and the general population are not possible. The average DHI scores for the patients in our study, however, were lower than those reported for 101 patients in another study.[38] Differences in scores between the two studies may be attributed to the stage of disease or different diagnostic groups of patients.[38] For example, 66% of the patients in Robertson and Ireland's study[38] had peripheral vestibular dysfunction, whereas 86% of the patients in our study had peripheral vestibular dysfunction. Thus, the case mix must be considered when interpreting the extent of the perceived disability.

Summary and Conclusions

Health-related quality-of-life questionnaires, in addition to impairment and human performance tests, may provide physical therapists with information to determine true treatment efficacy. Both the DHI and the SF-36 demonstrated good between-day reliability in patients with vestibular dysfunction. Based on relatively low correlations, the DHI and the SF-36 appear to provide different but complementary information about the health status of patients with vestibular dysfunction. Overall, the DHI total score was more responsive than the PCS-36 and the MCS-36. As in previous studies, however, the disease-specific instrument was not always more responsive than the generic instrument in all domains. Relative to a normative database, patients referred for vestibular rehabilitation have a poor perception of their health status. These health status assessments were highly reproducible 24 to 48 hours apart, and the patients' health status was improved after 6 to 8 weeks of vestibular rehabilitation. Whether vestibular rehabilitation contributed to that improvement warrants further study.

Acknowledgments

We thank Dr Jay Rubinstein for his assistance with confirming the patients' vestibular classification. We thank Mary Lohse Shepherd, PT, and the Department of Otolaryngology, University of Iowa Hospitals and Clinics, Iowa City, Iowa, for subject recruitment and questionnaire administration. We acknowledge Carol Leigh for her assistance with the preparation of the manuscript.

References

1 Sloane P, Blazer D, George L. Dizziness in a community elderly population. *J Am Geriatr Soc.* 1989;37:101–108.

2 Nedzelski J, Barber H, McIlmoy L. Diagnosis in a dizziness unit. *J Otolaryngol.* 1986;15:101–104.

3 Kroenke K, Lucas C, Rosenberg M, Schrokman B. Psychiatric disorders and functional impairment in patients with persistent dizziness. *J Gen Intern Med.* 1993;8:530–535.

4 McGee S. Dizzy patients: diagnosis and treatment. *West J Med.* 1995;162:37–42.

5 Baloh RW. *Dizziness, Hearing Loss, and Tinnitus: The Essentials of Neurotology.* Philadelphia, Pa: FA Davis Co; 1984:159–187.

6 Yardley L, Masson E, Verschuur C, et al. Symptoms, anxiety, and handicap in dizzy patients: development of the vertigo symptom scale. *J Psychom Res.* 1992;36:731–741.

7 Yardley L, Putman J. Quantitative analysis of factors contributing to handicap and distress in vertiginous patients: a questionnaire study. *Clin Otolaryngol.* 1992;17:231–236.

8 Yardley L, Todd AM, Harter-Lacoudraye MM, Ingham R. Psychosocial consequences of recurrent vertigo. *Psychology and Health.* 1992;6:85–96.

9 Boult C, Murphy J Sloane P, et al. The relation of dizziness to functional decline. *J Am Geriatr Soc.* 1991;39:858–861.

10 Cohen H, Kane-Wineland M, Miller L, Hatfield C. Occupation and visual/vestibular interaction in vestibular rehabilitation. *Otolarngol Head Neck Surg.* 1995;112:526–532.

11 Norre ME, Beckers A. Vestibular habituation training: exercise treatment for vertigo based upon the habituation effect. *Otolarngol Head Neck Surg.* 1989;101:14–19.

12 Shumway-Cook A, Horak FB. Vestibular rehabilitation: an exercise approach to managing symptoms of vestibular dysfunction. *Seminars in Hearing.* 1989;10:196–208.

13 Horak FB, Jones-Rycewicz C, Black FO, Shumway-Cook A. Effects of vestibular rehabilitation on dizziness and imbalance. *Otolarngol Head Neck Surg.* 1992;106:175–180.

14 Krebs DE, Gill-Body KM, O'Riley P, Parker SW. Double-blind, placebo-controlled trial of rehabilitation for bilateral vestibular hypofunction: preliminary report. *Otolarngol Head Neck Surg.* 1993;109:735–741.

15 Mruzek M, Marin K, Nichols D, et al. Effects of vestibular rehabilitation and social reinforcement on recovery following ablative vestibular surgery. *Laryngoscope.* 1995;105:686–692.

16 Jacobson GP, Newman CW. The development of the dizziness handicap inventory. *Arch Otolarngol Head Neck Surg.* 1990;116:424–427.

17 Patrick DL, Deyo RA. Generic and disease-specific measures in assessing health status and quality of life. *Med Care.* 1989;27:S217–S232.

18 Ware JE Jr. Methodological considerations in the selection of health status assessment procedures. In: Wenger N, Mattson M, Furberg C, Elinson J, eds. *Assessment of Quality of Life in Clinical Trials of Cardiovascular Therapies.* New York, NY: Le Jacq Publishing Inc; 1984:87–111.

19 Guyatt G, Feeny D, Patrick DL. Issues of quality of life measurement in clinical trials. *Control Clin Trials.* 1991;12:81S–90S.

20 Kantz ME, Harris W, Levitsky K, et al. Methods for assessing condition-specific and generic functional status outcomes after total knee replacement. *Med Care.* 1992;30:MS240–MS252.

21 Patrick DL, Deyo RA, Atlas SJ, et al. Assessing health-related quality of life in patients with sciatica. *Spine.* 1995;20:1899–1909.

22 Ware JE Jr, Sherbourne CD. The MOS 36-Item Short-Form Health Survey (SF-36), I: conceptual framework and item selection. *Med Care.* 1992;30:473–481.

23 Deyo RA, Diehr P, Patrick DL. Reproducibility and responsiveness of health status measures: statistics and strategies for evaluation. *Control Clin Trials.* 1991;12:142S–158S.

24 Jette AM. Using health-related quality-of-life measures in physical therapy outcomes research. *Phys Ther.* 1993;73:528–537.

25 Wagner E, LaCroix A, Grothaus L, Hecht J. Responsiveness of health status measures to change among older adults. *J Am Geriatr Soc.* 1993;41:241–248.

26 McHorney CA, Ware JE Jr, Rachel Lu JF, Sherbourne CD. The MOS 36-Item Short-Form Health Survey (SF-36), III: tests of data quality, scaling assumptions, and reliability across diverse patient groups. *Med Care.* 1994;32:40–66.

27 Ware JE Jr, Snow K, Kosinski M, Gandek B. *SF-36 Health Survey: Manual and Interpretation Guide.* Boston, Mass: The Health Institute, New England Medical Center; 1993.

28 Guyatt G, Walter S, Norman GO. Measuring change over time: assessing usefulness of evaluative instruments. *J Chronic Dis.* 1987;40:171–178.

29 Ware JE Jr, Kosinski M, Keller SD. *SF-36 Physical and Mental Health Summary Scales: A User's Manual.* Boston, Mass: The Health Institute, New England Medical Center; 1994.

30 Newman CW, Jacobson GP. Application of self-report scales in balance function handicap assessment and management. *Seminars in Hearing.* 1993;14:363–376.

31 McHorney CA, Tarlov AR. Individual-patient monitoring in clinical practice: Are available health status surveys adequate? *Qual Life Res.* 1995;4:293–307.

32 Bombadier C, Melfi C, Paul J, et al. Comparison of a generic and a disease-specific measure of pain and physical function after knee replacement surgery. *Med Care.* 1995;33:AS131–AS144.

33 Haley SM, McHorney CA, Ware JE Jr. Evaluation of the MOS SF-36 physical functioning (PF-10), 1: unidimensionality and reproducibility of the Rasch item scale. *J Clin Epidemiol.* 1994;47:671–684.

34 Streiner DL, Norman GO. *Health Measurement Scales: A Practical Guide to Their Development and Use.* Oxford, England: Oxford University Press; 1995:104–126.

35 Brazier JE, Harper R Jones NMB, et al. Validating the SF-36 health survey questionnaire: new outcome measure for primary care. *BMJ.* 1992;305:160–164.

36 Jette DU, Downing J. Health status of individuals entering a cardiac rehabilitation program as measured by the Medical Outcomes Study 36-Item Short-Form Survey (SF-36). *Phys Ther.* 1994;74:521–527.

37 Vickrey BG, Hays RD, Harooni R, et al. A health-related quality-of-life measure for multiple sclerosis. *Qual Life Res.* 1995;4:187–206.

38 Robertson D, Ireland D. Dizziness handicap inventory correlates of computerized dynamic posturography. *J Otolaryngol.* 1995;24:118–124.

Appendix 1.
Dizziness Handicap Inventory[16]

Patient Instructions: The purpose of this scale is to identify difficulties that you may be experiencing because of your dizziness or unsteadiness. Please answer "yes," "no," or "sometimes" to each question.

Functional Scale	Physical Scale	Emotional Scale
Because of your problem, do you have difficulty getting into or out of bed?	Does looking up increase your problem?	Because of your problem, do you feel frustrated?
Does your problem restrict your participation in social activities such as going out to dinner, going to the movies, dancing, or going to parties?	Do quick movements of your head increase your problem?	Because of your problem, are you afraid to leave your home without having someone accompany you?
	Does turning over in bed increase your problem?	Because of your problem, have you been embarrassed in front of others?
Because of your problem, do you have difficulty reading?	Does walking down a sidewalk increase your problem?	Because of your problem, are you afraid that people may think that you are intoxicated?
Because of your problem, do you avoid heights?	Does bending over increase your problem?	Because of your problem, is it difficult for you to concentrate?
Because of your problem, is it difficult for you to do strenuous housework or yardwork?	Does performing more ambitious activities such as sports, dancing, or household chores (eg, sweeping or putting away dishes) increase your problem?	Because of your problem, are you afraid to stay home alone?
Because of your problem is it difficult for you to walk around your house in the dark?		Because of your problem, do you feel handicapped?
Does your problem interfere with your job or household responsibilities?		Has your problem placed stress on your relationship with members of your family or friends?
Because of your problem, do you restrict your travel for business or recreation?		Because of your problem, are you depressed?

Appendix 2.
Summary of Medical Outcome Study 36-Item Short-Form Health Survey[27,29] (SF-36) Scales

Scale	Low Score Meaning	High Score Meaning
Physical function	Limited a lot due to health in performing all physical activities, including walking, dressing, and bathing	Ability to perform all types of activities, including the most vigorous activities without limitations due to health
Role limitation due to physical problems	Problems with work or other daily activities due to physical health	No problems with work or other daily activities as a result of physical health
Bodily pain	Very severe and limiting pain	No pain or limitations due to pain
General health	Evaluates personal health as poor and believes that it is likely to get worse	Evaluates personal health as excellent
Social function	Extreme and frequent interference with social activities due to emotional or physical problems	Performs normal social activities without interference due to physical or emotional problems
Vitality/energy	Feels tired and worn out all the time	Feels full of energy all the time
Role limitation due to emotional problems	Problems with work or other activities due to emotional problems	No problems with work or other daily activities as a result of emotional health
Mental health	Feelings of nervousness and depression all of the time	Feels peaceful, calm, and happy all the time
Physical component summary	Substantial limitations in self-care and physical, social, and role activities: severe bodily pain, frequent tiredness, health rated as "poor"	No physical limitations, disabilities, or decrements in well being; high energy level; health rated as "excellent"
Mental component summary	Frequent psychological distress, substantial social and role disability due to emotional problems; health in general rated as "poor"	Frequent positive affect; absence of psychological distress and limitation in usual social or role activities due to emotional problems; health rated as "excellent"

Use of the "Fast Evaluation of Mobility, Balance, and Fear" in Elderly Community Dwellers: Validity and Reliability

Background and Purpose. Identifying elderly community dwellers who are at risk for falling was assessed using a comprehensive screening tool referred to as the "Fast Evaluation of Mobility, Balance, and Fear" (FEMBAF). The purpose of this study was to evaluate the concurrent validity and reliability of scores on the FEMBAF. **Subjects.** Thirty-five elderly persons living in the community (4 men, 31 women), with a mean age 79.9 years (SD=8.5, range=60–92), participated. **Methods.** Subjects were tested using the FEMBAF and three other instruments—the balance subscale of the Tinetti Performance-Oriented Mobility Assessment (B-POMA), the Clinical Test of Sensory Interaction on Balance (CTSIB), and the Timed Up and Go Test. Scores on the FEMBAF were compared with scores on each the other instruments using Spearman rank-order correlation coefficients and analysis of covariance (with age as the covariate) for living status and diagnostic category. A comparison of the number of subjects classified as being at risk for falling was done descriptively for the FEMBAF, B-POMA, and CTSIB. **Results.** Associations ($r>.35$) were found between the FEMBAF and each of the other instruments in the areas of FEMBAF risk-factor count, task completion, mobility, and strength. The FEMBAF classified a greater number of subjects as being at risk for falling (89%) compared with the B-POMA (43%) and the CTSIB (63%). The mean chance-corrected percentage of agreement between raters on the FEMBAF was $\kappa=.95$ (SD=.15) for assessment of risk factors and $\kappa=.96$ (SD=.12) for task completion. **Conclusion and Discussion.** The FEMBAF provides valid and reliable measurements of risk factors, functional performance, and factors that hinder mobility. [Di Fabio RP, Seay R. Use of the "Fast Evaluation of Mobility, Balance, and Fear" in elderly community dwellers: validity and reliability. *Phys Ther.* 1997;77:904–917.]

Key Words: *Assessment, Balance, Falling, Function, Risk.*

Richard P Di Fabio

Rebecca Seay

Falls are the leading cause of accidental death in the home,[1] and they are a contributing factor in 40% of the admissions to nursing homes.[2] Identifying elderly persons who are at risk for falling through the use of appropriate screening tools and referring elderly persons who are prone to falls for physical therapy for gait, balance, and strength deficits are important because this intervention appears to be effective in reducing the risk of falling.[3]

In spite of the social and medical consequences of falls and mobility restrictions for many older persons, primary care physicians do not always refer community-dwelling elderly clients for rehabilitation.[4] One reason for the lack of appropriate referral may be that the needs of older persons living in the community are not always clearly delineated by health care professionals. Identifying elderly community dwellers who are at risk for falling could be done by using a comprehensive screening tool that examines known risk factors, assesses physical performance, and evaluates the patient's fear of falling. The ideal tool would be easy to administer and would apply to persons with a wide range of medical conditions (eg, those with orthopedic or neurologic deficits).

Clinical tools that measure some aspect of balance or mobility in elderly people have received much attention in the literature.[5–18] Recent studies[19–24] have also addressed the influence of fear of falling on balance and mobility. None of the instruments described in the peer-reviewed literature, however, in our opinion, enable clinicians to integrate risk-factor assessment, evaluation of physical performance, and self-assessment of the factors that impair the performance of activities of daily living.

Clinical balance and mobility assessment tools that can be used in the home usually involve either a performance-oriented assessment of balance and mobility[7,9,12,14,25] or an assessment of the underlying mechanisms that might contribute to balance dysfunction.[5,6,26] Performance-oriented balance assessments[7,9,10,12,27] require people to perform various activities (eg, stand from a sitting position, turn while standing) while the therapist rates the level of performance based on a predetermined time or distance requirement[7,8,12] or determines a score based on a qualitative index of performance (eg, "normal," "adaptive," "abnormal").[10] In contrast to rating the performance of functional activities, the impairments underlying balance or mobility deficits can be evaluated by assessing the patterns of sensory dependence for balance derived from timed stance tests during distortion of the sensory environment (eg, the Clinical Test of Sensory Interaction on Balance [CTSIB]).[5,6]

Some performance-oriented balance assessments[12,28,29] as well as the CTSIB[6] are predictive of falls among elderly community dwellers. Tinetti et al[28] assessed the frequency of falls in 336 older persons living in the community (mean age=78.0 years, SD=5.1) through phone contacts every other month for a year. Thirty-two percent of the subjects (n=108) had fallen at least once during the study period. An increase in the number of

---

RP Di Fabio, PhD, PT, is Professor, Program in Physical Therapy, Department of Physical Medicine and Rehabilitation, University of Minnesota, UMHC Box 388, 420 Delaware St SE, Minneapolis, MN 55455 (USA) (difab001@maroon.tc.umn.edu). Address all correspondence to Dr Di Fabio.

R Seay is a graduate student in the advanced master's degree program at the University of Minnesota.

This study was approved by the University of Minnesota Human Subjects Committee.

This article was submitted August 30, 1996, and was accepted March 5, 1997.

abnormalities in balance or gait determined from a performance-oriented mobility assessment (eg, unsteady sitting, turning, or loss of balance following a nudge to the sternum) contributed to an increase in the relative risk of falling. *Relative risk* is the likelihood that someone with a balance or mobility deficit will fall compared with someone without the deficit. A relative risk of 1.0 means that the balance or mobility deficit does not increase the risk of falling. The relative risk was 1.0 with 0 to 2 abnormalities, 1.7 with 3 to 5 abnormalities, and 2.5 with 6 to 7 abnormalities. Berg et al[29] found similar results in a longitudinal study of a performance-oriented balance assessment with 113 elderly subjects (mean age=83.5 years, SD=5.3). They reported a relative risk of 2.7 for multiple falls over the next 12 months if subjects scored less than 45 points on the Berg Balance Scale. Duncan et al[12] reported that elderly men who were unable to reach 15.2 cm (6 in) were likely to have fallen two or more times within 6 months of testing. Twenty-six of 191 subjects in their cohort were classified as recurrent fallers, and the odds ratio adjusted for age, depression, and cognitive impairment was 8.07.[12] The odds ratio provides an estimate of relative risk. Di Fabio and Anacker[6] studied 47 elder persons (mean age=80.5 years, SD=9.0, range=65–96), using the CTSIB. Thirty-four percent of the subjects (n=16) fell at least twice within 6 months prior to data collection. For those subjects who scored below an average of 81 seconds during trials involving stance on a foam pad, the estimated relative risk of falling was reflected by an age-adjusted odds ratio of 8.67.

Although tests of physical performance and the underlying sensory interaction for balance are predictive of fall risk, the narrow focus of each of these tests limits the assessment of fall risk to unidimensional entities (eg, "physical performance," "sensory integration"). This limitation creates a problem for health care professionals assessing fall risk, because known risk factors for falling[3,28] or restricted mobility[20,30] are not measured. In addition, it is difficult to develop a comprehensive care program that targets the multiple causes of falls without a broad survey of risk factors. The use of several instruments to separately assess physical performance,[10,12,27] strength,[31,32] sensory systems,[33,34] and the influence of fear of falling on mobility[19–22,24] or other responses about performing mobility tasks—while a potential solution to the problem—is cumbersome and time consuming. A comprehensive screening tool developed by Arroyo and colleagues[35] was designed to address this problem by integrating risk-factor assessment, an evaluation of physical performance, and the patient's response to mobility performance.

Arroyo et al[35] introduced a tool referred to as the "Fast Evaluation of Mobility, Balance, and Fear" (FEMBAF) baseline questionnaire. The FEMBAF consists of three components: (1) an assessment of 22 factors that could place a person at risk for falling, (2) evaluation of the ability to complete 18 functional tasks, and (3) reports of fear, pain, mobility difficulty, and the perception of strength deficits for each of the 18 items in the performance-oriented assessment (Appendix). A preliminary analysis of fall risk among 241 elderly community dwellers (mean age=77.5 years, SD=7.9) was done using the FEMBAF in a case-controlled experimental design study.[35] Fifty-nine percent of the subjects (n=142) reported falling at least once in the year preceding the study. Arroyo and colleagues found that elderly persons with a previous history of falling had more complaints of fear, pain, lack of strength, and mobility difficulty during the 18-item performance-oriented balance assessment compared with elderly persons with no recent history of falling. Each activity in the performance-oriented assessment was scored on a three-point scale, and a maximum score of 54 indicated the best possible performance. Arroyo et al suggested that scores between 35 and 45 represented "moderate fall risk," whereas scores below 35 were proposed as the range of "severe fall risk."

The components of the FEMBAF are integrated to form a single tool that can be administered in about 15 minutes. The validity and reliability of measurements obtained with the FEMBAF, however, have not been reported. In addition, it is not known how the assessment of fall risk on the FEMBAF compares with other tests of mobility or sensory integration for balance.[6,28] The purpose of our study was to evaluate the concurrent validity and reliability of scores on the FEMBAF as a clinical index of functional ability and fall risk.

Method

Subjects

Participants were chosen sequentially from the referrals for home care services to a home health agency located in the Minneapolis-St Paul (Minn) area. Referrals were received from local clinics and hospitals. Once the referral for a physical therapy evaluation was received, the patients were evaluated at their residence. All patients meeting the following inclusion criteria were invited to participate: (1) over 65 years of age, (2) living at home or in a community-based assisted living facility, (3) ambulatory (with or without assistive device), (4) not enrolled in a hospice program, and (5) having a Folstein Mini-Mental State Examination[36] score greater than 20. Folstein and Folstein developed the Mini-Mental State Examination to evaluate the cognitive aspects of mental function.[36] This tool is suited to on-site use in patient's home. Standardization of the test on 206 people with and without cognitive impairment indicated that scores of 20 or less was found in patients with dementia,

Table 1.
Characteristics of the Subjects

		Age (y)				Folstein Mini-Mental State Examination[36]			
	N	$\bar{X}$	SD	Median	Range	$\bar{X}$	SD	Median	Range
All subjects	35	79.9	8.5	81.9	60–92	29.2	1.2	30	25–30
Gender									
Male	4	68.3	3.0	67.6	66–73	30.0	0	30	0
Female	31	81.3	7.8	82.5	60–92	29.1	1.2	30	25–30
Living status (alone)									
Yes	18	82.2	8.4	83.9	66–92	29.2	1.4	30	25–30
No	17	77.4	8.1	81.0	60–88	29.3	0.9	30	27–30
Diagnosis									
Neurologic	9	74.9	7.1	74.2	66–84	29.3	0.9	30	28–30
Orthopedic	16	80.1	8.1	82.3	68–91	29.5	1.3	30	25–30
Weakness	10	82.8	8.9	83.8	60–92	28.7	1.2	29	27–30

delirium, schizophrenia, or affective disorders and not in elderly people without mental disorders or people with neurosis and personality disorders.

Thirty-five of the 40 patients who were interviewed met the inclusion criteria. Five patients had Folstein Mini-Mental State Examination scores below 20 and were excluded from the study. We were seeking older persons without cognitive impairment. Elderly persons with impaired cognitive ability represent a different population that is already known to be at risk for falling and sustaining serious injury from falls.[37]

The characteristics of the patients who met the inclusion criteria and participated in the study are summarized in Table 1. Patients with a primary diagnosis of neurologic deficit included those with stroke (n=6), multiple sclerosis (n=1), and tumor or brain injury (n=2). The orthopedic category (Tab. 1) included patients with hip fracture (n=6), rib or humeral fracture (n=2), hip arthroplasty (n=2) or knee arthroplasty (n=3), and fractured vertebra secondary to osteoporosis (n=3). Each subject signed an informed consent form prior to the initiation of testing.

Raters and Reliability
All tests were administered by a single physical therapist who had 8 years of experience (7 years in the home care field). Testing of intrarater or interrater reliability using a test-retest design was not feasible because the subjects generally could not tolerate repeated examinations on the same day. Testing subjects on different days was not considered a viable option because of the potential effects of maturation. Interrater reliability, therefore, was assessed with the physical therapist and a physical therapist assistant (with 4 of 5 years of experience in home care). Five subjects were randomly selected from the sample. The physical therapist administered and scored the test while the physical therapist assistant observed and simultaneously scored the test during the same session. There was no discussion between raters during the evaluation. The testers were blind to the determination of fall risk derived from any of the tests that were given to each subject.

Outcome Assessment
The FEMBAF was used as the outcome measure, and the following components were assessed: (1) number of risk factors, (2) task completion and risk of falling, and (3) fear, pain, mobility, and strength.

Number of risk factors. The subjects were evaluated on 22 items, which were scored in a dichotomous fashion ("yes" or "no") (Appendix). All affirmative conditions were tallied, and this count provided a relative index of the number of risk factors that could contribute to falling. The risk-factor assessment was based on observation, patient report, and information in the medical chart.

Task completion and risk of falling. Each subject was then asked to perform 18 tasks. Each task was scored according to the subject's ability to complete the task (3=task successfully completed without imbalance, 2=task initiated but unsteady or partially completed, 1=unable to perform or initiate task). The best possible score was 54. The assessment of fall risk suggested by Arroyo et al[35] was normal (>45), moderate fall risk (35–45), and severe fall risk (<35).

Assessments of fear, pain, mobility, and strength. During each task, the subjects were asked whether fear (Are you fearful of falling?), pain (Does this movement hurt you?), difficulty moving (Is it difficult for you to get started and keep moving?), or lack of strength (Do you feel weak during the motion?) hindered task perfor-

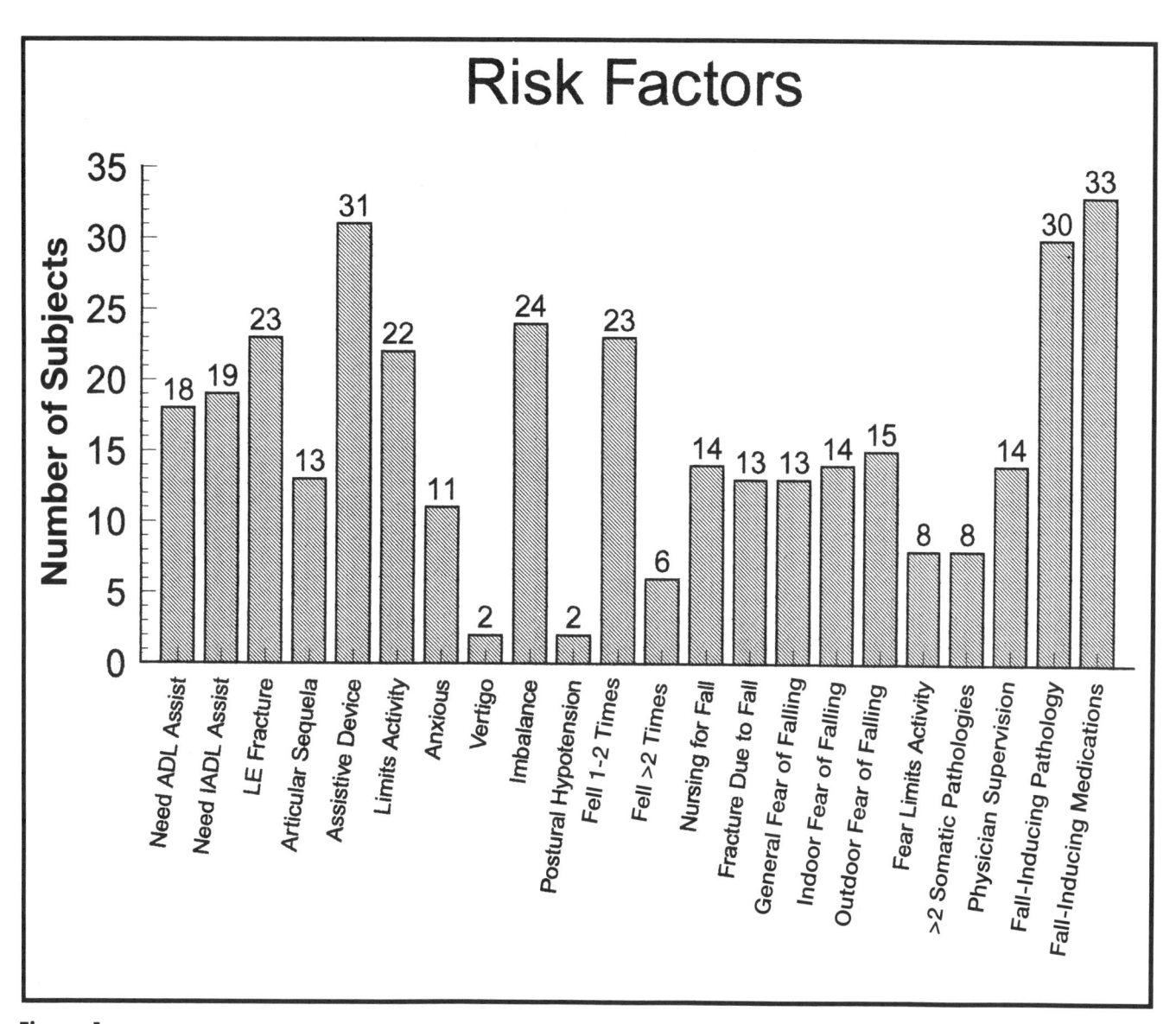

Risk Factors

Figure 1.
Risk factors acquired from the Fast Evaluation of Mobility, Balance, and Fear[35] for a cohort of 35 elderly persons living in the community and referred to a home health agency for physical therapy services. ADL=activities of daily living, IADL=instrumental activities of daily living, LE=lower extremity.

mance. Each affirmative answer was tallied as a "complaint" that potentially affected the subject's ability to complete the task. The number of "complaints" within each category (fear, pain, mobility, and strength) were evaluated as separate outcome variables.

Other Measures of Balance Ability

Three other measures of balance ability were used to evaluate the concurrent validity of the FEMBAF: (1) the balance subscale of the Tinetti Performance-Oriented Mobility Assessment[10] (B-POMA), (2) the CTSIB, and (3) the Timed Up and Go Test.[11]

B-POMA. This test consists of 13 tasks that are scored based on preestablished qualitative criteria.[10] The score for each task can be 2 (normal), 1 (adaptive), or 0 (abnormal). For example, the rating of a patient's response to a nudge on the sternum could be "steady, able to withstand pressure (normal)," "needs to move feet but able to maintain balance (adaptive)," or "begins to fall or needs assistance from examiner to maintain balance (abnormal)." Interrater reliability for aggregate scores on the gait and balance subscales of the Tinetti Performance-Oriented Mobility Assessment is $r=.95$.[38] Regarding validity, the B-POMA is highly predictive of falls and fall-related injuries in elderly community dwellers.[28,39,40] Five of the B-POMA tasks were the same as tasks that were included in the FEMBAF (Appendix). The B-POMA, however, had criteria developed specifically for each test item, whereas the FEMBAF used one rating system for all test items. Those items from the B-POMA that were identical to the FEMBAF, therefore, were scored twice (first using FEMBAF criteria for task completion to avoid a bias from exposure to the

B-POMA ratings). That is, a single attempt at completing the task received two scores.

CTSIB. The CTSIB is a timed balance test that requires the patient to stand on a firm or compliant (foam) surface with eyes open, with eyes closed, or with the head inside a "visual dome."[5,6] There is a maximum score of 30 seconds per trial, 90 seconds per condition (summed across three trials), and 540 seconds for the composite score summed across all conditions and trials. The CTSIB is a reliable tool and provides valid measurements reflecting the sensory influences on postural control among elderly community dwellers.[5,6] Anacker and Di Fabio[5] reported a test-retest correlation for the CTSIB of $r=.75$, with 95% agreement of the composite score between sessions. The kappa (κ) for the composite score was reported to be .77.[26] Di Fabio and Anacker[6] reported that the composite score for identifying fallers (cut-point=260 seconds) had a sensitivity of 44% and a specificity of 90%. When the average score of compliant-surface conditions was used as the boundary of normal/abnormal sensory integration, the sensitivity was 75% and the specificity was 65%. With an average score below 81 in the compliant-surface conditions, the estimated relative risk of falling was 8.67. We, therefore evaluated the FEMBAF against the CTSIB score averaged for the three compliant-surface stance conditions.

Timed Up and Go Test. A version of the Up and Go Test using qualitative descriptions of performance[41] was found to have weak concurrent validity.[5] We decided, therefore, to use the timed version of the test.[11] The Timed Up and Go Test requires a patient to stand up from sitting in a chair, walk 3 m, turn around, return to the chair, and resume a sitting position.[11] Intrarater and interrater reliability have been reported as excellent (intraclass correlation coefficient=.99 for each type of reliability). Berg et al[25] demonstrated concurrent validity by correlating the Up and Go Test with the Berg Balance Scale ($r=-.76$) in a group of 31 elderly subjects living in residential care facilities. The Up and Go Test was the same as one item included in the FEMBAF performance-oriented assessment (Appendix). The Timed Up and Go Test, however, is a timed test, whereas the FEMBAF uses a three-point rating scale (described earlier) to evaluate task performance. The tester, therefore, scored the item twice, first using the FEMBAF criteria to avoid bias from exposure to the results of the Timed Up and Go Test.

Procedure
The testing was always done in the same order. The Folstein Mini-Mental Examination was given initially, followed by the FEMBAF. The Timed Up and Go Test and five items of the B-POMA were nested within the FEMBAF task-completion section as already described.

Table 2.
Spearman Rank-Order Correlation Coefficients for Each Component of the Fast Evaluation of Mobility, Balance, and Fear[35] (FEMBAF) Versus the Other Measures of Balance Ability (N=35)

FEMBAF	B-POMA[a]	CTSIB[b]	Timed Up and Go Test[11]
Risk factors	−.69[c]	−.46[c]	.37[c]
Task completion	.91[c]	.54[c]	−.38[c]
Fear complaints	−.26	−.32	−.02
Pain complaints	−.01	−.18	.01
Mobility complaints	−.58[c]	−.24	.60[c]
Strength complaints	−.84[c]	−.56[c]	.42[c]

[a] B-POMA=balance subscale of the Tinetti Performance-Oriented Mobility Assessment.[10]
[b] CTSIB=Clinical Test of Sensory Interaction on Balance[5,6] (compliant-surface [foam] stance conditions only).
[c] $P<.05$.

Equipment needed for the FEMBAF were a chair with armrests, stairs, and cardboard 10 cm wide × 15 cm high.

The CTSIB was administered last. The testing was done on a hard surface of either linoleum or wood. The participants removed their shoes and assumed a posture of standing with malleoli touching, forefeet turned out 30 to 40 degrees, and arms crossed over the chest. Three conditions were timed in the following order: stance with eyes open, stance with eyes closed, and stance wearing a "visual dome." Each condition was then repeated during stance on high-density foam (7.62 × 50.8 × 50.8 cm, with a specific weight of 32.04 kg/m^3 and a compression of 31.75 kg). *Compression* is the amount of weight that will compress the pad to 75% of the original height. To assist in uniform foot placement during the compliant-surface stance conditions, an outline of feet was used on the foam to delineate proper foot position. Some participants had difficulty achieving this position because of posture changes secondary to cerebrovascular accident, so a posture as close to the one described was attempted. Stance was timed up to 30 seconds. If the subjects successfully completed the trial, they received 30 points (seconds) for each of the remaining trials. If the subjects moved the arms off the chest, took a step, flexed one or both knees, or moved heels or toes off the foam base, the timer was stopped and trials 2 and 3 were initiated.

Data Analysis

Description of risk factors. The number of patients with each risk factor (Appendix) was plotted for descriptive analysis.

Concurrent validity. Concurrent validity of each component of the FEMBAF was established by calculating Spearman rank-order correlation coefficients between

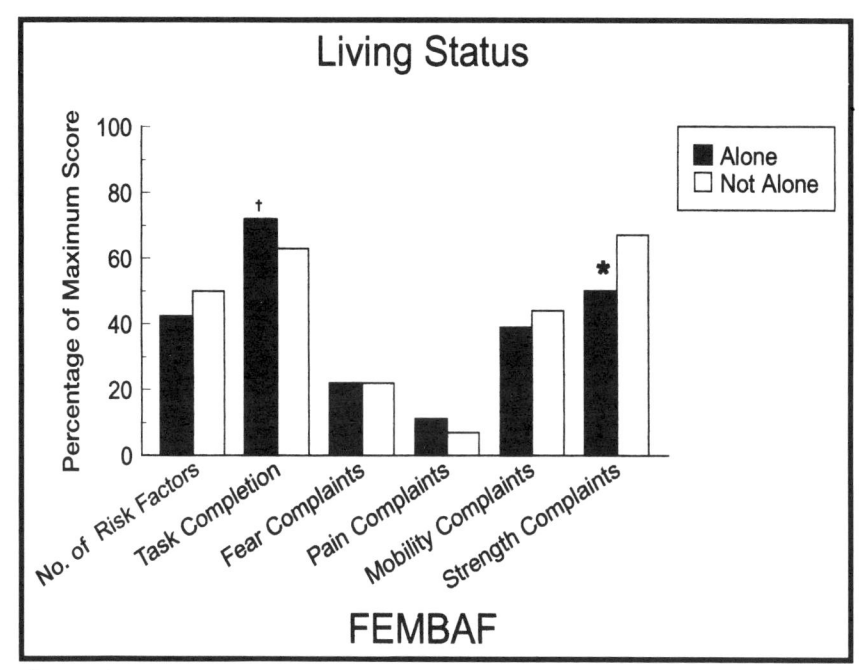

Figure 2.
Percentage of maximum score for the means on each component of the Fast Evaluation of Mobility, Balance, and Fear[35] (FEMBAF) for subjects living alone (n=18) and subjects not living alone (n=17). Asterisk (*) indicates significantly lower difference (P<.05); dagger (†) indicates trend toward higher scores (P=.058).

scores from the FEMBAF and scores from the other measures of balance ability (B-POMA, CTSIB, and Timed Up and Go Test). The statistical significance of the correlation coefficients (H₀: $r=0$) was evaluated by converting the coefficient to a t statistic.[42] This procedure allowed us to test the null hypothesis of $r=0$ on a two-tailed t distribution with n−2 degrees of freedom. The smallest correlation coefficient that would still be significantly different from 0 was $r=.35$ ($P<.05$). All correlation coefficients equal to or greater than .35, therefore, were statistically significant.

Balance, living status, and diagnostic category. To determine whether the differences detected by the other three measures of balance ability within selected stratifications of the cohort were also detected by the FEMBAF, subjects were grouped according to living status (living alone or not alone) and diagnostic category (Tab. 1). A one-way analysis of covariance (ANCOVA) was done across each stratification for each outcome measure. The subjects' age was used as a covariate because a previous study[5] showed that stance duration on timed balance tests decreases (linearly) as age increases among nondisabled elderly community dwellers.

Descriptive comparison of fall risk. The score on the task-completion section of the FEMBAF was used to assign subjects to a fall-risk category. The three-level risk classification suggested by Arroyo et al[35] (ie, normal, moderate, severe) was collapsed to form a dichotomous variable (normal versus at risk) so that direct comparisons could be made with other balance assessments. Scores on the task-completion component of the FEMBAF greater than 45 were considered normal, and scores less than or equal to 45 were considered to indicate a risk for falling. This "cut-point" placed all subjects with moderate or severe fall risk (using Arroyo and colleagues' original classification[35]) into a "risk" category.

Tinetti et al[28] identified seven activities in their performance-oriented assessment that showed the greatest prevalence in their study group and reflected the highest relative risk of falling. They collapsed a three-point scale (ie, normal, adaptive, abnormal) to create a dichotomous assessment of performance on each activity (normal versus abnormal). Abnormalities on zero to two activities showed no relative risk of falling (1.0), whereas abnormalities on three to five activities had a relative risk of falling of 1.7. Three of the seven activities involved an assessment of gait and were not included in our study. We therefore used the remaining four activities (sitting down, stance on one leg, turning, and a nudge to the sternum) to estimate fall risk. A fall-risk index was estimated from the B-POMA by determining the number of abnormal responses and assigning risk categories as normal (zero to two abnormalities) or at risk (three or four abnormalities).[28] For the CTSIB, it was previously determined that an average stance duration score of less than 81 seconds for three compliant-surface (foam) conditions distinguished fallers from nonfallers.[6] We therefore used this cut-point to classify subjects who were at risk for falling. The number of subjects classified as "at risk" and "not at risk" was plotted to provide a descriptive comparison of fall risk for each tool.

Reliability. Kappa coefficients were calculated to determine the chance-corrected percentage of agreement between raters for each test item. Kappa coefficients were averaged to provide a composite reliability coefficient for the risk-factor and task-completion components of the FEMBAF.

Results

Description of Risk Factors

The prevalence of risk factors obtained from the FEMBAF is summarized in Figure 1. Eighty-nine percent

Table 3.
Means and Standard Deviations of Outcome Variables by Living Status and Diagnostic Category

	Living Status				Diagnostic Category					
	Not Alone		Alone		Neurologic		Orthopedic		Weakness	
	X̄	SD	X̄	SD	X̄	SD	X̄	SD	X̄	SD
FEMBAF[a]										
Risk factors	11.3	3.4	9.1	5.0	13.3	2.6	9.5	4.8	8.4	4.1
Task completion	34.2	6.4	39.3	6.8	29.8	5.5	39.4	6.0	39.0	5.7
Fear complaints	4.2	3.8	3.9	4.0	5.8	4.9	3.2	3.8	3.8	2.7
Pain complaints	1.7	3.6	1.8	2.6	2.0	4.1	2.6	3.1	0.1	0.3
Mobility complaints	8.0	5.4	6.6	5.3	9.4	6.4	7.8	4.9	4.6	4.2
Strength complaints	12.5	3.4	8.6	5.0	15.1	2.9	8.5	4.2	9.5	3.8
Other measures of balance ability										
B-POMA[b]	16.5	6.2	19.5	4.6	11.7	4.9	19.9	4.5	20.8	2.5
CTSIB[c]	51.9	32.9	57.0	33.1	29.0	30.1	61.5	31.2	66.4	23.8
Timed Up and Go Test[11,d]	25.9	22.3	30.8	19.7	32.3	32.0	24.6	14.3	30.8	20.0

[a] FEMBAF=Fast Evaluation of Mobility, Balance, and Fear.[35] Risk factors=number of risk factors tallied. Task completion=score on 18 functional tasks, with each task rated from 1 (worst performance) to 3 (best performance). Fear, pain, mobility, and strength complaints=number of complaints tallied during each functional task.
[b] B-POMA=balance subscale of the Tinetti Performance-Oriented Mobility Assessment.[10] Values are total scores on the B-POMA, with each of the 13 items rated from 0 (worst performance) to 2 (best performance).
[c] CTSIB=Clinical Test of Sensory Interaction on Balance,[5,6] measured as stance time (in seconds) averaged for three compliant-surface (foam) conditions.
[d] Timed Up and Go Test measured as time (in seconds) to stand from a sitting position, walk 3 m, and resume sitting in a chair.

of the subjects (n=31) used assistive devices for ambulation, and 83% of the subjects (n=29) reported falling at least one time during the past year. In addition, 86% of the subjects (n=30) had pathology that was likely to induce falls, and 94% of the subjects (n=33) were taking medications that were potentially dangerous with regard to falls. Although 63% of the subjects (n=22) limited their activities to basic activities of daily living at home, only 23% of the subjects (n=8) reported that fear of falling was the limiting factor.

Concurrent Validity

The correlations between the FEMBAF and the other measures of balance ability are summarized in Table 2. Higher scores on task completion, indicating greater proficiency, correlated with higher (better) scores on the B-POMA (Tab. 2). As the number of risk factors or the number of tasks performed poorly due to perceived lack of strength or mobility problems increased, the B-POMA score decreased, indicating a decrement in balance function (Tab. 2).

Longer stance duration on the CTSIB (average of scores for the compliant-surface stance conditions) also had an association with better task-completion scores (Tab. 2). In contrast, shorter stance duration (indicating a decrement in balance function) was associated with a greater number of risk factors or an increase in the number of tasks performed poorly due to perceived lack of strength (Tab. 2).

The magnitude of the association between the scores from the Timed Up and Go Test and the scores from the FEMBAF was low, overall, compared with the magnitude of association between the other measures of balance ability and the FEMBAF, but several relationships still achieved statistical significance. There was a positive association between the Timed Up and Go Test score and the number of risk factors, mobility, and strength complaints (ie, longer transit time during the Timed Up and Go Test was associated with more risk factors or complaints). In addition, a low proficiency in the FEMBAF task completion was associated with a prolonged duration for completing the Timed Up and Go Test.

Balance, Living Status, and Diagnostic Category

FEMBAF and living status. When corrected for age, the number of strength deficits perceived to affect performance was lower for subjects who lived alone than for subjects who did not live alone (F=5.57; df=1,32; P=.03; Fig. 2). The task-completion scores were higher for subjects who lived alone than for subjects who did not live alone (F=3.86; df=1,32; P=.058; Fig. 2). There were no differences in the number of risk factors, fear, pain, or mobility complaints between subjects who lived alone and subjects who did not live alone (Tab. 3, Fig. 2).

Other measures of balance ability and living status. There were no differences in B-POMA, CTSIB, or Timed Up and Go Test scores between subjects who lived alone and subjects who did not live alone (Tab. 3, Fig. 3).

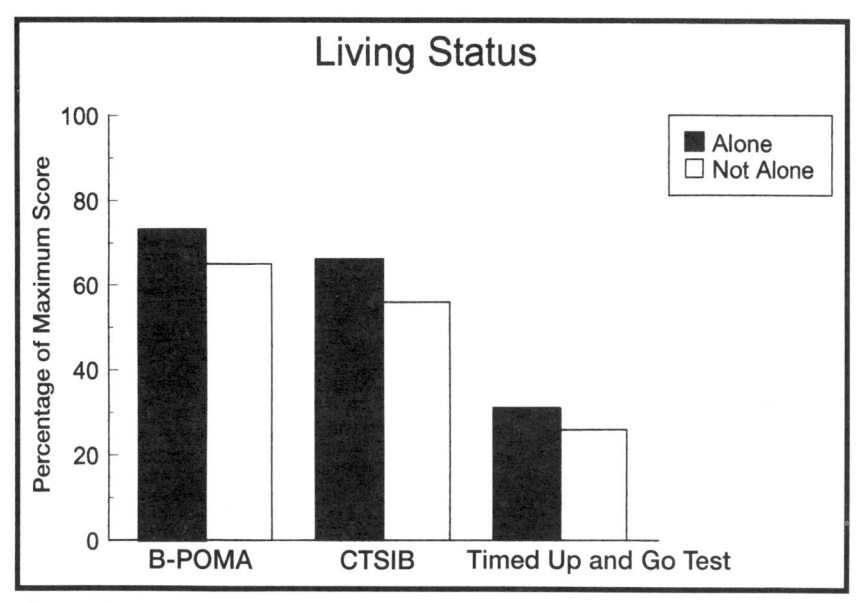

Figure 3.
Percentage of maximum score for the means on each measure of balance ability (balance subscale of the Tinetti Performance-Oriented Mobility Assessment[10] [B-POMA], Clinical Test of Sensory Interaction on Balance[5,6] [CTSIB], Timed Up and Go Test[11]) for subjects living alone (n=18) and subjects not living alone (n=17). Note: for purposes of illustration, the Timed Up and Go Test score was normalized to 100 seconds.

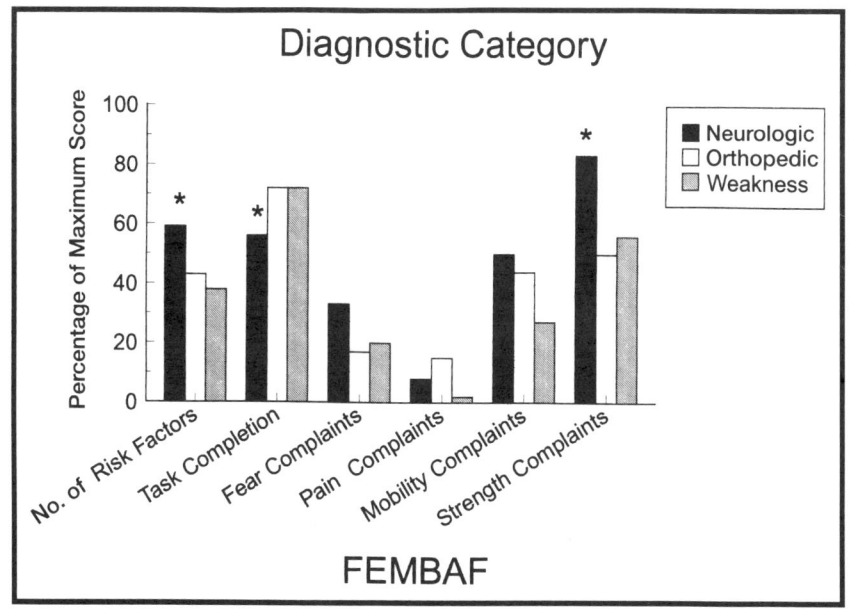

Figure 4.
Percentage of maximum score for the means on each component of the Fast Evaluation of Mobility, Balance, and Fear[35] (FEMBAF) for each diagnostic category (neurologic, n=9; orthopedic, n=16; generalized weakness, n=10). Asterisk (*) indicates significantly different at $P<.05$.

FEMBAF and diagnostic category. When corrected for age, the outcomes across diagnostic categories showed that the number of risk factors (F=3.35; $df=2,31$; $P=.048$) and the number of perceived strength deficits (F=7.69; $df=2,31$; $P<.001$) were greatest for subjects with neurologic diagnoses compared with subjects with orthopedic conditions or generalized weakness (Fig. 4).

The rate of task completion was lower in the neurologic category (F=7.51; $df=2,31$; $P=.002$) than in all other diagnostic categories. There were no differences in the number of complaints of fear, pain, or mobility deficit across diagnostic categories.

Other measures of balance ability and diagnostic categories. The B-POMA scores were lower (F=15.14; $df=2,31$; $P<.001$) and stance duration during the CTSIB was shorter (F=7.79; $df=2,31$; $P<.001$) for subjects with neurologic conditions than for subjects with orthopedic conditions or subjects with generalized weakness (Fig. 5). There were no differences among diagnostic categories with respect to the Timed Up and Go Test scores.

Descriptive Comparison of Fall Risk
The FEMBAF classified 31 of 35 subjects as being at risk for falling. The B-POMA and the CTSIB classified 15 and 22 subjects, respectively, as being at risk for falling (Fig. 6).

Reliability
There was high interrater agreement on the determination of risk factors (mean $\kappa=.95$, SD=.15) and task completion (mean $\kappa=.96$, SD=.12).

Discussion
The FEMBAF appears to provide valid and reliable measurements of balance, mobility, and fall risk in a group of elderly community dwellers who did not have cognitive impairments. There were correlations between several components of the FEMBAF (number of risk factors, task completion, strength, and mobility complaints) and the other measures of balance ability (Tab. 2). The number of fear or pain complaints during task performance did not show an association with any of the other measures of balance ability (Tab. 2).

A general fear of falling was expressed by 37% of the cohort, but only 23% of the subjects indicated that fear limited their activities (Fig. 1). The disassociation of "fear of falling" from functional performance has been documented by Tinetti et al.[19] In a study of more than 1,000 elderly persons living in the community, Tinetti and colleagues found that fear of falling was not associated with impairments of higher-level physical or social functioning (eg, home repair, yard work, sports participation) and that fear of falling was only marginally associated with activities of daily living.

It was clear that multiple factors influence mobility proficiency and fall-avoidance behavior, because the number of risk factors identified by the FEMBAF had a relationship to the outcome on each of the other measures of balance ability (Tab. 2). These findings support the notion that multiple factors contribute to fall risk.[28,39] One implication of these findings is that the FEMBAF might be a useful screening tool because it accounts for the "additive" effects of multiple disabilities on falling.

The identification of modifiable risk factors is an important aspect of developing effective strategies for therapeutic interventions to improve mobility and prevent injurious falls.[3,43] Tinetti et al[3] described several modifiable risk factors, and many of these factors are "scored" on the FEMBAF (ie, postural hypotension; use of sedatives; impairments in balance, gait, and strength). The risk-factor component of the FEMBAF identified and provided a count of the factors that might contribute to falling, but fall risk was determined by the task-completion score on the FEMBAF (Appendix). More subjects were identified as being at risk for falling on the FEMBAF compared with the B-POMA or CTSIB (Fig. 6). One possible reason for these differences might be that the FEMBAF incorporates more challenging balance tasks (eg, jumping, climbing stairs, standing from a kneeling position) than does the B-POMA or the CTSIB. The "ceiling" effect that might be expected with activities that do not challenge balance, therefore, was minimized with the FEMBAF.

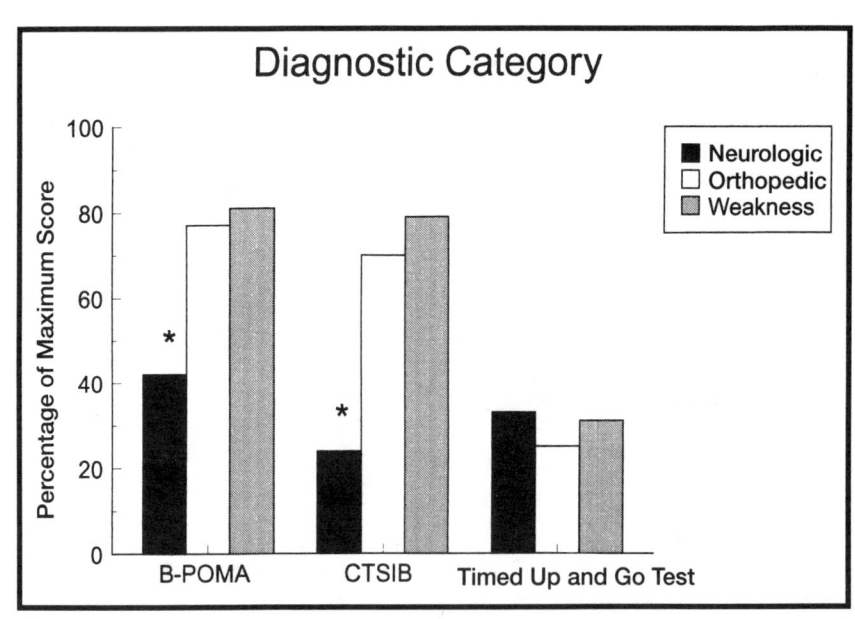

Figure 5.
Percentage of maximum score for the means on each measure of balance ability (balance subscale of the Tinetti Performance-Oriented Mobility Assessment[10] [B-POMA], Clinical Test of Sensory Interaction on Balance[5,6] [CTSIB], Timed Up and Go Test[11]) for each diagnostic category (neurologic, n=9; orthopedic, n=16; generalized weakness, n=10). Note: for purposes of illustration, the Timed Up and Go Test score was normalized to 100 seconds. Asterisk (*) indicates significantly different at $P<.05$.

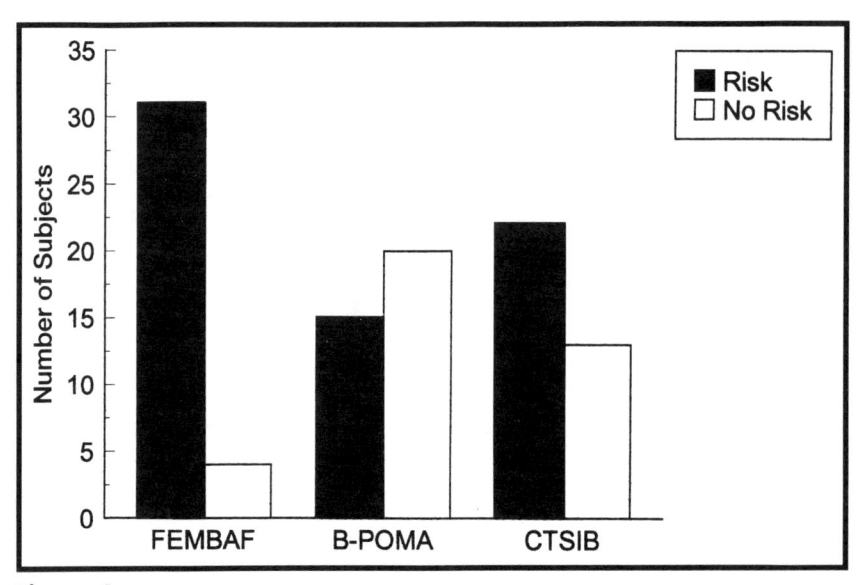

Figure 6.
Comparison of the number of subjects classified as being at risk for falling with the Fast Evaluation of Mobility, Balance, and Fear[35] (FEMBAF), the balance subscale of the Tinetti Performance-Oriented Mobility Assessment[10] (B-POMA), and the Clinical Test of Sensory Interaction on Balance[5,6] (CTSIB).

When the cohort was stratified according to living status, there was a reduction in the number of strength complaints (Fig. 2) and the task-completion scores tended to be higher for subjects who lived alone than for subjects who did not live alone (Fig. 2). These findings suggest that independent living requires a high level of functional competence. There were no differences when outcomes on the other measures of balance ability were evaluated with respect to living status. The comparison measures, however, tended to show better scores for subjects who lived alone than for subjects who did not live alone (Fig. 3). The scores of the measures of balance ability indicating better performance for subjects who lived alone (Fig. 3), therefore, were in the same direction as the FEMBAF task-completion scores for this group of subjects (Fig. 2).

Elderly persons who return home from the hospital following inpatient treatment for a neurological deficit may have up to three times the risk for falling compared with elderly persons without neurological deficits living in the community.[44] With respect to diagnostic category, the FEMBAF, B-POMA, and CTSIB showed poorer outcomes for subjects with primarily neurologic dysfunction than for subjects with orthopedic-related disorders or generalized weakness (Figs. 4, 5). The consistency of findings from the FEMBAF and each of the other measures of balance ability across diagnostic categories provides additional support for the validity of the FEMBAF.

Limitations

This study was a preliminary demonstration of the usefulness of a new screening tool that can be used to identify risk factors and functional deficits in elderly persons living in the community. Whether this tool will help clinicians modify the care of clients living in the community in order to prevent injury due to falls remains to be determined. The level of disease severity of the subjects in our study required us to limit the rigor of the reliability test. The design for evaluating reliability was restricted to interrater reliability, and one of two raters was required to score the test strictly as an observer. Additional research is needed to show the predictive capacity of the FEMBAF. In addition, one rater did not interact with the person being measured, which eliminated a source of error that would be present when the instrument is normally used. A more complete description of reliability (eg, in the form of a test-retest design) was not feasible.

Conclusions

Concurrent validity of the measurements from the FEMBAF was evident from associations with each of the other measures of balance ability in the areas of risk-factor assessment, task completion, mobility, and strength complaints. Differences in performance across diagnostic categories were detected by the measures of balance ability as well as by the FEMBAF. The interrater reliability of the measures was excellent, with interrater chance-corrected agreement on the order of 95%. The FEMBAF may enable practitioners to identify patients who are at risk for falling or mobility dependence, and it provides a format for delineating risk factors that are known to respond to treatment.

References

1 Lamb K, Miller J, Mernadez M. Falls in the elderly: causes and prevention. *Orthopedic Nursing*. 1987;6:45–49.

2 Kellogg International Work Group on the Prevention of Falls by the Elderly. *Dan Med Bull*. 1987;34(suppl 4):1–24.

3 Tinetti ME, Baker DI, McAvay G, et al. A multifactorial intervention to reduce the risk of falling among elderly people living in the community. *N Engl J Med*. 1994;331:821–827.

4 Hoenig H, Mayer-Oaks SA, Siebens H, et al. Geriatric rehabilitation: What do physicians know about it and how should they use it? *J Am Geriatr Soc*. 1994;42:341–347.

5 Anacker SL, Di Fabio RP. Influence of sensory inputs on standing balance in community-dwelling elders with a recent history of falling. *Phys Ther*. 1992;72:575–581.

6 Di Fabio RP, Anacker SL. Identifying fallers in community-living elders with a clinical test of sensory interaction for balance. *Eur J Phys Med Rehabil*. 1996;6:61–66.

7 Rossiter-Fornoff JE, Wolf SL, Wolfson LI, et al. A cross-sectional study of the FICSIT common database static balance measures. *J Gerontol*. 1995;50A:M291–M297.

8 Berg K, Wood-Dauphinee S, Williams JI. The balance scale: assessment with elderly residents and patients with acute stroke. *Scand J Rehabil Med*. 1995;27:27–36.

9 Mahoney FI, Barthel DW. Functional evaluation: the Barthel index. *Md Med J*. 1965;14:61–65.

10 Tinetti ME. Performance-oriented assessment of mobility problems in elderly patients. *J Am Geriatric Soc*. 1986;34:119–126.

11 Podsiadlo D, Richardson S. The timed "up & go": a test of basic functional mobility for frail elderly persons. *J Am Geriatr Soc*. 1991;39:142–148.

12 Duncan PW, Studenski S, Chandler J, Prescott B. Functional reach: predictive validity in a sample of elderly male veterans. *J Gerontol*. 1992;47:M93–M98.

13 Gabell A, Simons MA. Balance coding. *Physiotherapy*. 1983;68:286–288.

14 MacKnight C, Rockwood K. A hierarchical assessment of balance and mobility. *Age Ageing*. 1995;24:126–130.

15 Di Fabio RP. Reliability and validity of functional assessment in patients with stroke. *Journal of Neurologic Rehabilitation*. 1990;4:145–152.

16 Harada N, ChiU V, Damron-Rodriquez J, et al. Screening for balance and mobility impairment in elderly individuals living in residential care facilities. *Phys Ther*. 1995;75:462–469.

17 Hu MH, Woollacott MH. Multisensory training of standing balance in older adults, II: kinematic and electromyographic postural responses. *J Gerontol*. 1994;49:M62–M71.

18 Wolfson LI, Whipple RH, Amerman P, et al. Stressing the postural response: a quantitative method for testing balance. *J Am Geriatr Soc*. 1986;34:845–850.

19 Tinetti ME, Mendes de Leon CF, Doucette JT, Baker DI. Fear of falling and fall-related efficacy in relationship to functioning among community-living elders. *J Gerontol*. 1994;3:M140–M147.

20 Howland J, Peterson EW, Levin WC, et al. Fear of falling among the community-dwelling elderly. *Journal of Aging and Health*. 1993;5:229–243.

21 Powell LE, Myers AM. The activities-specific balance confidence (abc) scale. *J Gerontol.* 1995;50A:M28–M34.

22 Tinetti ME, Richman D, Powell LE. Falls efficacy as a measure of fear of falling. *J Gerontol.* 1990;45:P239–P243.

23 Maki BE, Holliday PJ, Topper AK. Fear of falling and postural performance in the elderly. *J Gerontol.* 1991;46:M123–M131.

24 Arfken CL, Lach HW, Birge SJ, Miller JP. The prevalence and correlates of fear of falling in elderly persons living in the community. *Am J Public Health.* 1994;84:565–570.

25 Berg KO, Maki BE, Williams JI, et al. Clinical and laboratory measures of postural balance in an elderly population. *Arch Phys Med Rehabil.* 1992;73;1073–1080.

26 Di Fabio RP, Badke MB. Relationship of sensory organization to balance function in patients with hemiplegia. *Phys Ther.* 1990;70:542–548.

27 Berg KO, Wood-Dauphinee SL, Williams JI, Gayton D. Measuring balance in the elderly: preliminary development of an instrument. *Physiotherapy Canada.* 1989;41:304–311.

28 Tinetti ME, Speechley M, Ginter SF. Risk factors for falls among elderly persons living in the community. *N Engl J Med.* 1988;319:1701–1706.

29 Berg KO, Wood-Dauphinee SL, Williams JI, Maki BE. Measuring balance in the elderly: validation of an instrument. *Can J Public Health.* 1992;83:s7–s11.

30 Gill TM, Williams CS, Tinetti ME. Assessing risk for the onset of functional dependence among older adults: the role of physical performance. *J Am Geriatr Soc.* 1995;43:603–609.

31 Wolfson L, Judge J, Whipple R, King M. Strength is a major factor in balance, gait, and the occurrence of falls. *J Gerontol.* 1995;50A(Special Issue):64–67.

32 Judge JO, King MB, Whipple R, et al. Dynamic balance in older persons: effects of reduced visual and proprioceptive input. *J Gerontol.* 1995;50A:M263–M270.

33 Lord SR, Ward JA, Williams P, Anstey K. Physiological factors associated with falls in older community-dwelling women. *J Am Geriatr Soc.* 1994;42:1110–1117.

34 Lord SR, Clark RD, Webster IW. Visual acuity and contrast sensitivity in relation to falls in an elderly population. *Age Ageing.* 1991;20:175–181.

35 Arroyo JF, Herrmann F, Saber H, et al. Fast evaluation test for mobility, balance, and fear: a new strategy for the screening of elderly fallers. *Arthritis Rheum.* 1994;37:S416. Abstract.

36 Folstein MF, Folstein SE, McHugh PR. Mini-Mental State: a practical method for grading the cognitive state of patients for the clinician. *J Psychiatr Res.* 1975;12:189–198.

37 Nevitt MC, Cummings SR, Hudes ES. Risk factors for injurious falls: a prospective study. *J Gerontol.* 1991;46:M164–M170.

38 Tinetti ME, Baker DI, Garrett PA, et al. Yale FICSIT: risk factor abatement strategy for fall prevention. *J Am Geriatr Soc.* 1993;41:315–320.

39 Tinetti ME, Williams TF, Mayewski R. Fall risk index for elderly patients based on number of chronic disabilities. *Am J Med.* 1986;80:429–434.

40 Robbins AS, Rubenstein LZ, Josephson KR, et al. Predictors of falls among elderly people: results of two population-based studies. *Arch Intern Med.* 1989;149:1628–1633.

41 Mathias S, Nayak USL, Isaacs B. Balance in elderly patients: the "Get-up and Go" Test. *Arch Phys Med Rehabil.* 1986;67:387–389.

42 Glass GV, Stanley JC. *Statistical Methods in Education and Psychology.* Englewood Cliffs, NJ: Prentice-Hall; 1970:316.

43 Overstall PW. Falls after strokes. *BMJ.* 1995;311:74–75.

44 Forster A, Young J. Incidence and consequences of falls due to stroke: a systemic inquiry. *BMJ.* 1995;311:83–86.

Appendix.
Modified Fast Evaluation of Mobility, Balance, and Fear (FEMBAF) Baseline Questionnaire[a]

Name _____ Age _/_/_ Gender ____ Height ____ Weight ____ Blood Pressure ____ Lives at Home, Alone ____
Lives With Somebody ____ Lives in Institution ____

RISK FACTORS

1. Needs aid for two (or more) basic activities of daily living (washing, cooking, dressing, walking, continence, feeding)	yes	no
2. Needs aid for two (or more) instrumental activities of daily living (money management, shopping, telephone, medications)	yes	no
3. Has had a fracture or articular problems at hips, knees, ankles, feet	yes	no
4. Has visible articular sequela in the mentioned joints	yes	no
5. Uses a walking device (eg, cane, walker)	yes	no
6. Limits physical activity to basic activities of daily living at home	yes	no
7. Self-defines as anxious	yes	no
8. Complains of vertigo	yes	no
9. Complains of imbalance	yes	no
10. Makes complaints suggesting an existing postural hypotension	yes	no
11. Fell one or two times in the current year	yes	no
12. Fell more than twice in the current year	yes	no
13. Required nursing after the fall	yes	no
14. Had a fracture after the fall	yes	no
15. Is afraid of falling in general	yes	no
16. Is afraid of falling indoors (eg, bathtub, kitchen)	yes	no
17. Is afraid of falling outdoors (eg, bus, stairs, street)	yes	no
18. Avoids going outside for fear of falling	yes	no
19. Presents three or more somatic pathologies that require regular medical supervision	yes	no
20. The pathologies require home-based medical-social supervision	yes	no
21. Shows a specific pathology likely to induce falls:	yes	no

    —neurological (eg, cancer, peripheral neuropathy, multiple sclerosis, lupus)
    —cardiovascular (eg, postural hypotension)
    —musculoskeletal (eg, total joint replacements, arthritis)
    —sensory (eg, visual impairment)
    —other (amputation, Parkinson's disease, Alzheimer's disease)

22. Takes medications that are potentially dangerous in regard to falls:	yes	no

    —hypotensives
    —neuroleptics
    —hypnotics/anxiolytics
    —antiarrythmics
    —antiparkinsonians
    —analgesics/anti-inflammatory drugs
    —various vasoregulators

Risk Factors (=total of "yes" answers): ____

Appendix. Continued.

TASK COMPLETION   **TASK SCORE (3, 2, 1)***

1. Sitting on a chair, with folded arms, raises both legs horizontally   —
   __fear   __pain   __mobility difficulties   __lack of strength

**2. Sitting on a chair with armrests, stands up without aid, without using banister   —
   __fear   __pain   __mobility difficulties   __lack of strength

***3. Sitting on a chair, stands up without aid, walks five steps, turns around, goes back and sits down   —
   __fear   __pain   __mobility difficulties   __lack of strength

**4. One-footed standing (left foot): stands on left foot without aid during 5 seconds minimum   —
   __fear   __pain   __mobility difficulties   __lack of strength

5. Repeat with one-footed standing (right foot)   —
   __fear   __pain   __mobility difficulties   __lack of strength

**6. Romberg Test: stands with heels together, eyes closed, remains steady for 10 seconds   —
   __fear   __pain   __mobility difficulties   __lack of strength

7. Squatting down: without aid, squats down until buttocks reach knee level, then stands up   —
   __fear   __pain   __mobility difficulties   __lack of strength

**8. Picking up a pencil from the ground without aid or support   —
   __fear   __pain   __mobility difficulties   __lack of strength

9. Standing jumping without losing balance, over a distance equal to one's own foot   —
   __fear   __pain   __mobility difficulties   __lack of strength

10. Stepping over an obstacle (foam or cardboard, 10 cm wide × 15 cm high) without touching it; the foot to arrive past the obstacle at a distance equal to its own size (left)   —
    __fear   __pain   __mobility difficulties   __lack of strength

11. Repeat with overstepping to the right   —
    __fear   __pain   __mobility difficulties   __lack of strength

12. Shoving forward to trunk; subject to remain steady following a nudge between shoulder blades (examiner's arms stretched out, nudge realized by a sudden bending of hand on trunk)   —
    __fear   __pain   __mobility difficulties   __lack of strength

**13. Repeat with shoving backward (nudge on the sternum)   —
    __fear   __pain   __mobility difficulties   __lack of strength

14. Climbing stairs without losing balance, without aid or using banister (five steps minimum)   —
    __fear   __pain   __mobility difficulties   __lack of strength

15. Repeat with descending stairs (five steps minimum)   —
    __fear   __pain   __mobility difficulties   __lack of strength

16. Transfer from standing-kneeling (both knees on the ground); stable, no assistance for rising   —
    __fear   __pain   __mobility difficulties   __lack of strength

17. Managing the "eyes-closed forward fall"; the subject lets himself/herself fall, eyes closed, onto the examiner standing 50 cm from him/her   —
    __fear   __pain   __mobility difficulties   __lack of strength

18. Repeat with eyes-closed backward fall   —
    __fear   __pain   __mobility difficulties   __lack of strength

FEMBAF TOTAL TASK COMPLETION SCORE: —

FEMBAF TOTAL SUBJECTIVE COMPLAINT SCORES:

    fear __   pain __   mobility difficulties __   lack of strength __

[a] This tool was originally described by Arroyo et al.[35] Single asterisk (*) indicates task-completion score (3=successfully completed without imbalance, 2=task initiated but unsteady or partially completed, 1=unable to perform or initiate task). Double asterisk (**) indicates same task as the balance subscale of the Tinetti Performance-Oriented Mobility Assessment.[10] These items were scored twice, first using the FEMBAF criteria and then using the criteria described by Tinetti et al.[1] Triple asterisk (***) indicates that the time needed to complete this task was entered as the Timed Up and Go Test score.[11]